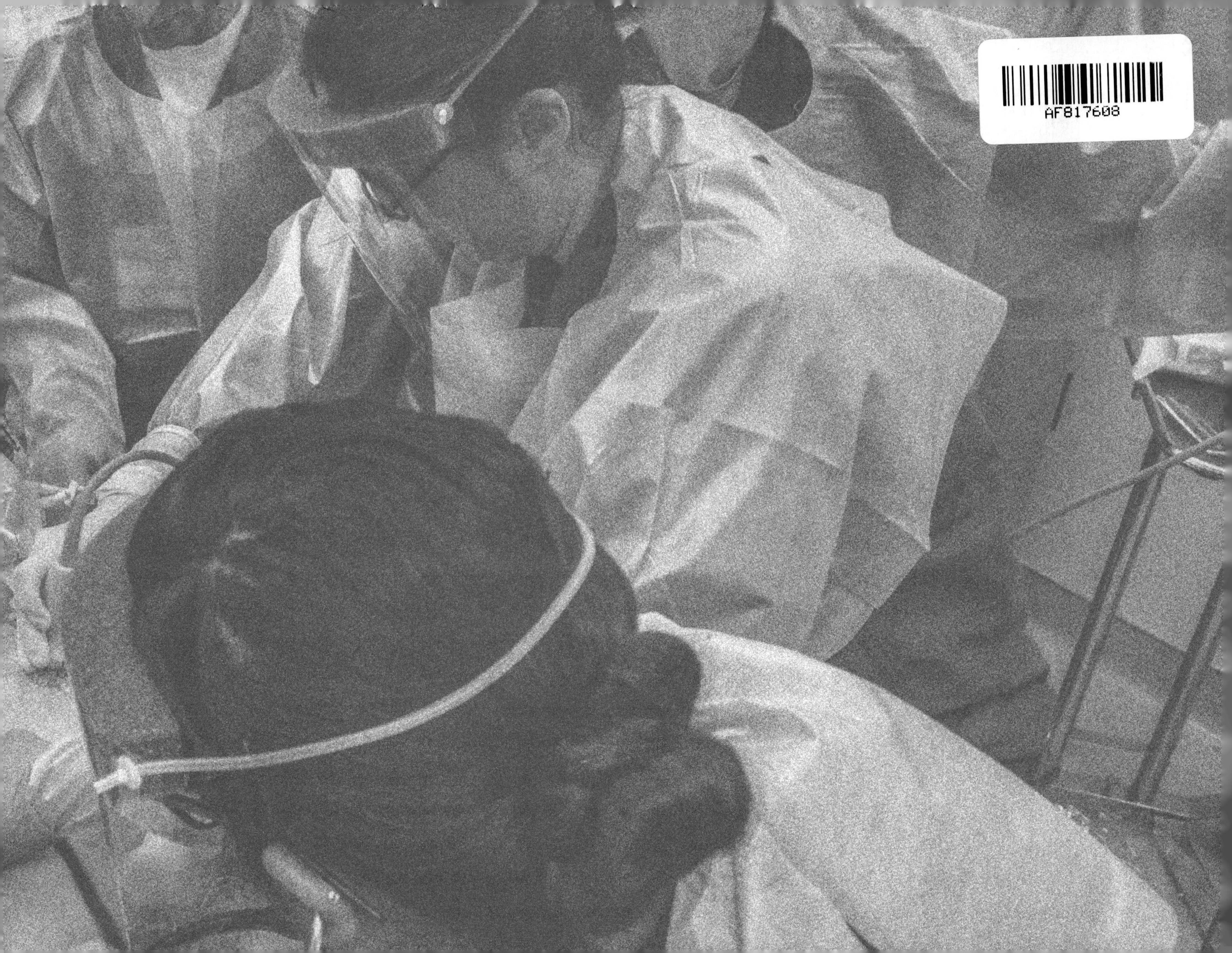

DEDICATION

For clinicians on the front line, who inspire us with their resolve, compassion, and unflinching commitment to their communities and their patients.

You represent all that is good in medicine — all that is good in humanity.

Publisher's Notice

The American College of Emergency Physicians (ACEP) makes every effort to ensure contributors and editors of its publications are knowledgeable subject matter experts and that they use their best efforts to ensure accuracy of the content. However, it is the responsibility of each reader to personally evaluate the content and judge its suitability for use in his or her medical practice in the care of a particular patient. Readers are advised that the statements and opinions expressed in this publication are provided as recommendations of the contributors and editors at the time of publication and should not be construed as official college policy. ACEP acknowledges that, as new medical knowledge emerges, best practice recommendations can change faster than published content can be updated. ACEP recognizes the complexity of emergency medicine and makes no representation that this publication serves as an authoritative resource for the prevention, diagnosis, treatment, or intervention for any medical condition, nor should it be the basis for the definition of or standard of care that should be practiced by all health-care providers at any particular time or place. To the fullest extent permitted by law, and without limitation, ACEP expressly disclaims all liability for errors or omissions contained within this publication and for damages of any kind or nature, arising out of use, reference to, reliance on, or performance of such information.

To contact ACEP, call 800-798-1822 or 972-550-0911 or write to PO Box 619911, Dallas, TX 75261-9911; or email bookstore@acep.org. Your comments and suggestions are always welcome.

American College of Emergency Physicians®
ADVANCING EMERGENCY CARE

ISBN: 978-0-9988912-7-9
First printing, October 2018

Library of Congress Cataloging-in-Publication Data

Names: Stader, Donald E., III, editor. | Donihoo, Rachel S., editor. | Brady, Mark F., editor. | American College of Emergency Physicians.
Title: Bring 'em all : chaos. Care. Stories from medicine's front line / Donald E. Stader, III, editor-in-chief ; Rachel S. Donihoo, co-editor, Mark F. Brady, co-editor.
Description: Dallas, Texas : American College of Emergency Physicians, 2018.
Identifiers: LCCN 2018027653 | ISBN 9780998891279
Subjects: | MESH: Allied Health Personnel | Autobiography
Classification: LCC R697.A4 | NLM WZ 112.5.A2 | DDC 610.73/7069--dc23
LC record available at https://lccn.loc.gov/2018027653

Printed in the United States of America at Walsworth

BRING 'EM ALL

Chaos. Care. Stories from Medicine's Front Line.

Photographs and interviews by Eugene Richards

Donald E. Stader III, MD, FACEP
Editor-in-Chief

Rachel S. Donihoo
Co-Editor

Mark F. Brady, MD, MPH, FACEP
Co-Editor

Contents

Foreword

If you've ever found yourself in an emergency department, it probably wasn't one of your better days. But if you looked past the rushing ambulance crews and through the blur of activity, you probably saw a coordinated team of emergency physicians, nurses, technicians, and other support staff — all there, carving order out of chaos. Odds are you underwent tests, were given a diagnosis, and received treatment for your condition.

It hasn't always been like this. Only a few decades ago, emergency care in the United States and across the globe was agonizingly poor. Although medicine had rapidly advanced in many areas, the care of the sickest patients inexplicably remained neglected. Emergency departments, which were regarded as "the weakest link" in trauma care, were commonly staffed by inexperienced physicians — or even medical students — who had no formal training in emergency care. The stories from this era are grim — unrecognized bleeding that led to the death of a child, failure to provide a lifesaving breathing tube to a patient in respiratory failure, a misdiagnosed fatal infection. Early ambulance services were often run by undertakers driving hearses. Emergency departments were disorganized, scary places.

As the public began to cry out for improvements, several forward-thinking doctors stepped up to do something about the sorry state of emergency care. In 1961, James Mills Jr., MD, president of the medical staff at the Alexandria Hospital in Virginia, recognized his emergency department was plagued by long waits, inadequate care, and the ire of an angry community. Mills committed to solving the problem himself — with a little help. He took the bold step of leaving a successful general practice, convincing three other risk-taking generalists to join him in staffing the emergency department full time. In doing so, they provided around-the-clock care in Alexandria's emergency department. As we reflect on it now, the arrangement seems amazingly simple, yet it was a revolutionary step in emergency care. In the next decade, many more "Alexandria Plan" practices popped up around the United States, many of them guided by Mills and his colleagues. The results were obvious and positive. Patients got better care and the emergency staff was grateful to finally have order.

Although the number of physicians in full-time emergency practice multiplied, the specialty had yet to achieve status as a "real" medical profession. There was a great need to improve educational programs for practicing emergency physicians, who yearned for more professional might in the house of medicine. Into this gap stepped John Wiegenstein, MD. In 1968, he and seven colleagues came together to create a tiny organization they somewhat presumptuously named the American College of Emergency Physicians (ACEP).

In a classic case of "if you build it, they will come," other emergency physicians from across the nation soon flocked to ACEP's early meetings, hungry for the opportunities and camaraderie it had to offer. The organization's members soon began to function as a larger and more influential body, and many realized there was much more to be done.

Physicians in any of the other twenty-two medical specialties were required to complete residency training before they could practice. Emergency medicine needed to catch up. The first emergency medicine residency program was established at the University of Cincinnati in 1970. Bruce Janiak, MD, whom you'll meet in this book, was the program's first resident. Other institutions soon followed; by 1975, thirty-five emergency medicine residencies were up and running.

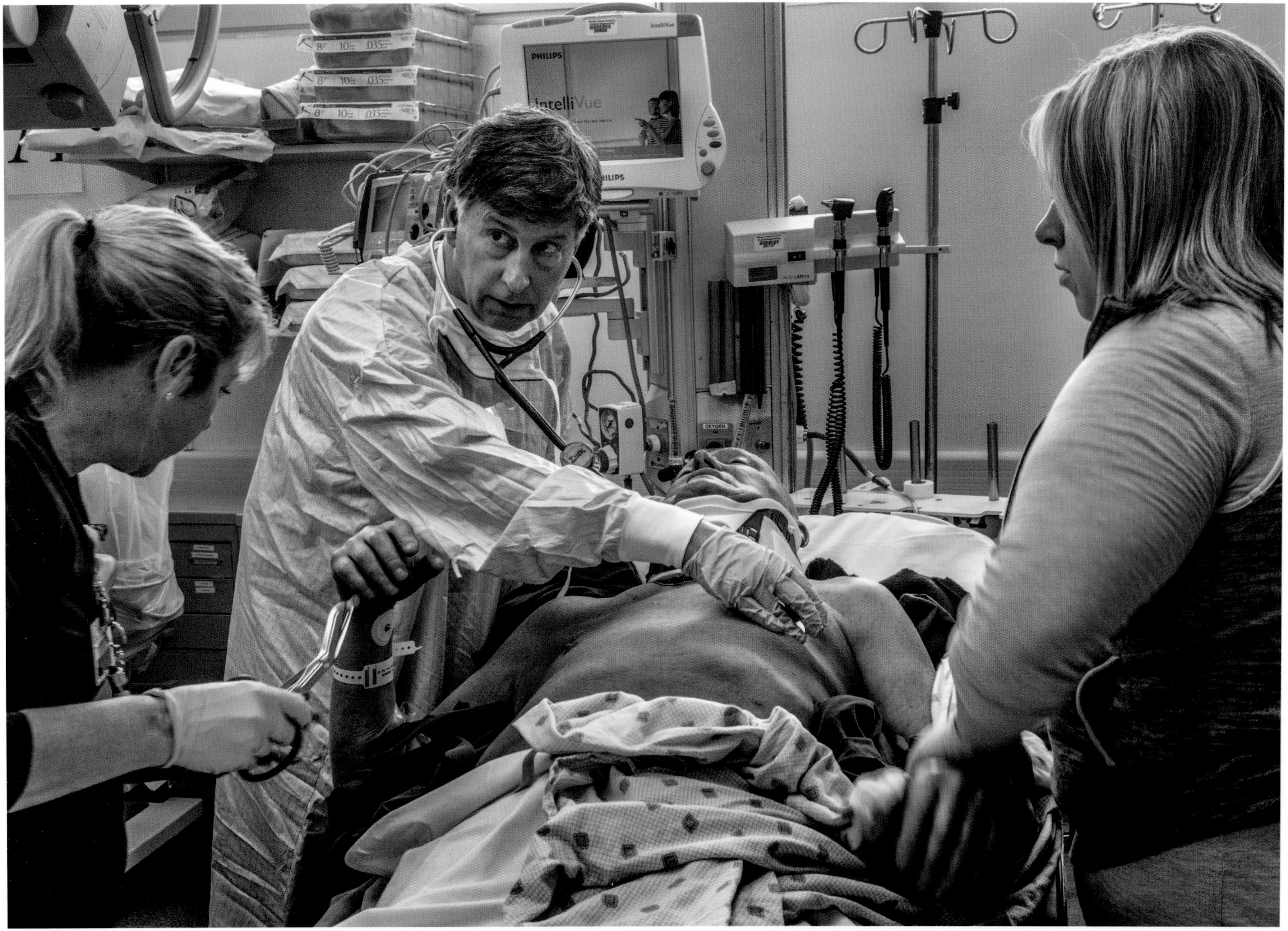

Brian Zink, MD

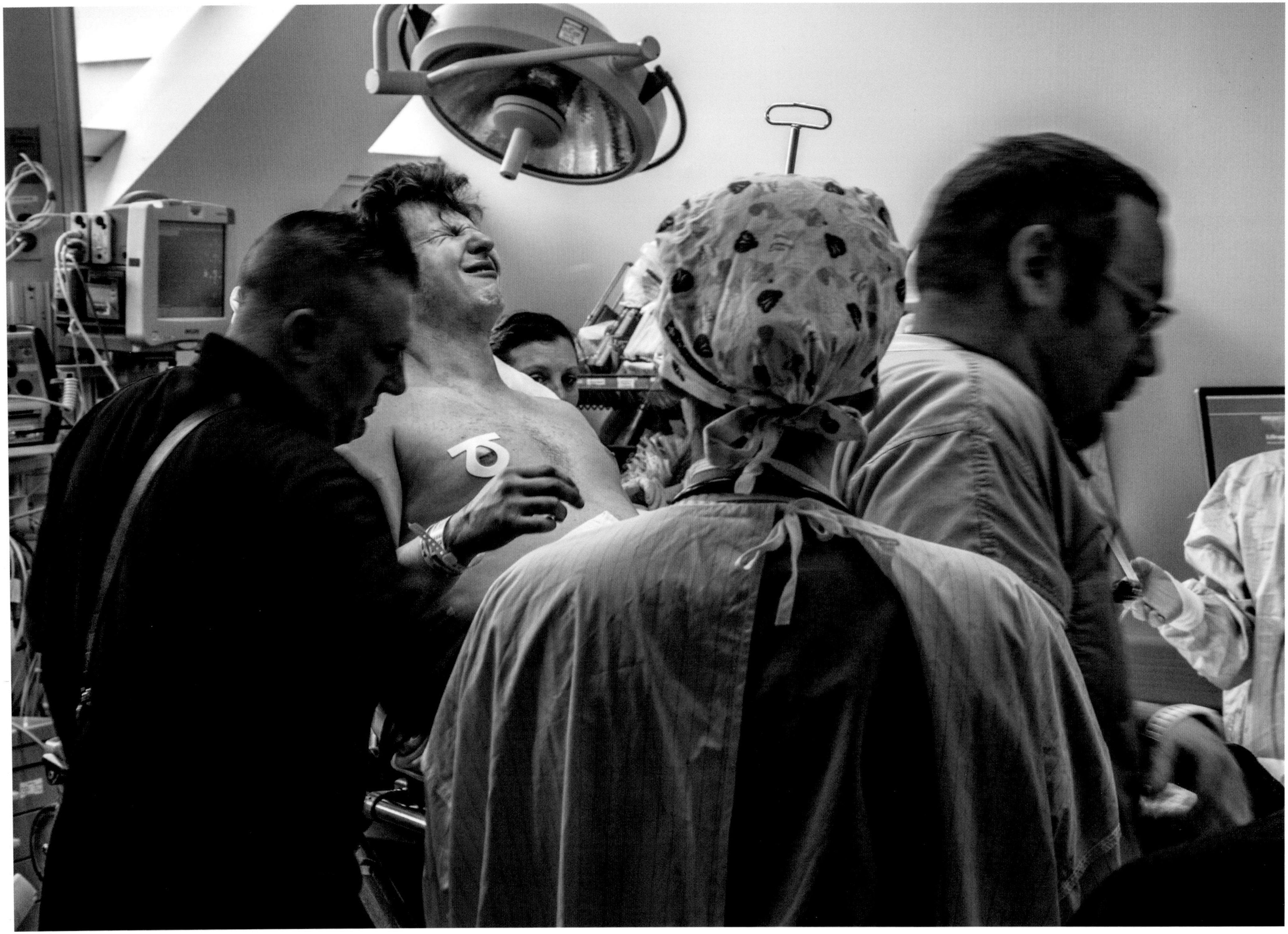

Most of the sentinel emergency medicine residency programs were born in the heartland of America. For many years, emergency medicine remained notably absent in the country's most prestigious medical schools, many of which held a dim view of this new realm of practice, and thought even less of those who chose to "waste a career" on its pursuit. These universities continued to staff their hospital emergency departments with unsupervised interns and residents, who were expected to take care of the sickest and most complex of patients. The specialty still had a long way to go.

ACEP knew if emergency physicians wanted to be regarded as true professionals in American medicine, they would need to be certified by a specialty board, yet none existed. In 1976, the organization began to build a framework that would become the American Board of Emergency Medicine (ABEM). It was a painstaking process that would involve years of horse trading and wrangling before the field would be sanctioned by the American Board of Medical Specialties (ABMS). ABEM became official in 1979, but the development wasn't viewed favorably by many in the medical establishment. To reduce the grumbling, a "modified conjoint" board provided ABEM seats to members of other major ABMS boards in fields such as pediatrics and surgery. The collaboration was fruitful; other experienced medical leaders came to appreciate this new specialty and provided sound advice that guided its future.

Fast-forward to the present. The specialty now boasts more than 32,000 ABEM-certified emergency physicians and more than 160 residency programs. Emergency medicine is now the third most popular specialty choice for graduating US medical students. Its leaders continue to serve at the top echelons of major medical organizations and government. Arguably, nothing has had a more positive impact on American medicine in the last fifty years than the improvement in emergency care.

The demand for emergency care has been unrelenting since the end of World War II. As the population swells, so has the number of cases — from preventable diseases like heart attacks and strokes to accidents and injuries triggered by our increasingly motorized world and from infectious diseases caused by globalization to the medical sequelae of crime and poverty.

David Wagner, MD, an early emergency medicine pioneer, remarked that ours is the only specialty created by the *people* rather than the medical establishment. This grassroots ambition would be tested in the ensuing years, however, as the emergency department became the safety net for a dysfunctional health-care system. The passage of the Emergency Medical Treatment and Labor Act in 1986 further codified what was already happening — emergency departments were required to accept any and every patient regardless of their condition or ability to pay.

The volume of patients who rely on emergency care has increased exponentially with each passing year; US emergency departments received more than 140 million visits in 2017 alone. You might ask why would anyone choose to work in such an unpredictable, high-stress environment. What would possess a clinician to take on the ills of society and endure this daily stream of tribulations and tragedies? The truth is, we love the rollercoaster ride. We gravitate toward crises and are trained to be at our best on your worst day. But we also suffer unmistakable pain — the unsuccessful cardiac resuscitation, the young life lost to the opioid epidemic, the horror of child abuse. We are pained by the random, unfathomable things that happen to nice, ordinary people. The toll of grief, however, is eased by the satisfaction that comes with true service. There is no feeling more authentic than working in the emergency department, fully immersed in the culture of your own community.

The diverse spectrum of clinicians you are about to meet is a testament to the men and women on whose backs this specialty was built. Their stories reflect the commitment we all share to those we serve.

Brian Zink, MD, FACEP

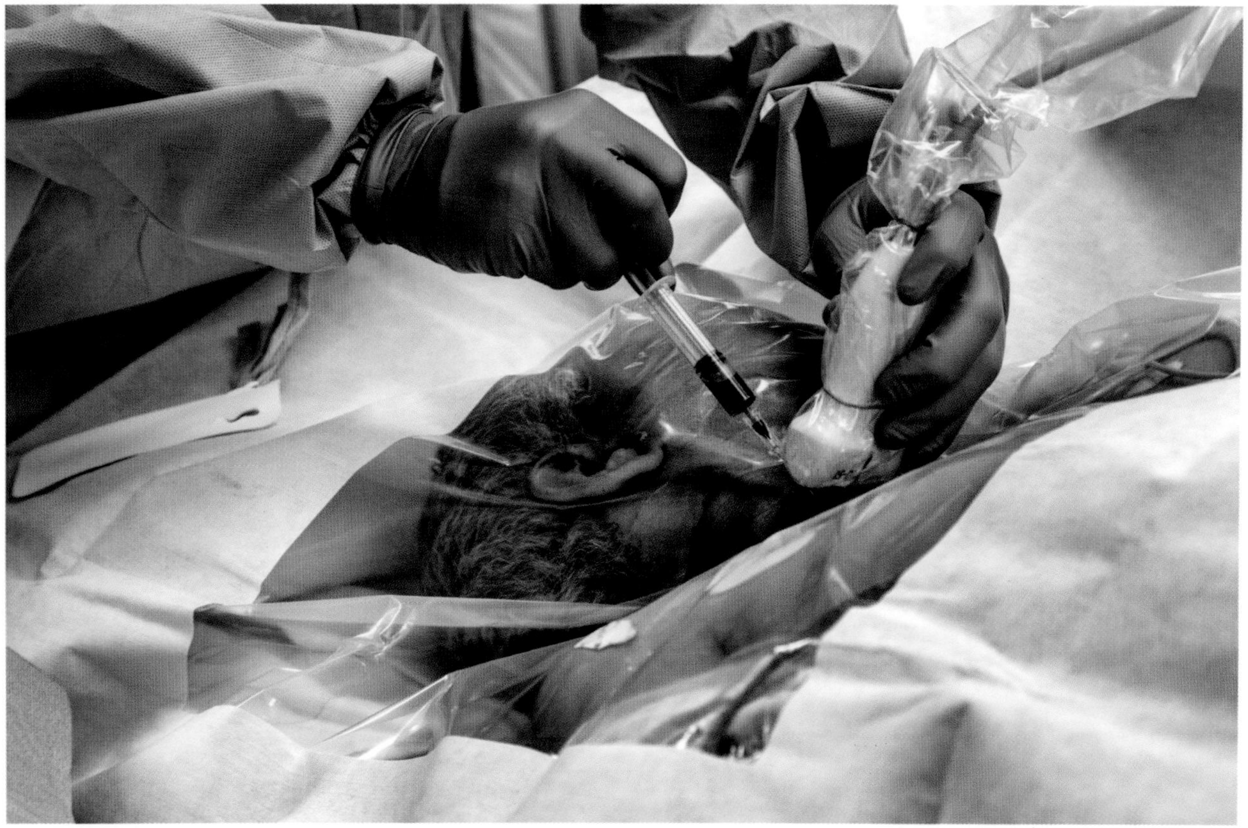

Preface

Shortly after midnight on June 20, 2012, a heavily armed gunman entered a movie theater in Aurora, Colorado. He lobbed two canisters of tear gas into a crowd of four hundred civilians and then — in rapid succession — fired seventy-six rounds of ammunition into the audience.

Two miles away, Aurora Medical Center charge nurse Jen Farris began receiving calls from 911 dispatchers, desperate to know where to transport the scores of victims. The emergency department's trauma bays and half of its treatment rooms were closed due to renovation, and the two on-duty physicians were already tending to an overflow of patients. Although she had several good reasons to refuse or accept only a limited number of victims, Jen provided an answer that epitomizes the spirit of emergency care. She told the dispatcher, *"Bring 'em all."*

Twenty-one patients were transported to Aurora within the span of an hour, many of whom were critically injured. In addition to the valiant efforts of Drs. Paige Archey and Kevin "Woody" McGlothlen, clinical staff poured in from across the hospital to care for the influx of victims. Some, including Dr. Gilbert Pineda, rushed from their homes upon hearing of the shooting. Amidst the horror, these clinicians went about their sacred duty to care for the injured and maimed. Although the rampage claimed twelve lives, wounded seventy, and rattled the nation, not a single person transported to Aurora Medical Center died.

Bring 'EM All. Chaos. Care. Stories from Medicine's Front Line pays homage to the heroic men and women of America's emergency care system, who work to preserve the health of their communities every second of every hour of every day, 365 days a year. This groundbreaking book was commissioned by the specialty's leading architect, the American College of Emergency Physicians (ACEP), in celebration of its fiftieth anniversary. We can think of no better way to commemorate this milestone than to present a work that honors and reflects what it means to be an emergency clinician.

The book is modeled after a typical emergency department shift. Every shift is, in essence, a tapestry of stories. The time spent with each patient is short; brevity is mandated by the intensity and demands of caring for so many. These temporal constraints force emergency clinicians to cut

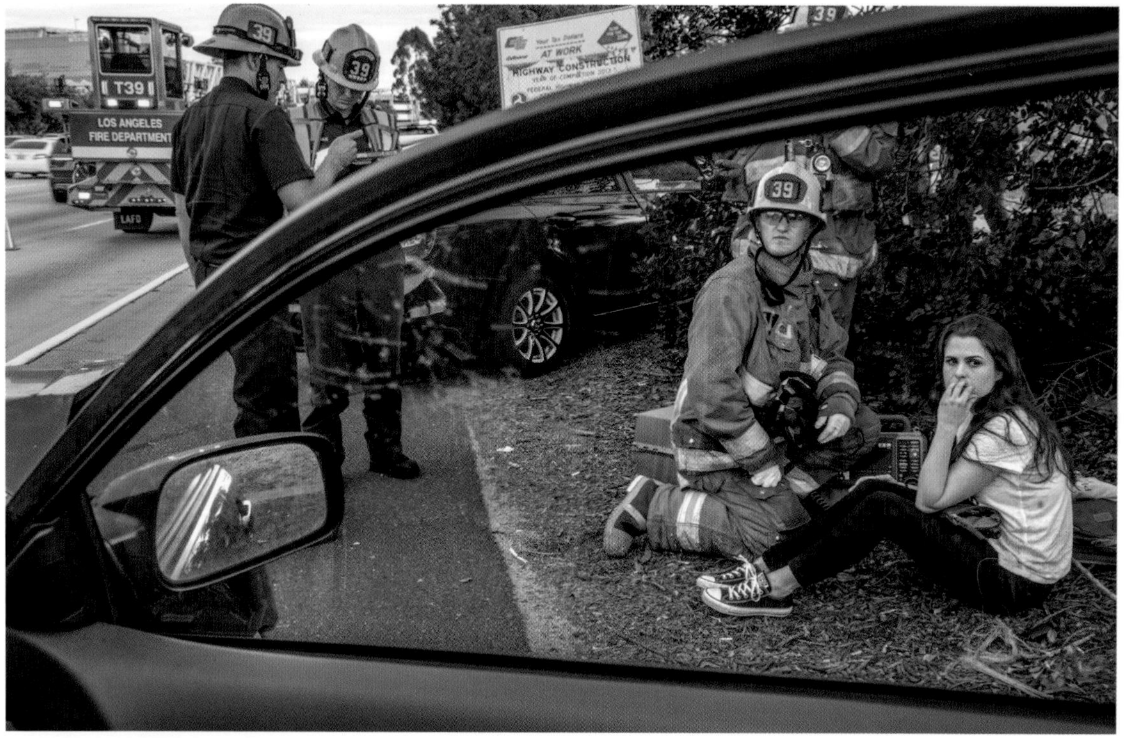

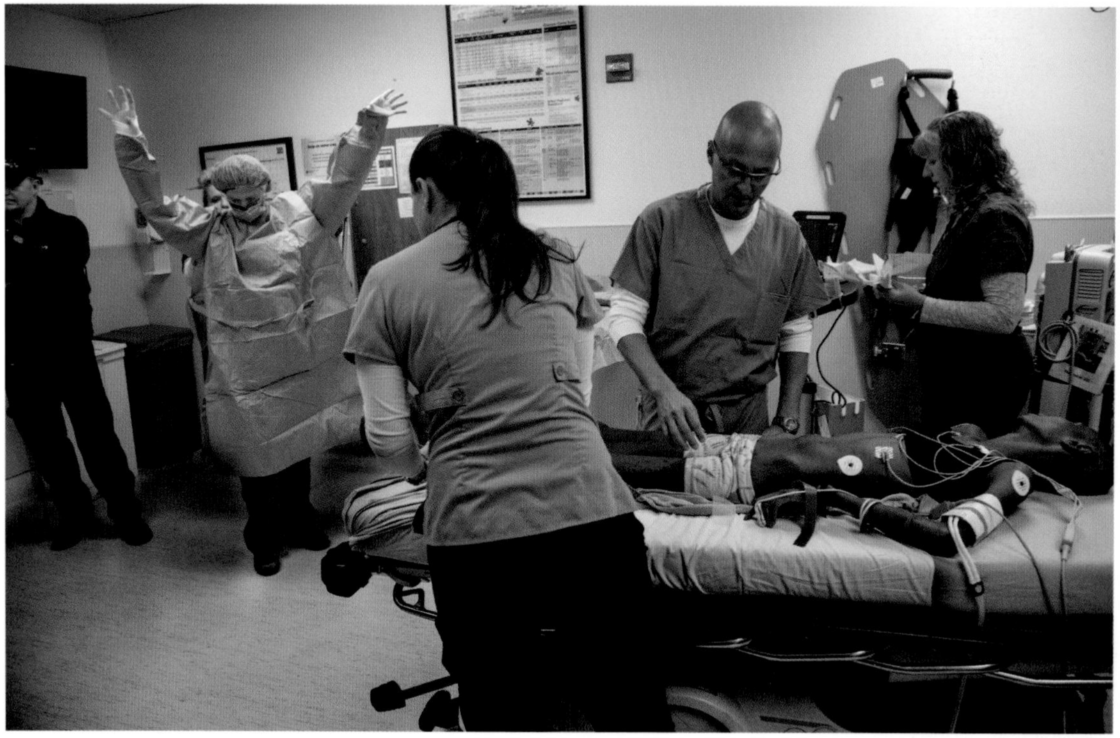

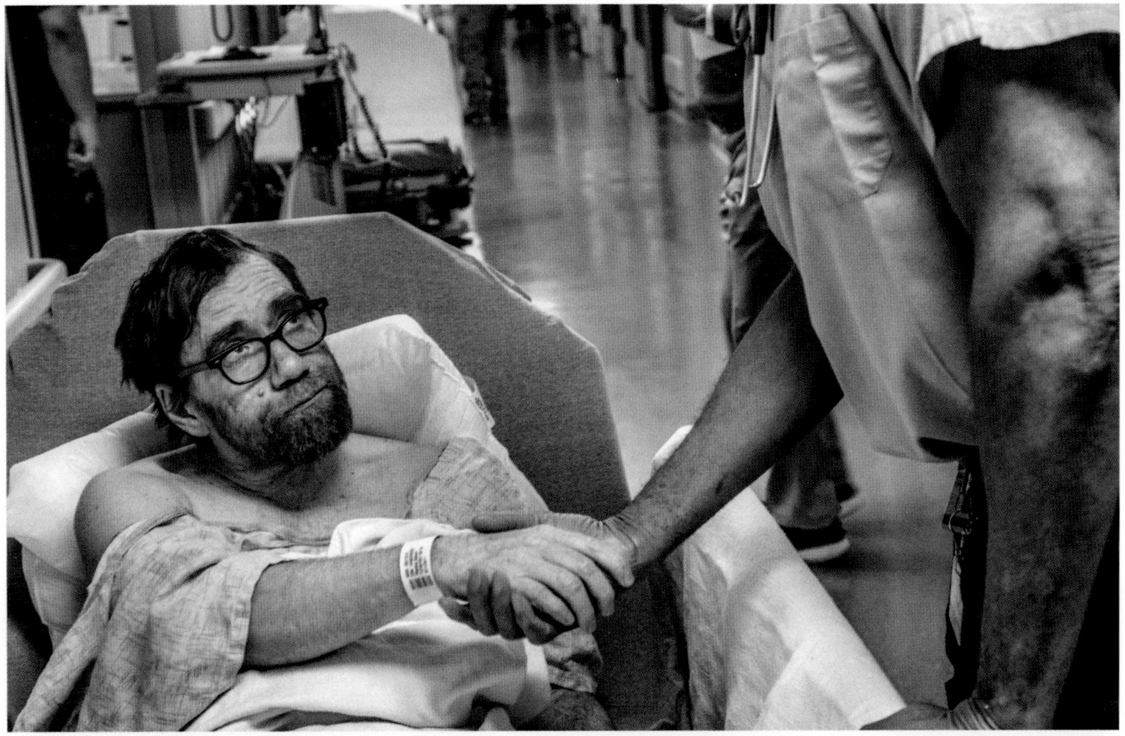

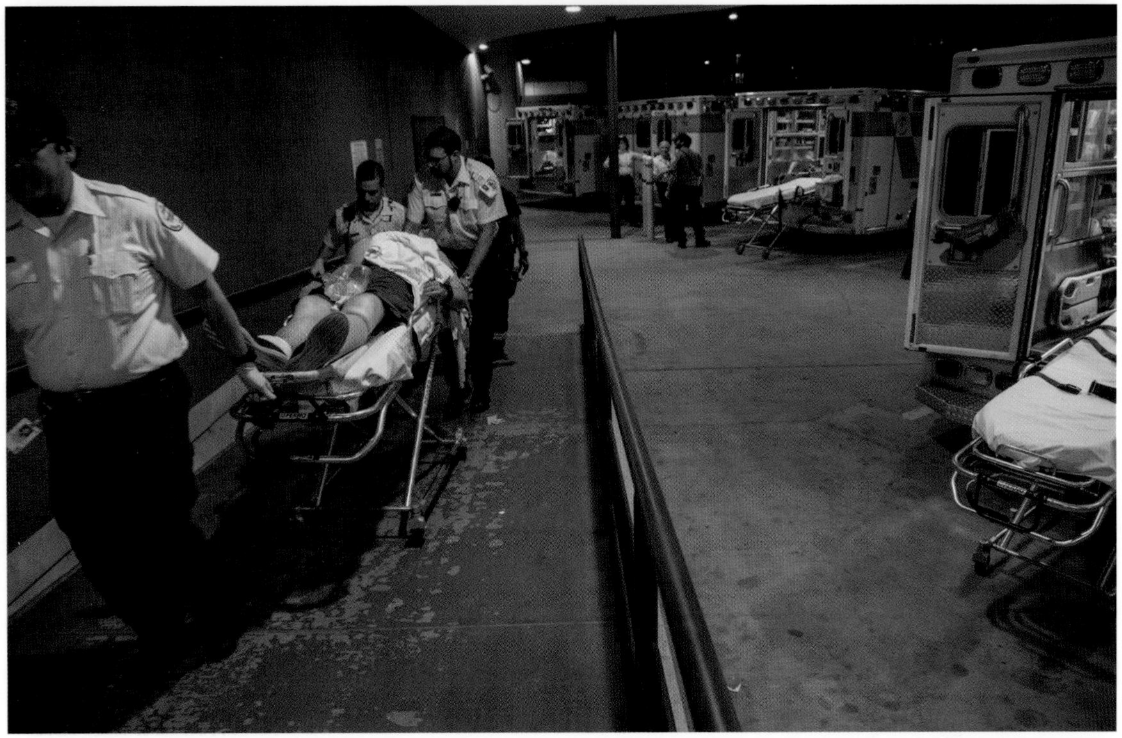

to the chase and demand we delve quickly into the core of a patient's health and history. The stories in this book reflect the cadence of those interactions — short, concise, powerful.

In the 1980s, a talented photojournalist was tasked with capturing life and death in an American emergency room. Eugene Richards quickly befriended the physicians, paramedics, and staff of Denver General — a kinship that resulted in his celebrated work, *The Knife and Gun Club: Scenes from an Emergency Room*. That book helped to define the specialty — for the public and for itself.

Now, nearly thirty years later, Richards has turned his lens on a new generation of caregivers. For more than two years, our production team traveled across the country — from rural Alaska to Atlanta, from Los Angeles to New York — to capture everyday life in the emergency department. Richards photographed and interviewed clinicians in a vast array of environments, ranging from major urban trauma centers to small community hospitals and from city streets to remote stretches of wilderness.

On these pages, you'll be introduced to both emergency medicine pioneers and young residents in the throes of training. You'll meet paramedics and firefighters who risk their lives to render aid and nurses and physician assistants who tend to their patients at the bedside with unrelenting care. Without exception, the first-person accounts found on these pages demonstrate the extraordinary spirit of this rare breed of medical providers, who dedicate their lives to confronting uncertainty and chaos with unwavering compassion. While tremendously diverse, they are unified by a central calling.

Through these powerful narratives and images, ACEP seeks to provide an intimate view of emergency care in America while honoring the profound sense of duty that motivates its providers. We are proud to provide this glimpse into the heart and soul of the specialty and what it means to serve on medicine's front line.

Donald E. Stader III, MD, FACEP
Editor-in-Chief

Acknowledgments

Many have called emergency medicine the ultimate team sport and for good reason. In emergency departments across the nation, clinicians work in unison to restore life, provide comfort, and serve as the guardians of their community's health. This book, inspired by the same spirit of collaboration and resolve, would not have been possible without the extraordinary people and institutions that supported and guided our vision.

To the patients we photographed — thank you for allowing us to capture your vulnerability, which so beautifully reveals the humanity of emergency medicine. To the clinicians who shared their stories — your candor, wit, and strength inspire us. To the hospitals and EMS agencies that generously opened their doors to our team — it is a privilege to highlight the care your dedicated clinicians provide. To our collaborators both within and outside of the American College of Emergency Physicians — thank you for your tireless work and commitment.

We extend our profound gratitude to the following people and institutions.

Janine Altongy
Lisa Bundy, MD, FACEP
Leslie Clark
Nick Jouriles, MD, FACEP
Christopher Kang, MD, FACEP
Linda Lawrence, MD, FACEP
Don Lum, MD, FACEP
Jana Nelson
Sam Richards
Carolyn Skei
Daniel Sullivan
Dean Wilkerson, JD, MBA, CAE
Brian Zink, MD, FACEP

Bellevue Hospital Center
Beth Israel Deaconess Medical Center
Bonneville County Sheriff's Office | Bonneville County Jail
Brooke Army Medical Center
Cleveland Clinic | Akron General Hospital
Denver Health Medical Center
Denver Health Paramedic Division
Drexel University | Hahnemann University Hospital
Grady Memorial Hospital
Henry Ford Health System
KentuckyOne Health | St. Joseph East Hospital
LifeMed Alaska
Los Angeles County + USC Medical Center
Los Angeles Fire Department
Mat-Su Regional Medical Center
Medical Center of Aurora
Museum of Science, Boston
Oregon Health & Science University
Philadelphia Sexual Assault Response Center
Rhode Island Hospital
STRATUS Center for Medical Simulation | Brigham and Women's Hospital
University of North Carolina

We also extend special thanks to the ACEP 50th Anniversary Task Force and ACEP Board of Directors for their stalwart support.

Introduction

The American College of Emergency Physicians (ACEP) was established in response to a growing public need for quality emergency care. With grit and determination, its founders pushed countless boundaries to create a robust, collaborative network that would come to define a brand-new specialty — emergency medicine.

From its humble beginning on August 16, 1968, when eight physicians convened in Lansing, Michigan, ACEP has grown to become the largest emergency medicine organization in the world. Our 38,000 members embody the college's rich history as the leading advocate for emergency physicians, their patients, and the public.

Year after year, ACEP has provided world-class medical education and research; resources for quality care and patient safety; management tools and guidelines for clinical practice; and support for residency training, EMS, and disaster response to clinicians across the globe. Throughout its five decades of leadership, the organization has exceeded the dreams of its founders by successfully championing better emergency care at the local, state, and national levels.

In keeping with that pioneering spirit, ACEP is enormously proud to present this compelling collection of images and stories, which so potently illustrate the dedication, humor, and compassion emergency clinicians bring to the front line. We believe our specialty is the backbone of health care — an essential right that should forever be available to every individual in every community. We consider it a calling and are privileged to serve alongside the accomplished clinicians featured on these pages.

Paul Kivela, MD, MBA, FACEP
President, ACEP

Nicholas J. Jouriles, MD, FACEP
Chair, ACEP 50th Anniversary Task Force

A Note from the Artist

The workday began pretty much the same way every time, every place. After being buzzed into the emergency department by public relations or security, I'd introduce myself, find a place to stand in the shadows of the farthest corner, and wait. The running joke was that the minute I walked into an ED, the world stopped, or at least slowed to a crawl; there would be no falls from high-up scaffolds, no stabbings, no multicar wrecks, fewer overdoses, fewer strokes, no failing hearts.

I often wouldn't take a single meaningful picture until very late in the day, when things had, in fact, quieted down. Then again, the quietest times weren't all that quiet. I'd hear patients moan, clear their throats, snore, beg to go home. I'd see doctors on their computers, searching through medical records, making decisions; nurses sprinting from room to room; patients waiting for I don't know what, their faces slack and full of resignation.

Each time a new patient was brought onto the ward, I'd grow anxious. The doctor or nurse need only look my way and off I'd go, trailing behind through the ward. There was seldom a moment I didn't feel like a stalker, waiting just outside a patient's room, a *sick* person's room, for a waving hand to motion me inside.

I made pictures any time I could . . . when patients were feeling better and there was time to talk . . . when a weary doctor was pronouncing a time of death . . . when the trauma room was so jammed with people — shoulder to shoulder, heads to shoulders — that I was afraid to move. I made pictures when it was pleasant and easy to do so, and even when I couldn't get rid of the feeling that everyone in the room was working to assist the patient except me. I kept shooting even when I couldn't shake my own feelings of helplessness, as I watched everyone working in unison to assist the patient — everyone except me.

The interviews with the doctors, nurses, physician assistants, and paramedics came after the shifts had ended. And if I'd forgotten, these conversations reminded me that pictures are one thing, spoken language another. Face to face with people I deeply admired, I didn't always know what to say. I'd blurt out, "Tell me what it was like for you as a child," causing most everyone to sit up and take a breath before leading me, each in their own way, through the innumerable twists and turns of their lives.

Eugene Richards

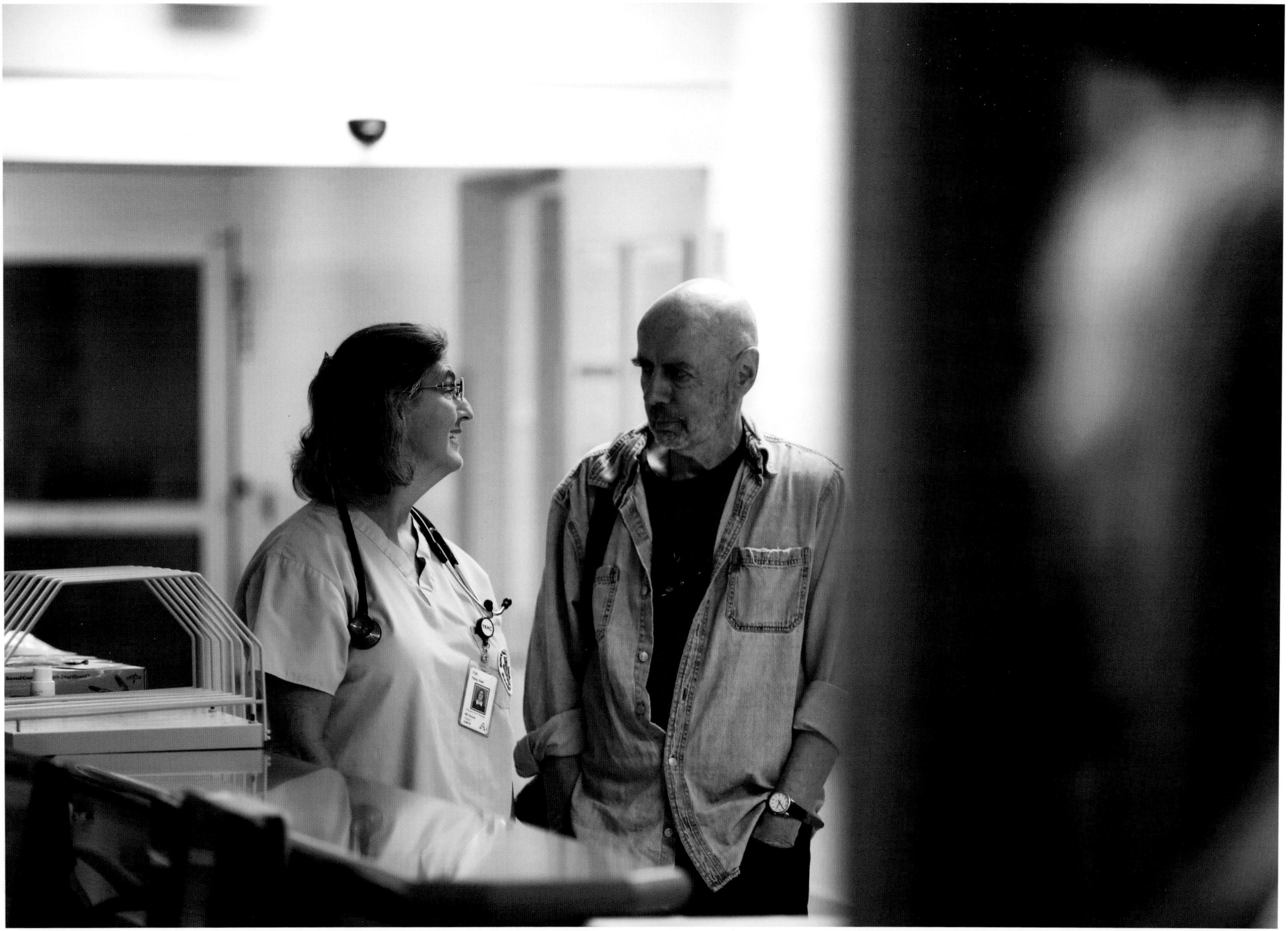

Eugene Richards

Paige Archey, MD | Gilbert Pineda, MD

Emergency Physicians
Aurora, Colorado

Paige: We started hearing things on the police blotter . . . something had happened at the movie theater. My charge nurse announced that shooting victims were on the way. The next thing I know, she was saying, "Just bring 'em all." I thought, *God, what all are we going to get?* And they started coming, one after another after another. Police cars were pulling up to the ambulance bay and we were unloading victims from the backseat. There was a patient with a leg wound, screaming in the hallway . . . the trauma surgeon was cracking the chest of a pregnant woman. One of our hospitalists was frantically trying to reach her son who'd been at the movies that night. There were people everywhere.

Gilbert: The phone rang just as I was falling asleep; it was 12:53 am. The voice on the other end said, "Gilbert, there's been a mass shooting in Aurora. You need to get to the hospital." I didn't ask any questions . . . I don't think I said yes or no . . . I just remember backing out of the driveway, still in a daze. I flipped on the EMS radio in my car and heard someone say there were six dead on scene and many more expected. I arrived at the ER as an ambulance was pulling up . . . they were unloading a twenty-something-year-old girl with a bullet in her head. I later found out she was a violinist.

Paige: Soon, staff started streaming in from other parts of the hospital. Our emergency department was under construction, so we were working with half an ER. We had no open beds, no major resuscitation bay, but we managed somehow. We just put our heads down and kept moving. We had to work through the logistical steps of managing this flood of high-acuity patients with very limited space.

Gilbert: I went from room to room to room. One of my colleagues was doing chest compressions . . . another was performing a thoracotomy. I heard a patient in the hallway screaming, "Help me!" . . . another was searching for his wife. I'm not one to sensationalize, but the injuries were graphic — and there were a lot of them. I didn't let my emotions get in the way, though. It was all about getting down to business. *Let's do it.* It was an impressive scene . . . everyone was being cared for.

Paige: It was strange, but the most critically ill were very serene. No tears . . . no screams . . . no demands. They just patiently waited for direction from us. Maybe it was the shock . . . I don't know . . . but I remember being impressed by their ability to hold it together. It was probably around 4:30 in the morning before I could tend to the other patients — the ones who'd arrived before the shooting. I kept apologizing for ignoring them, but, without fail, they all said, "You do what you need to do. We know what happened."

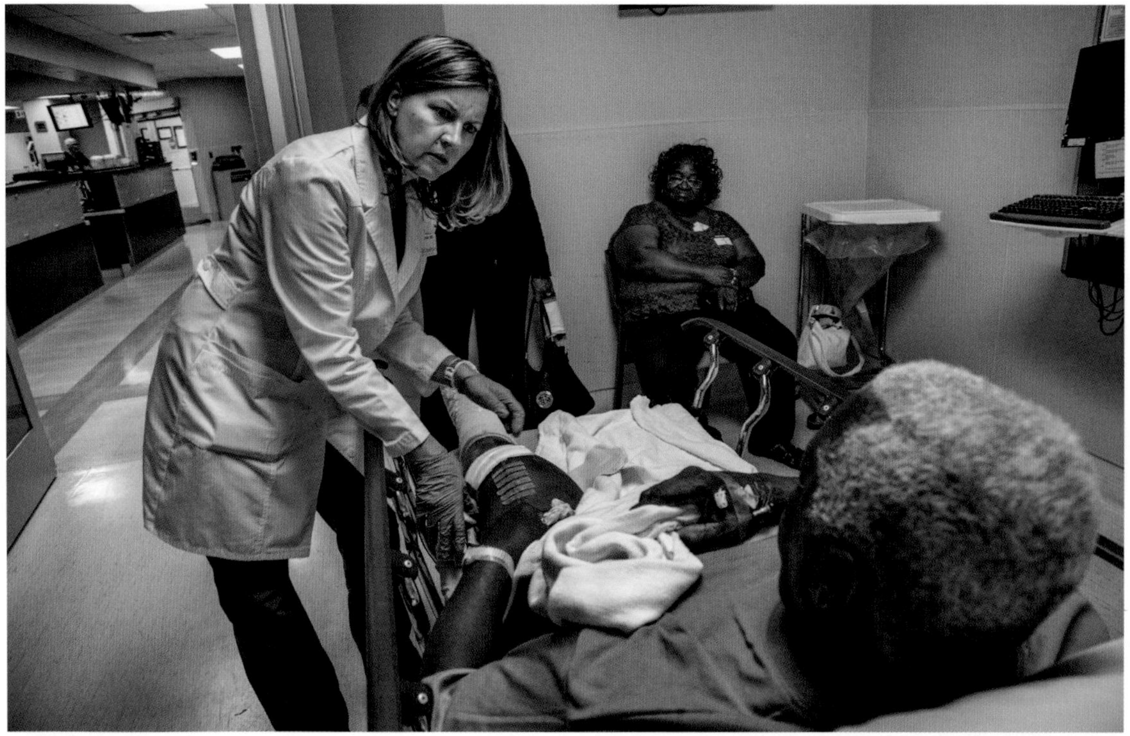

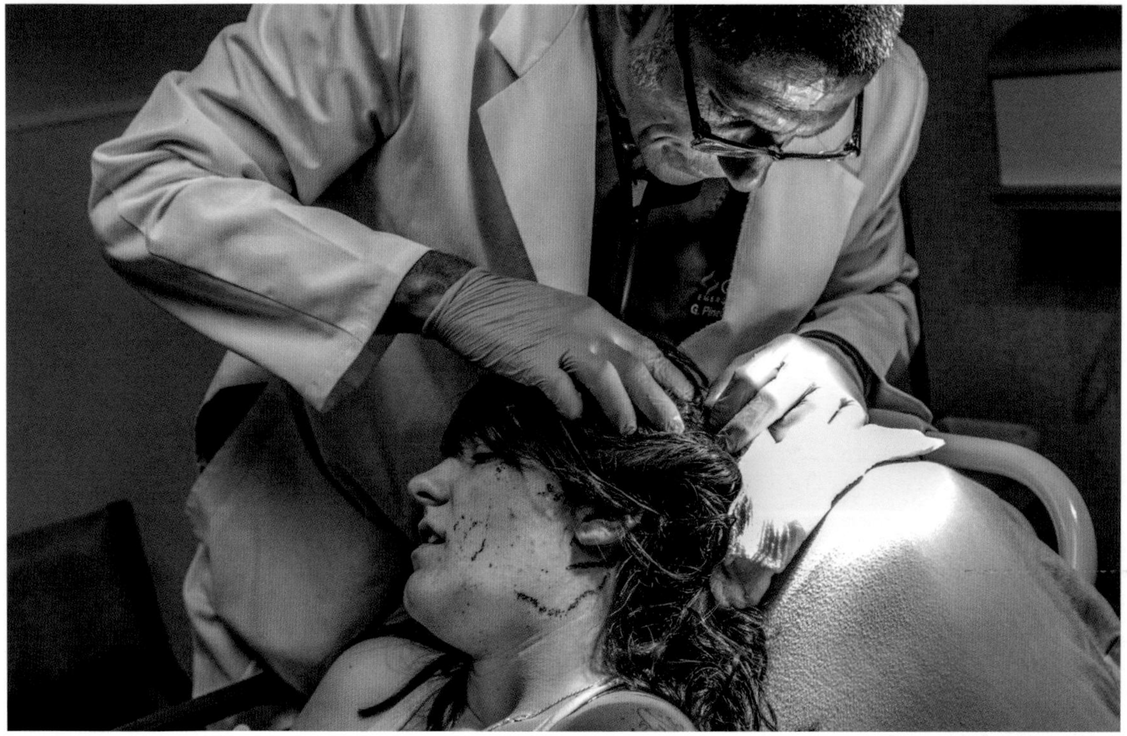

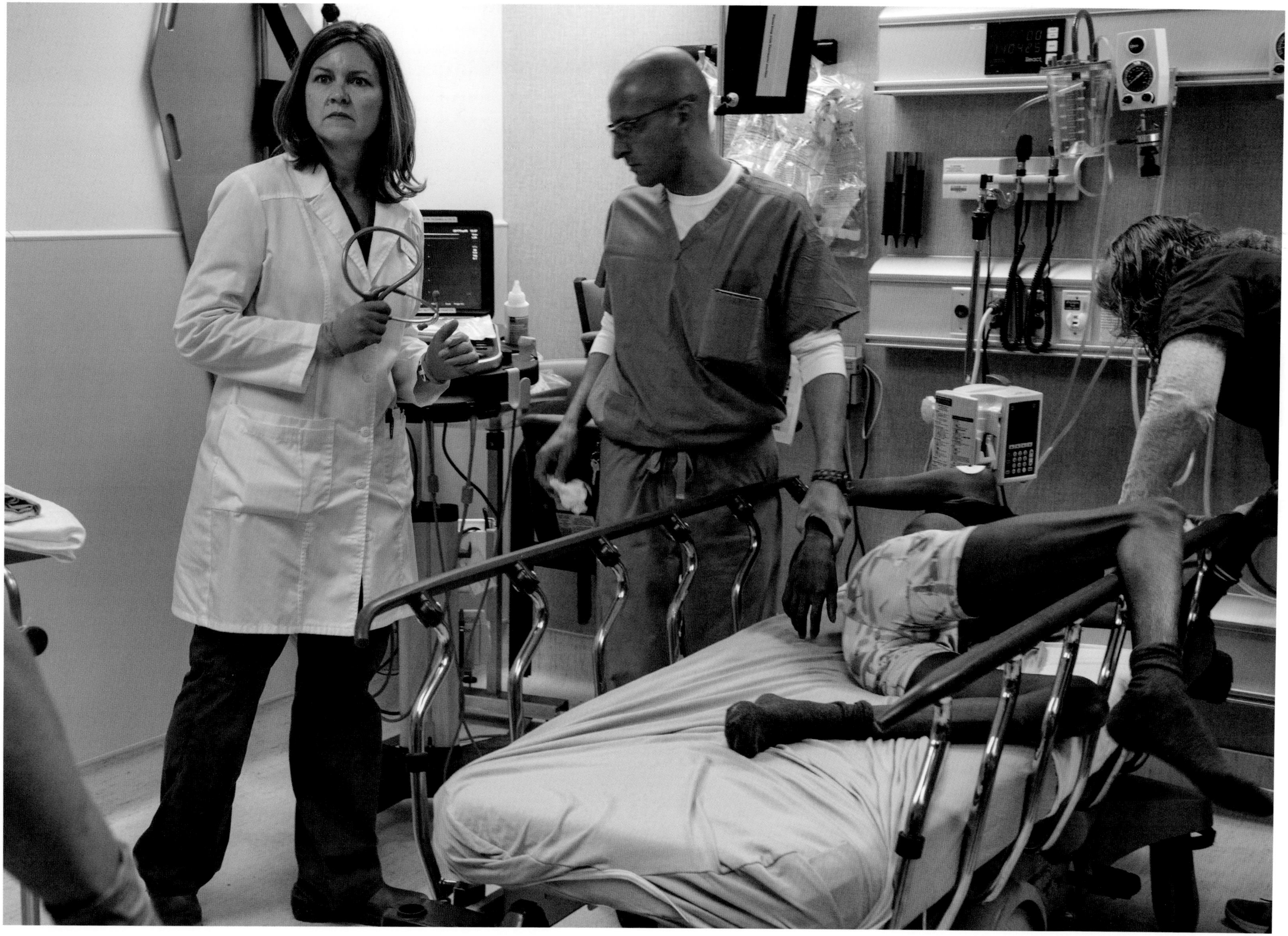

Paige Archey, MD | Gilbert Pineda, MD

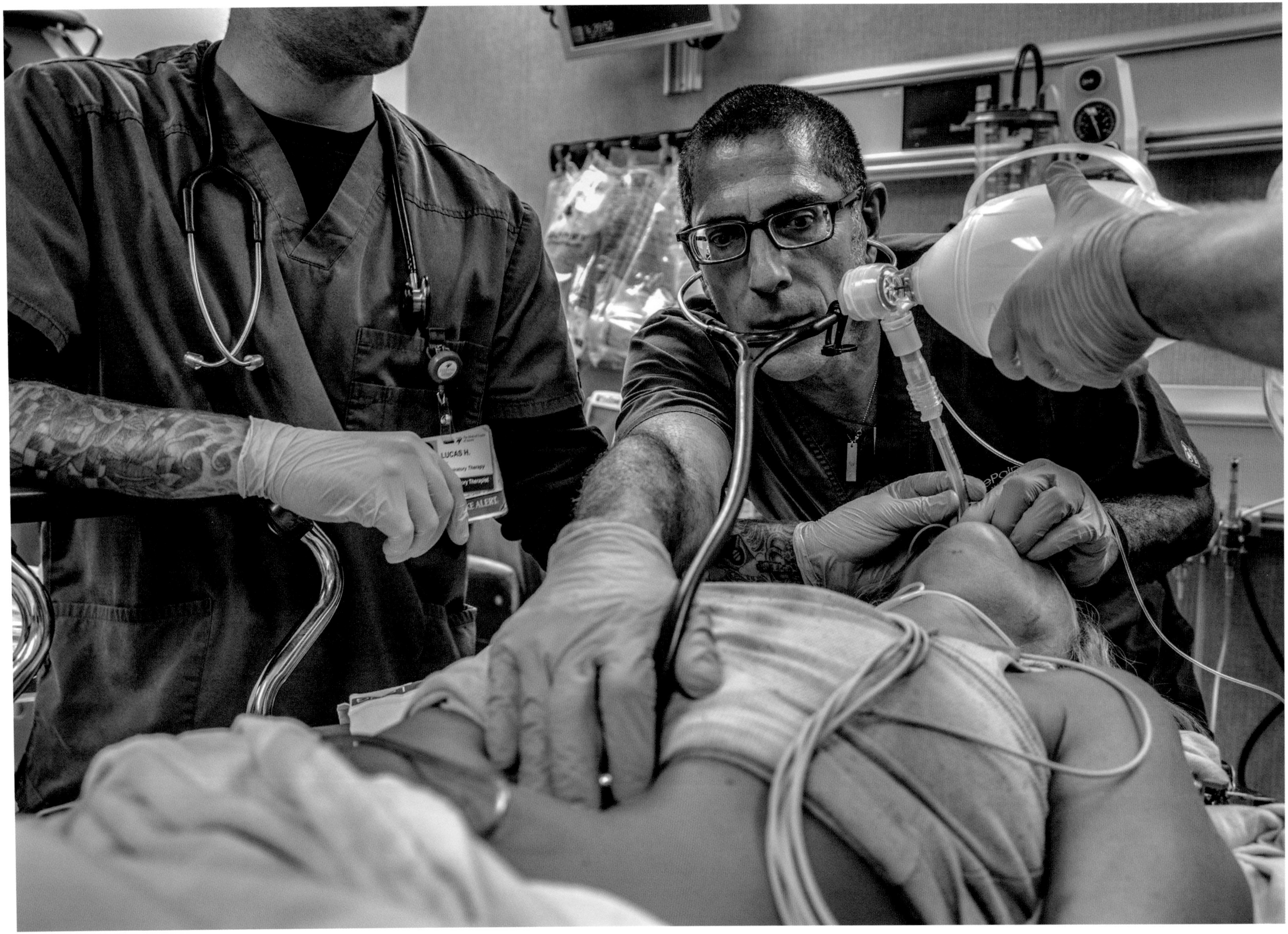
LUCAS H.

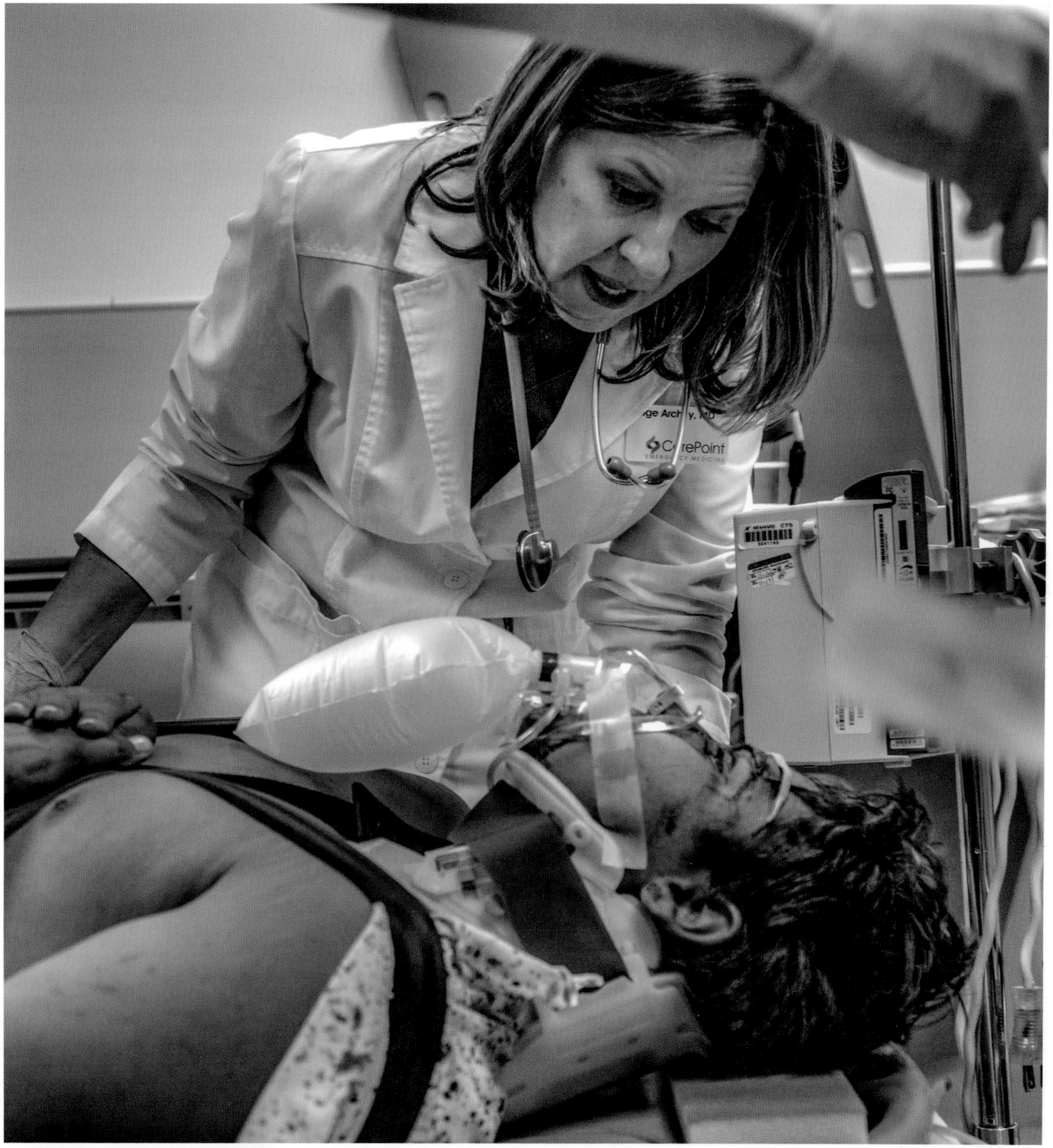
CarePoint

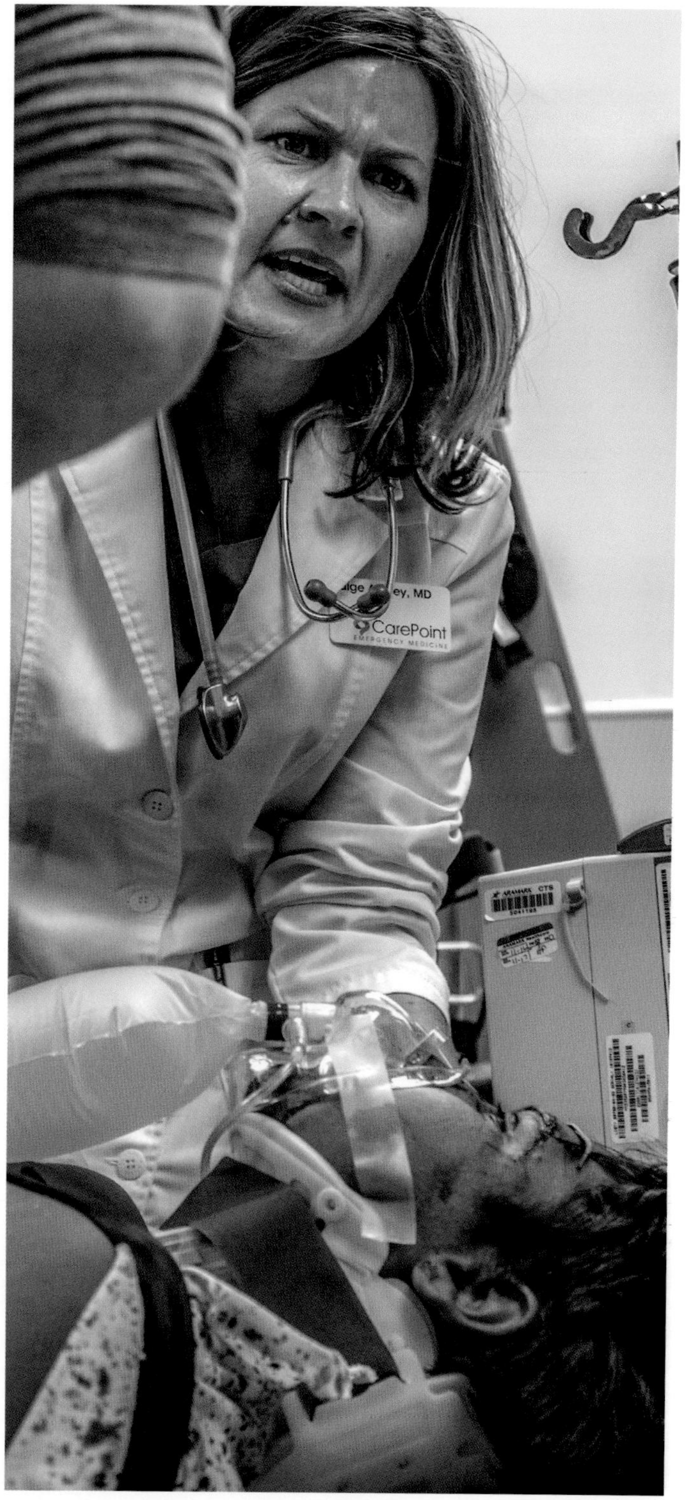
CarePoint

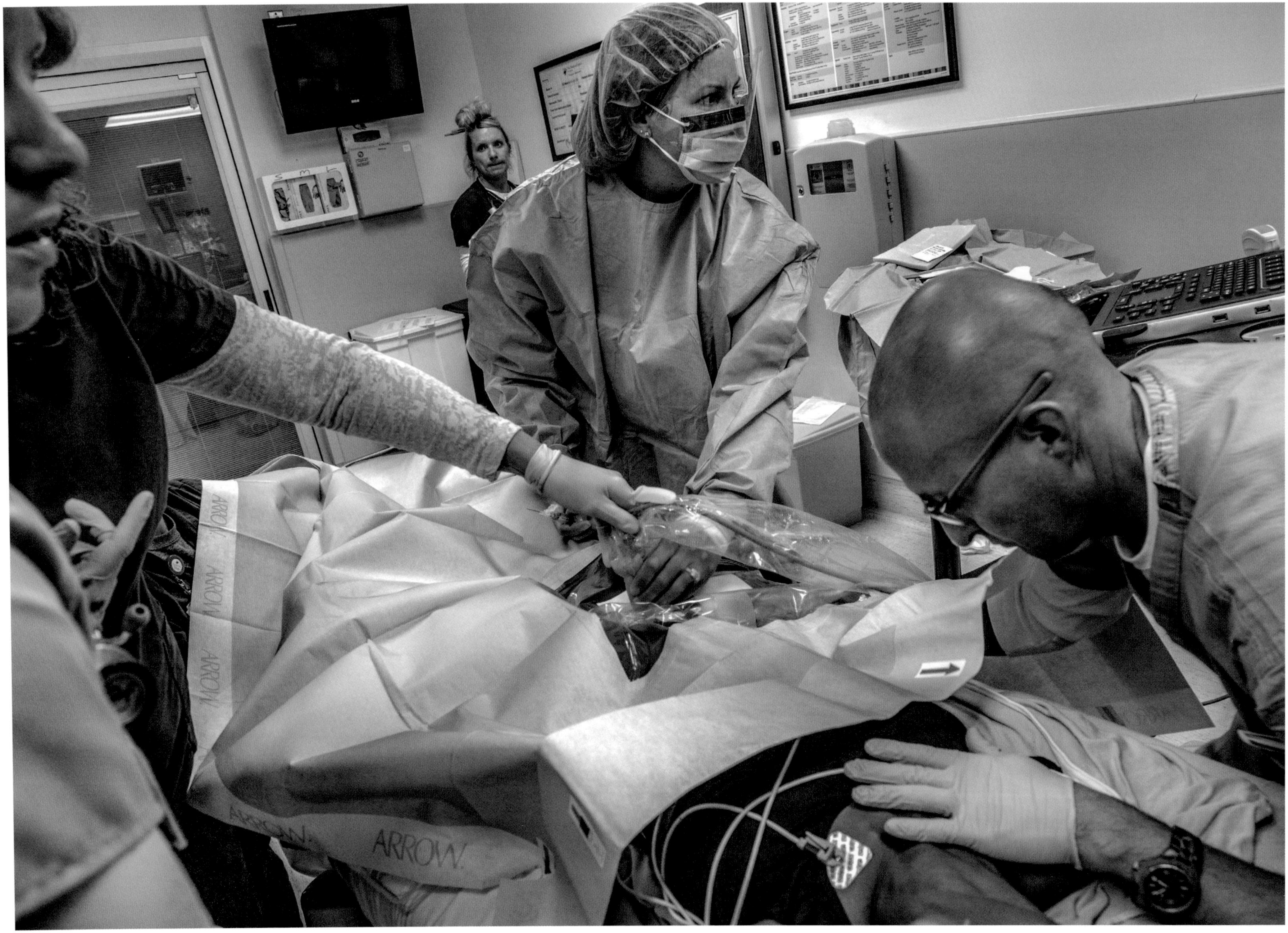
ARROW
ARROW
ARROW
ARROW
ARROW

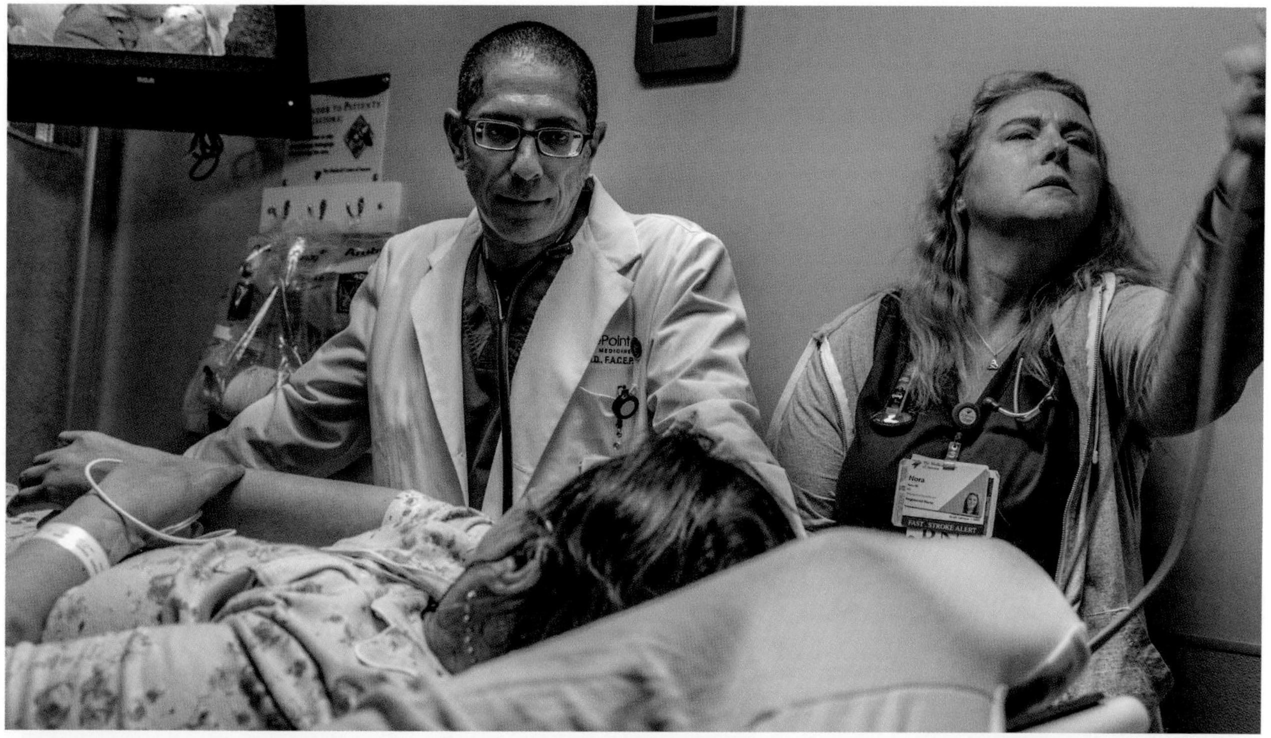

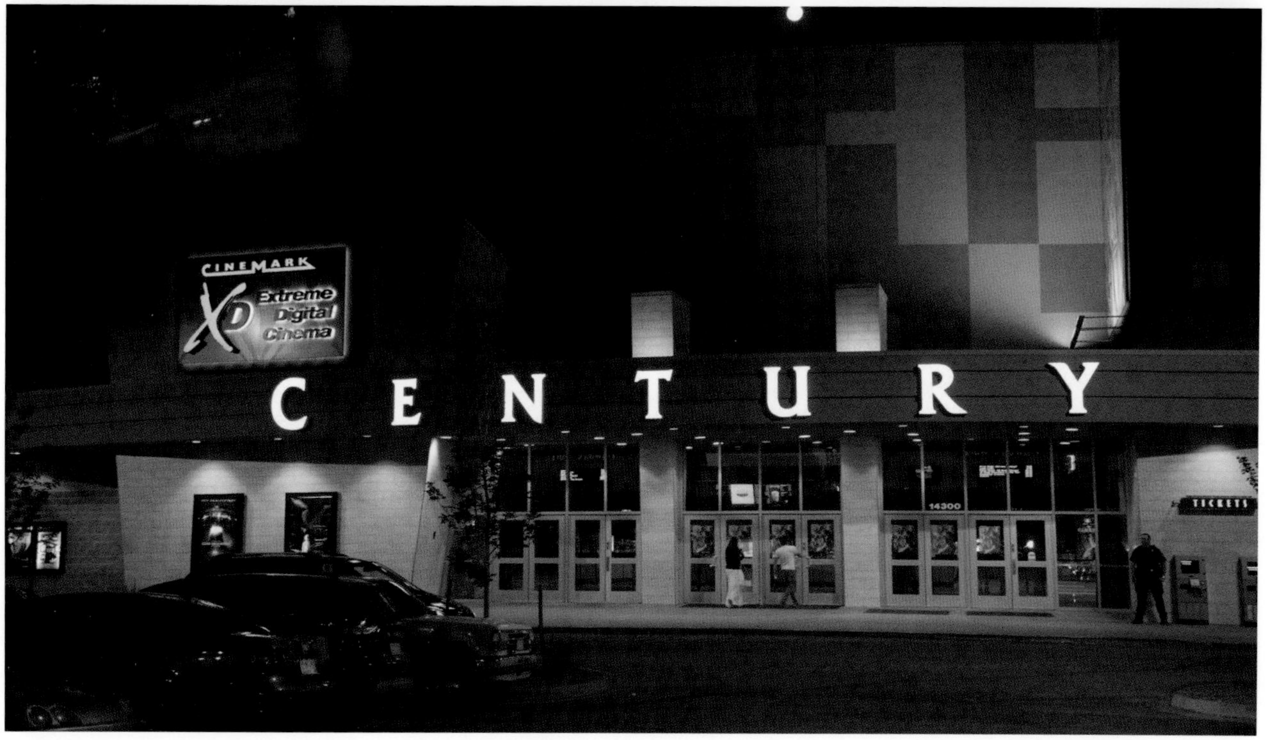

Gilbert: There's a drinking hole I go to right up the street from my house. I stop there a lot and have a beer on my way home from work. It's a quiet little place . . . nobody knows me or what I do for a living. One of the guys killed at the movie theater was a regular. I see his mug hanging on the wall, but that place is my little escape. The shooting is the last thing I want to talk about when I'm there. I've still never told anyone at the pub what I did that night . . . what I saw. I'd like to keep it that way.

Paige: I've had to file that night away . . . push it into a deep, dark place in the past. It's what you have to do if you ever want to get back on the bike. But I'll never forget it. It was horrific. Yet, in the middle of all that tragedy, we found something beautiful — the way we were able to work together to provide care to all these patients and the fact that everyone we treated survived. It's really pretty incredible. But, yeah, it was several years before I could go back to the movies.

Gilbert: I have very strong opinions about weapons, and not everyone wants to hear them. In that theater, the shooter managed to hit seventy people in four minutes . . . round after round . . . just firing away . . . *boom, boom, boom, boom.* Why do we need guns that can kill that many people in that short a period of time? *To protect ourselves! We're hunters!* What bullshit. The AR-15 was designed to accomplish one thing: mass maiming. I know all about testosterone, trust me, but maybe you'd feel the same way I do if you ever saw a six-month-old with a gunshot wound.

Paige: Emergency medicine gives you a unique perspective on life. It makes you appreciate what you have, but it can also make you fearful. You hug your children a little more tightly and strap your furniture to the wall. You see things around here and think, "That sure as hell isn't going to happen to *my* kids," but the reality is, there are some things you just can't prepare for. Every time I come home from a shift my little one asks me, "Mommy, who did you save?" They always want to hear the stories, but some are better left untold. They're too young to know that that kind of evil exists in the world. All I can do is teach them — to the best of my ability — how to be good human beings. I want them to embrace life. That desire is part of who I am, but it's also a reaction to this job. I know all too well that we're never guaranteed tomorrow.

Gilbert: Sometimes you get thrown into the deep end and just have to do the best you can. You either fail, flail, or sail. And I'd say we sailed that night. I felt lucky to be there in the ED . . . happy to help . . . and proud to be an emergency physician. ✚

Alyson McGregor, MD

Emergency Physician & Sex and Gender Researcher
Providence, Rhode Island

When you're an attending physician, you're leading the orchestra . . . it's up to you to create the energy in the room. People tell me I always look relaxed but inside, I'm on high alert. I just work hard to keep a calm exterior so people feel the situation is under control. If the conductor is calm, everyone — including the patients — can concentrate on the music.

Early on, emergency medicine was very male-dominated, probably because the personality of the specialty more closely aligned with traditional male attributes — intense, physical, adrenaline-fueled. Women are stereotypically perceived as kind and compassionate, so we're encouraged to pursue family-oriented specialties . . . like pediatrics.

Without a doubt, there are true biological variables between men and women — fundamental cellular differences. But there are equally powerful societal norms and expectations that can affect clinical care. The way men and women develop and describe disease is different in every way. It's shocking. The public assumes that researchers have always accounted for the fact men and women are different. But, in reality, women were historically considered a protected subject. For so long, we tried to fit a square peg into a round hole . . . we assumed what's good for one must be good for the other. Sex-related disparities weren't factored into the way we were taught to identify illness, or use diagnostic testing, or prescribe medications.

When men have a heart attack, they often present with chest pain, classically described as "an elephant sitting" on their chest. Doctors are told to look for that sign. Women, on the other hand, have a different anatomy and physiology. Their heart muscle and surrounding coronary arteries are influenced by a separate DNA and different hormones. This means a heart attack is going to feel different for women . . . they're not going to complain about the familiar male-pattern symptoms. We've defined disease based on how it feels to *men* — a shortsighted perspective that has affected outcomes for female patients. This inherent bias in research and education is partly to blame for the fact women with a heart attack or stroke simply do worse than their male counterparts.

We need to research men, of course, but we cannot assume those results are transferable to women. Aspirin is a classic example. Low-dose aspirin therapy has a protective effect in the primary prevention of myocardial infarction in men but not in women. Unfortunately, I see many patients whose primary care doctors don't understand these important indications.

I care deeply about this. My goal is for sex- and gender-related differences to become so ingrained in clinical practice they are addressed by every specialist, included in every lecture, and factored into every study. We also need to get the public involved by encouraging them to have these conversations with their doctors. Everyone needs to demand their care be based on their own sex.

I don't know if it will happen in my lifetime . . . and I know it's asking a lot . . . but I think we can transform the face of medicine by addressing sex and gender. We simply can't go back to the way things used to be. We need change . . . and I want to be a catalyst. ✚

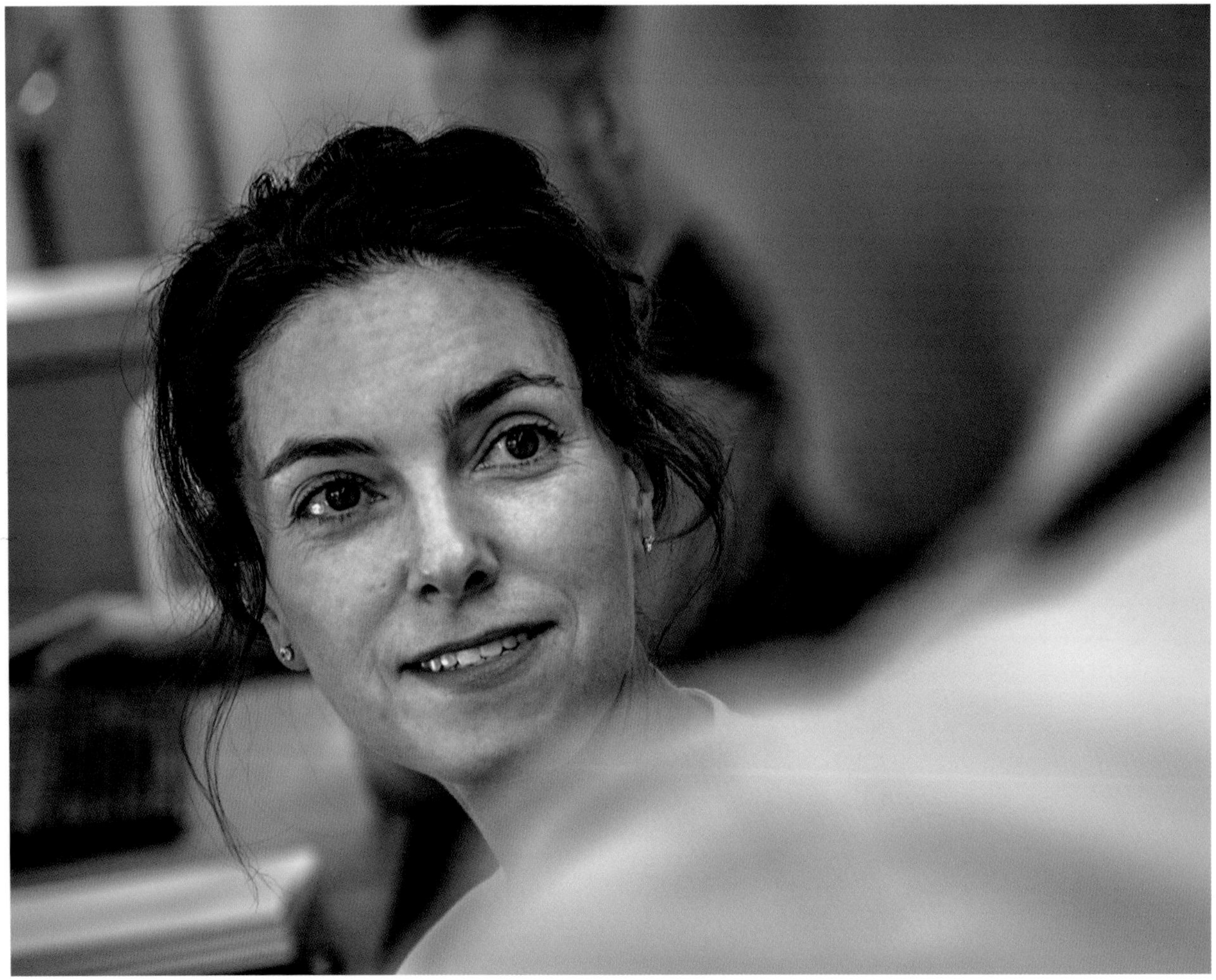

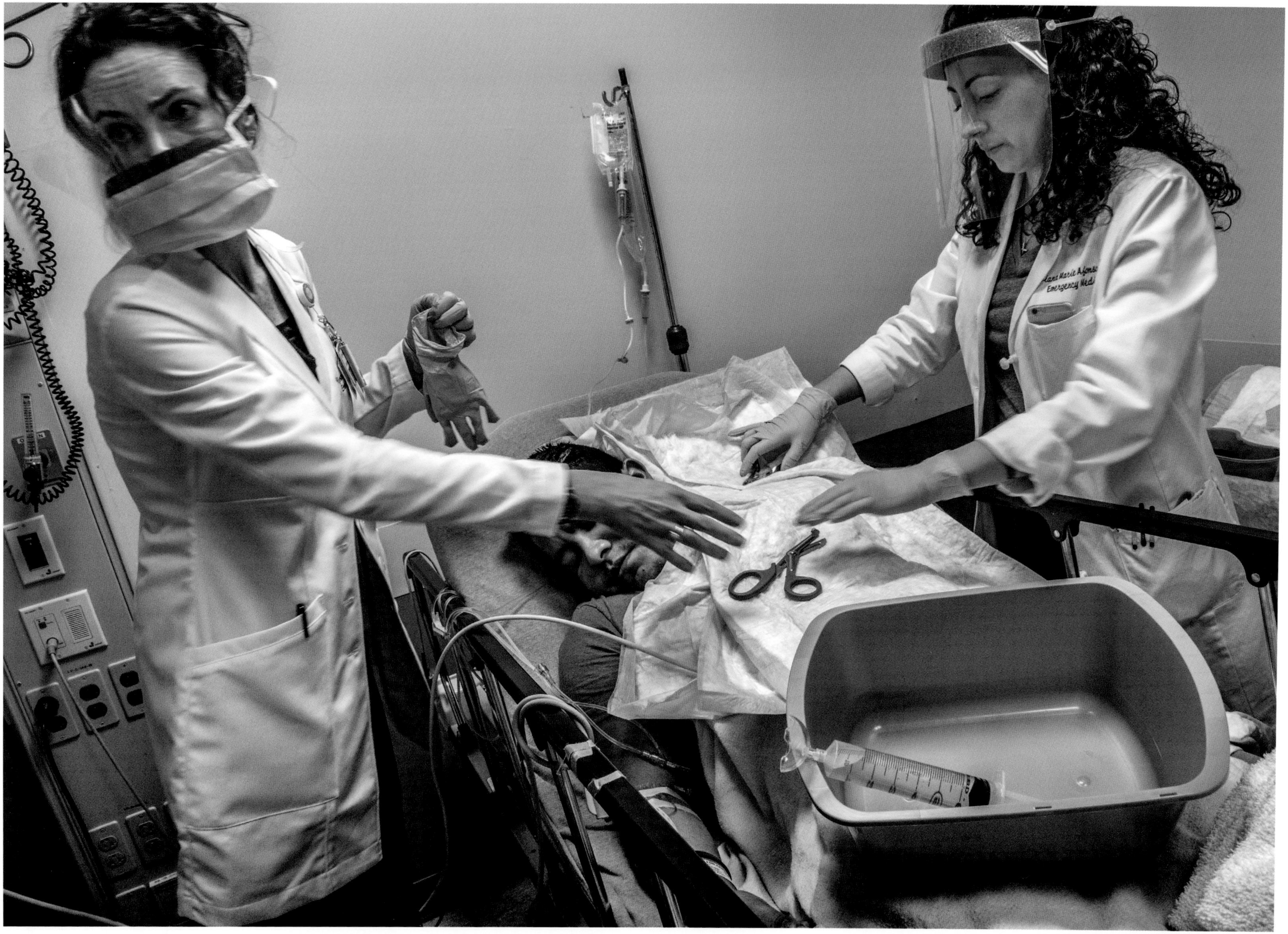

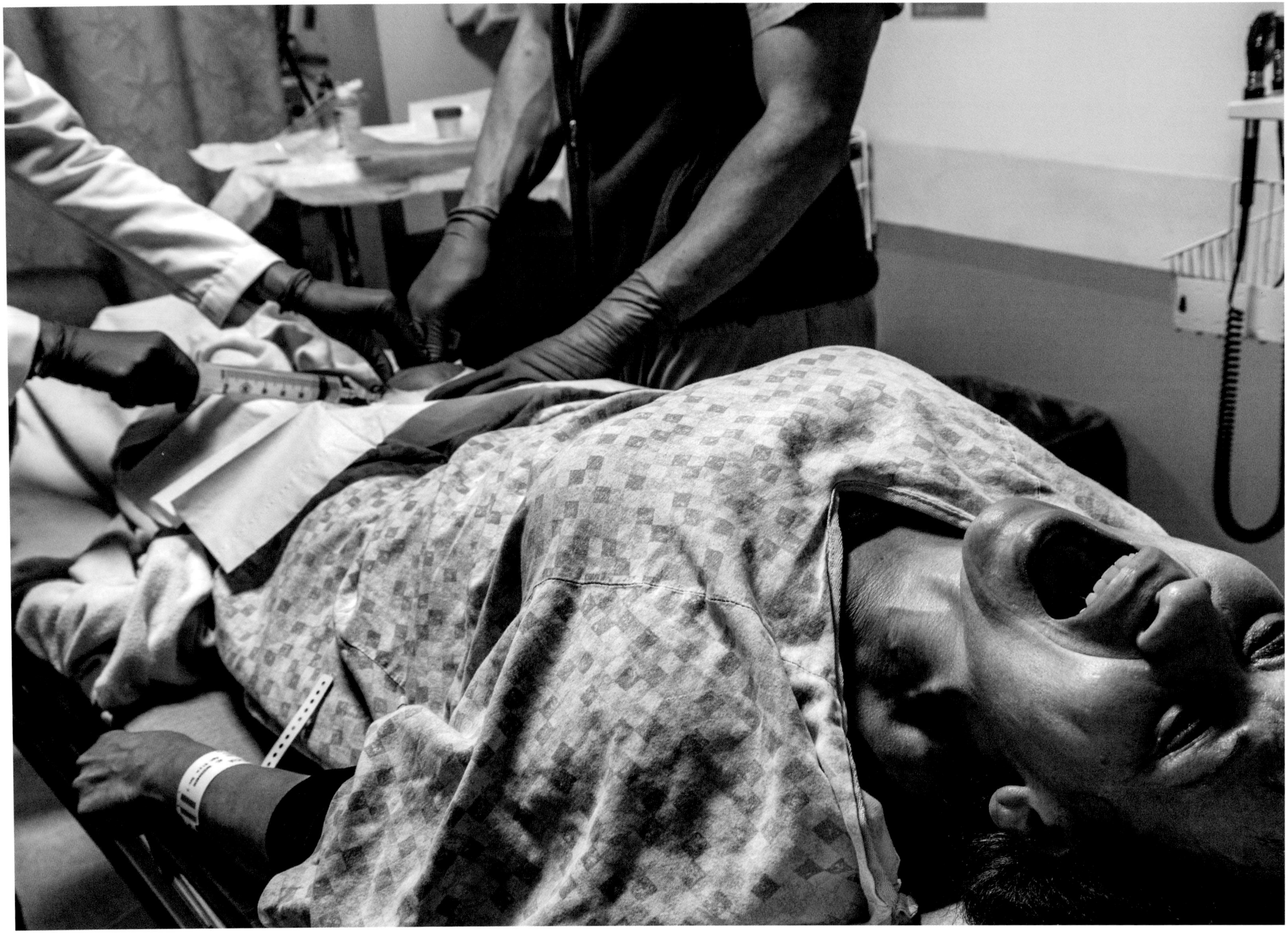

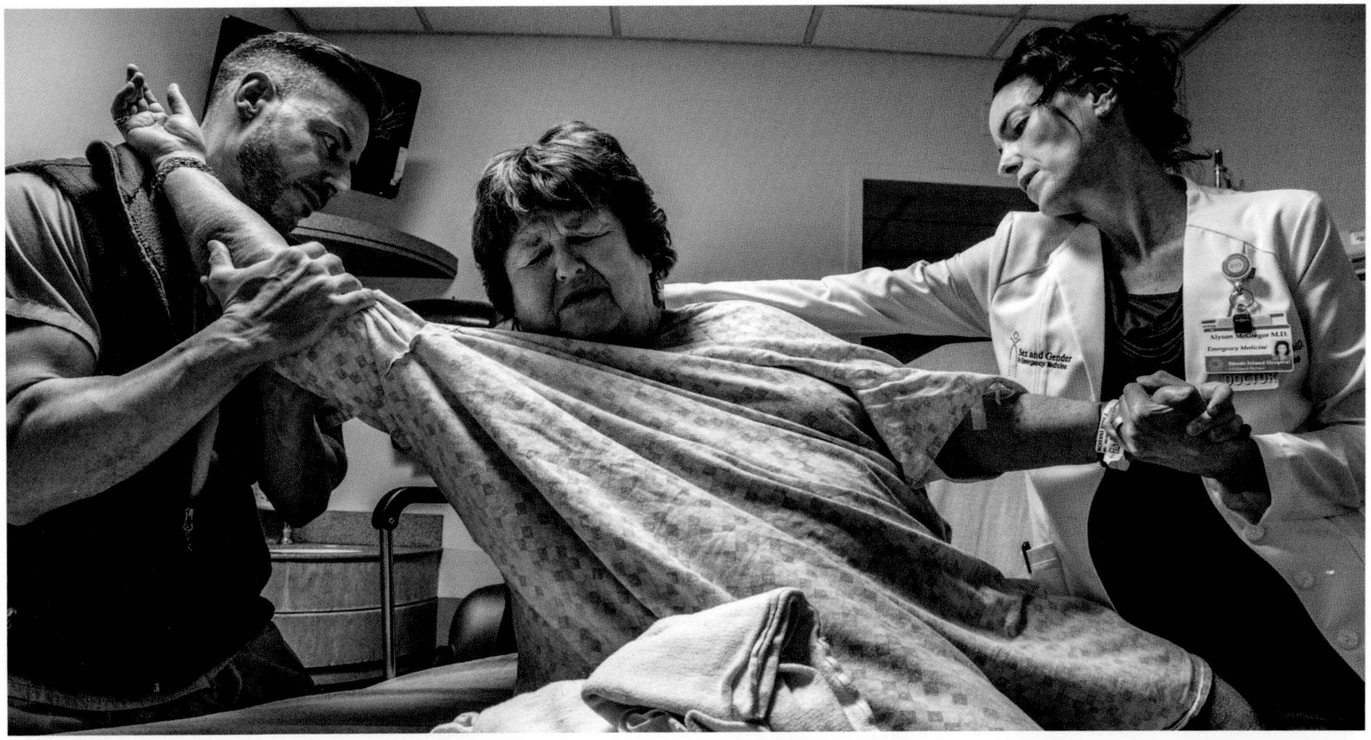
Sex and Gender in Emergency Medicine
Alyson McGregor M.D.
Emergency Medicine
DOCTOR

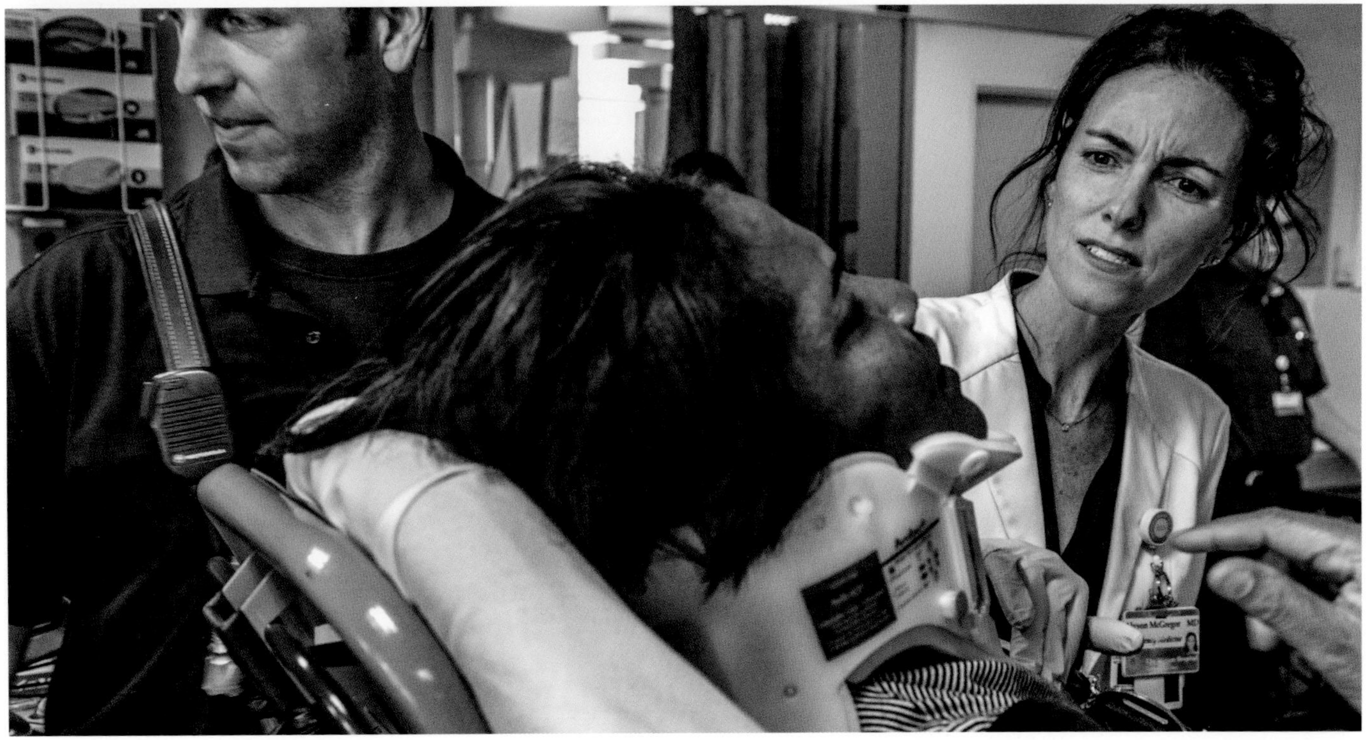

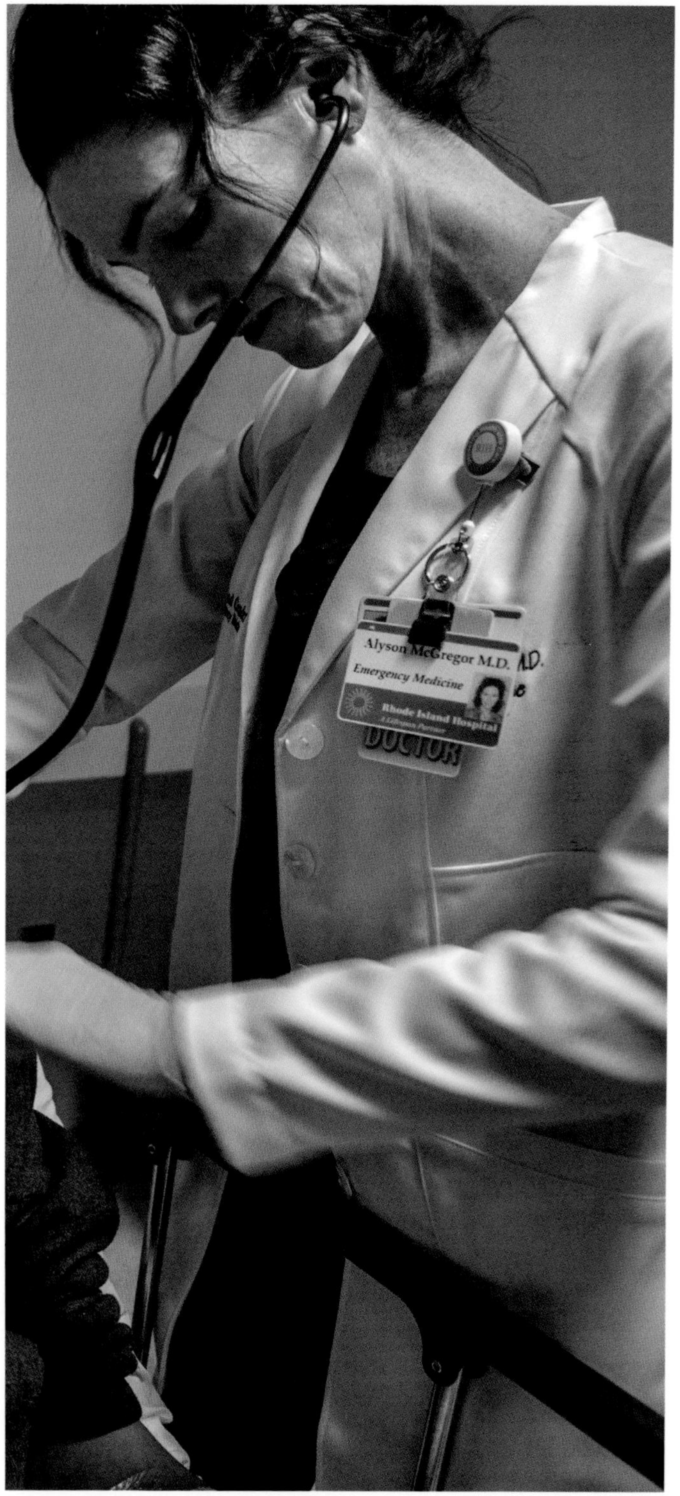
Alyson McGregor M.D.
Emergency Medicine
Rhode Island Hospital
DOCTOR

Christopher Hoyte, MD

Emergency Physician & Toxicologist
Denver, Colorado

So, this guy comes in for unexplained hair loss and a terrible burning pain in his legs. It seems like a medical problem — until we figure out his wife has been spiking his coffee with thallium. You know, marital strife. That's one of the things I love about toxicology . . . you see some wild stuff . . . the kind of stuff that "only happens on TV."

I've been an expert witness on cases where patients or their animals were poisoned. People come up with all kinds of creative ways to kill each other. The nurse who was offing her nursing home patients with huge hits of potassium chloride . . . the chemist who was slipping cyanide into his wife's soup . . . all true stories. It's a very complicated world, and it can be hard to tell the difference between a crime and a health condition.

A lot of the things we see are self-inflicted, of course. It's human nature to take risks, but sometimes I wish I could turn the clock back and ask, "Are you sure you really want to do this?" We had a guy who managed to get his hands on some aluminum phosphide, which is an extremely dangerous "critter killer" that releases a toxic gas if it comes into contact with water. He put it underneath his raised porch, probably to get rid of mice or something. Well, the next day he decides to cool the house down by spraying the exterior with a water hose. The gasses were released . . . and his family died at the scene . . . the dogs, too.

Our poison center covers six states, including Hawaii, so the calls we get run the gamut. Most of the poisonings we see are the result of household items — bleach, cleaners, automotive products, and other people's medications. We also see the consequences of designer drugs — bath salts, amphetamine strains, synthetic cannabinoids. There's always something new being sold on the streets. And then you get the snake bites, spider bites, scorpion stings, lionfish and jellyfish envenomations . . . the list goes on.

Toxicology's a very important piece of disaster preparedness, but it's often ignored. People talk a lot about how to take shelter from a hurricane or tornado, but we need to talk more about how to protect ourselves from a dirty bomb. Clinicians need to understand the individual roles they'd play during that kind of disaster and be prepared to perform amidst the chaos. Around here, we take our training seriously. We know we must be ready when and if that call comes in. ✚

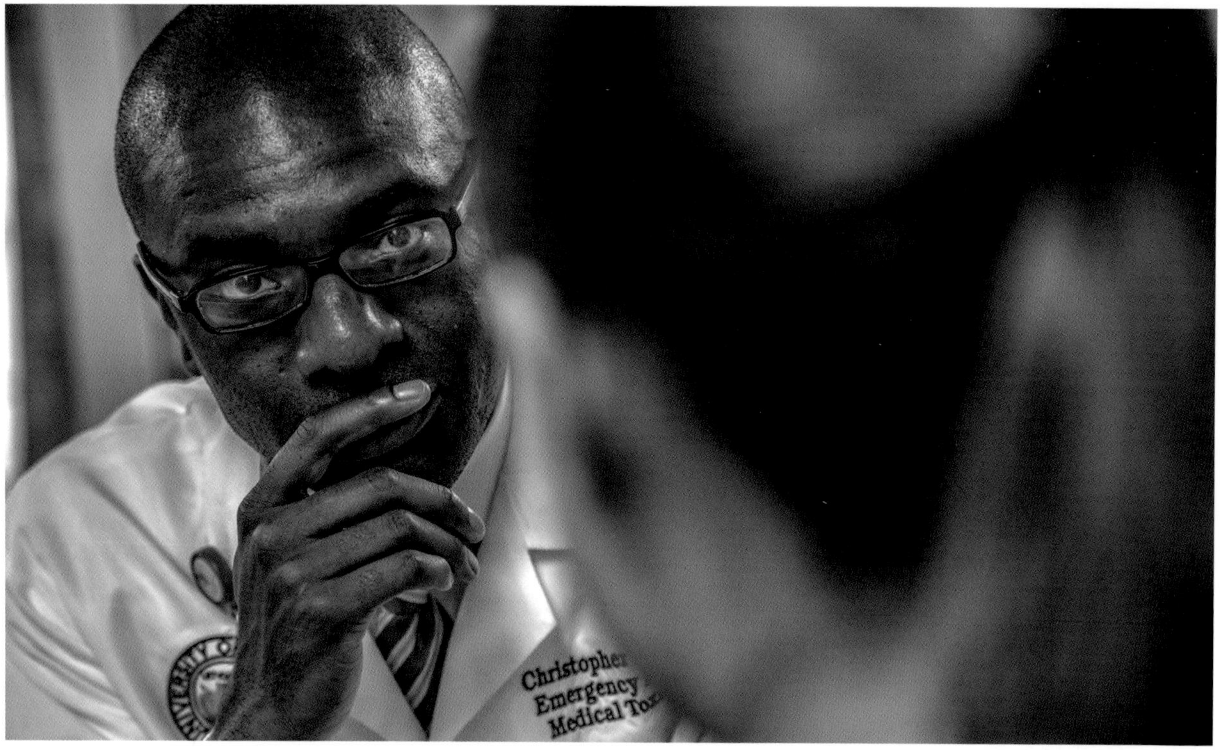

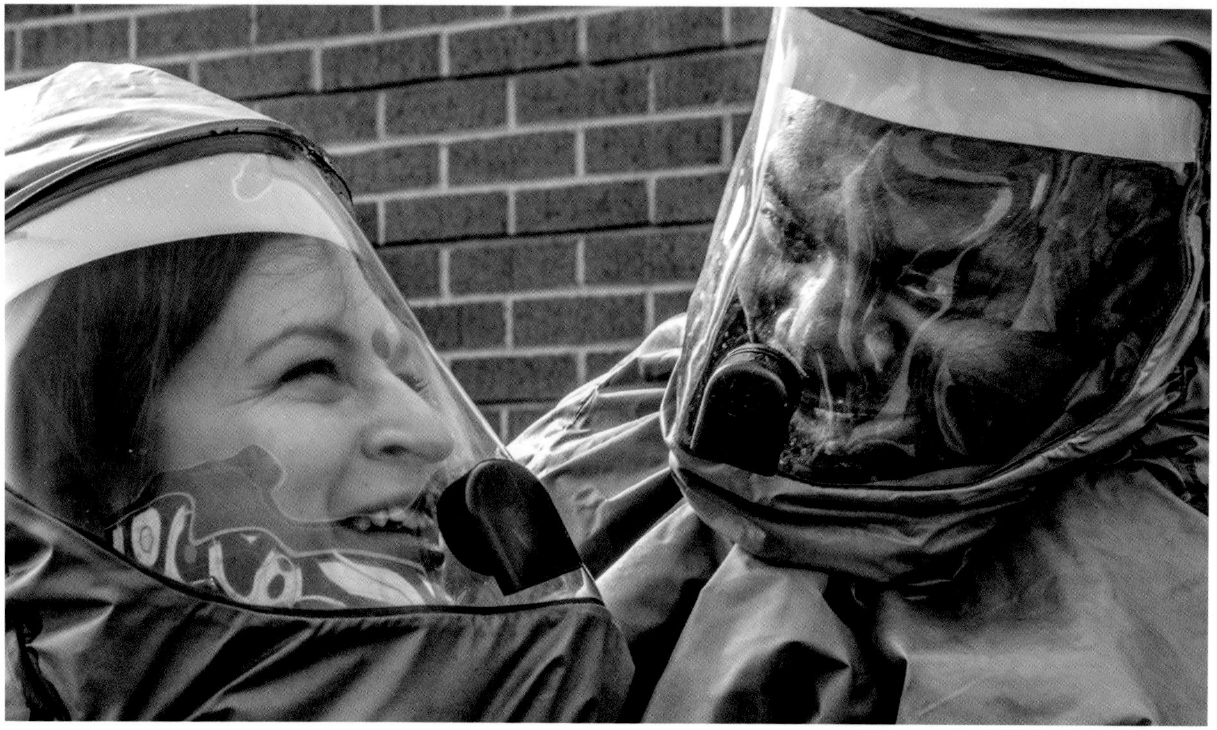

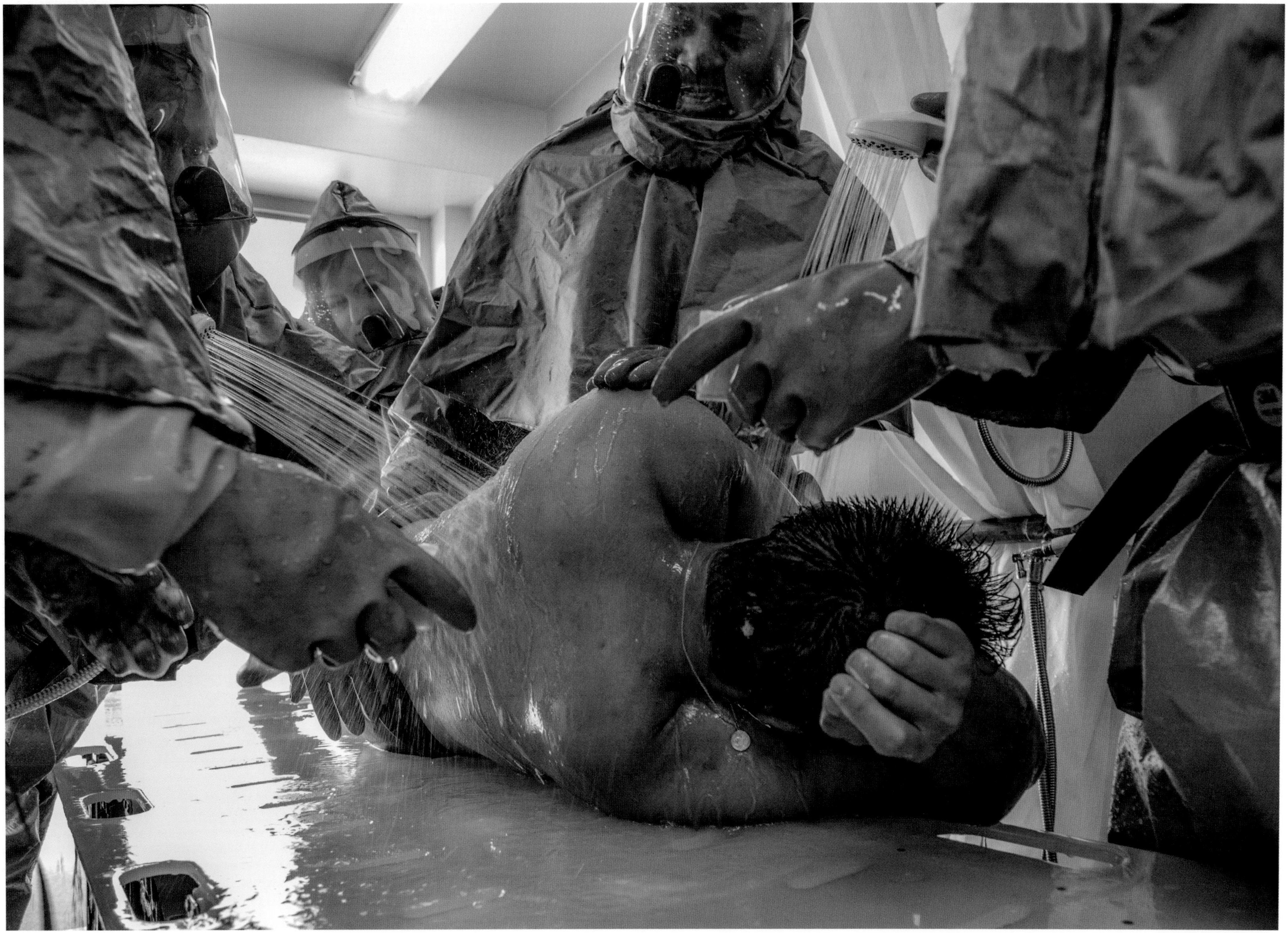

Steven Pine, RN

Emergency Nurse
Providence, Rhode Island

I was born to be an ER nurse. I'm not big on empowering myself to become the manager. I want to take care of people, that's why I signed up for this. I'm fifty-two, and other nurses will come up to me and say they can't believe I'm still here. And I've got one thing to say: I like what I'm doing.

Patients come in and play possum. Oh, they will lie, it's amazing. They'll fake abdominal pain, even seizures. We get the same chronic patients who come into the ER — the alcoholics, the drug users — and they will lie right to our faces. They might be trying to get medications, but sometimes they just don't have anywhere else to stay. Nurses are directly connected to the patients and their social issues. You have to feel your way through all that stuff, figure out what's going on in their heads.

I'm Portuguese and Italian. I make good favas. My grandfather shortened our name from *Pinero* to *Pine*, I guess because he thought it'd be easier to get a job in this country. I didn't realize it then, but we were pretty poor. I used to wear ripped clothes to school. I remember it all so well — the lunch tokens, Social Security lines, buckets of peanut butter and blocks of cheese, and food stamps. We were always happy, though.

I used to feed the fish in the classrooms while the other students would be fooling around in the woods smoking — you know, doing drugs. I got teased — I was a small kid and they used to call me "Shorty." I graduated when I was seventeen and joined the US Navy. I just wanted to travel. I figured it would be a big adventure, but I was seasick all the time. It was awful. I became a hospital corpsman on the ship, which was fun — sutures and sick calls. No one really got that sick because we were all pretty young and healthy, but I began to think it wouldn't be too bad to go to nursing school. I liked working with people.

I had some butterflies when I first started, so I understand new nurses feel intimidated at first, like they can't do the job. But I tell them, "Yes, you can. It just takes time, it takes practice. You have to do it over and over again, like anything else, and it'll come to you." Emergency nursing is different than many other areas of nursing. It's all about managing time skillfully and keeping patients safe. Unfortunately, there's a big turnover here because the stress is so high. We do get abused at times, but I've just gotten used to it.

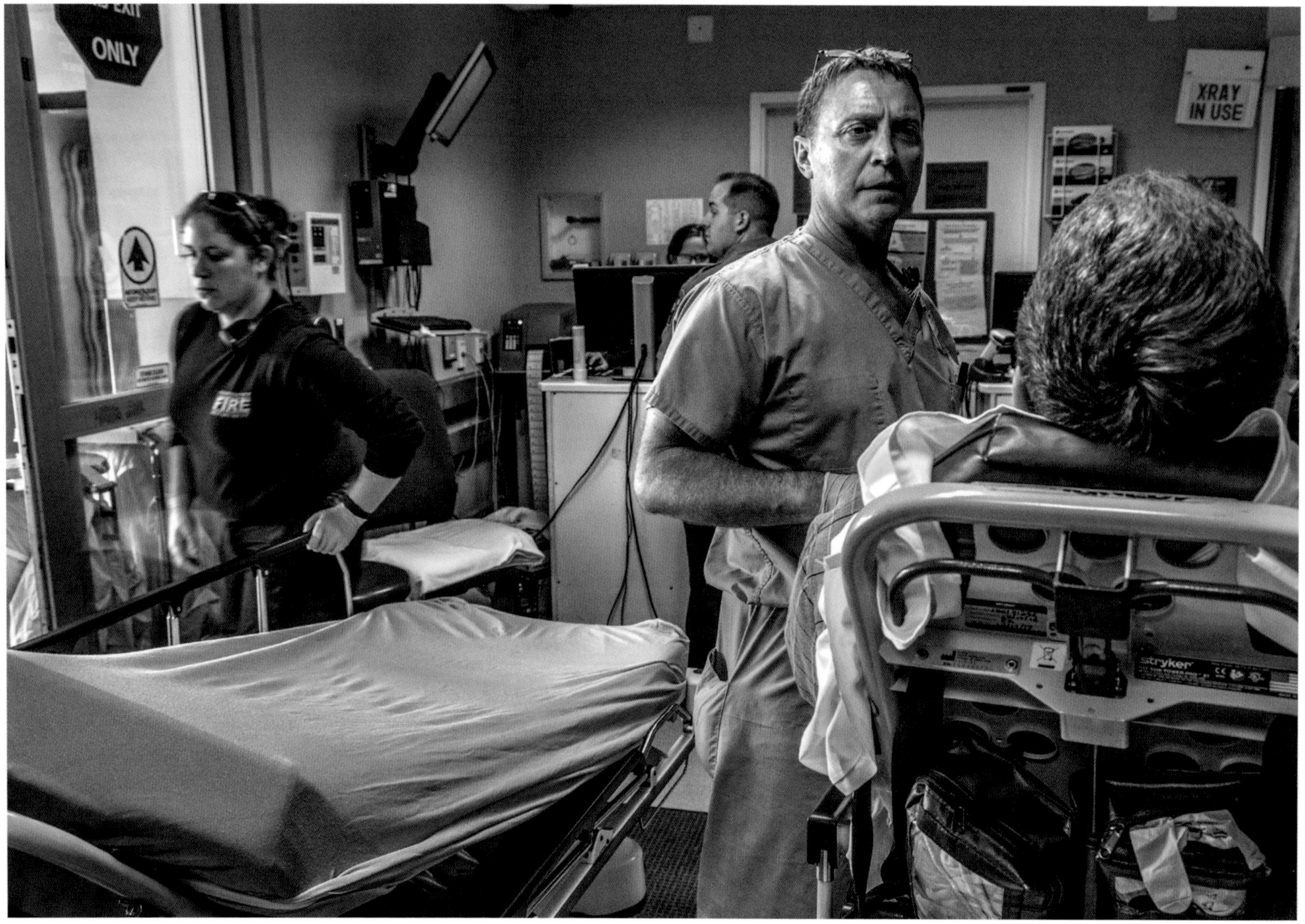

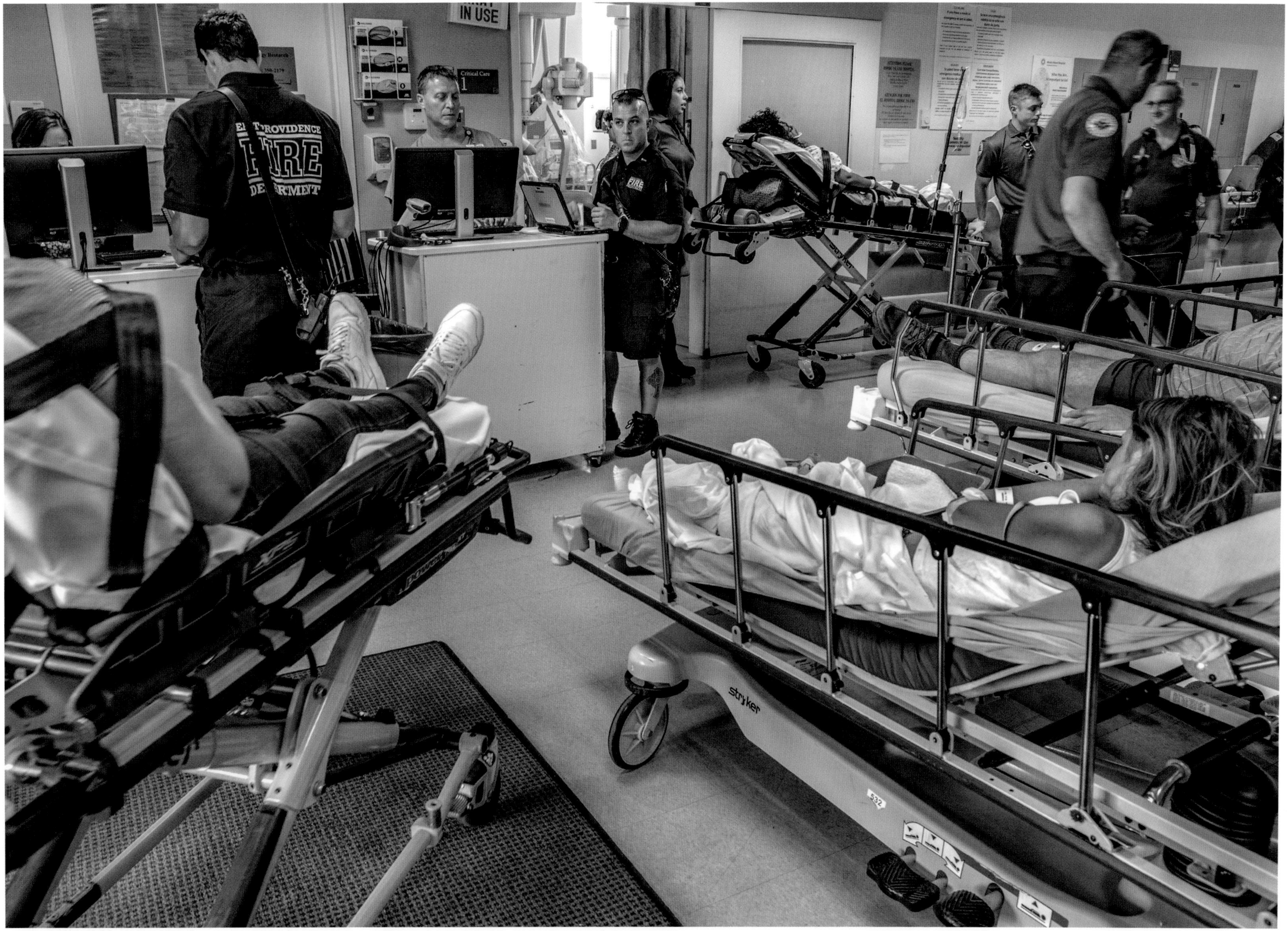

Steven Pine, RN

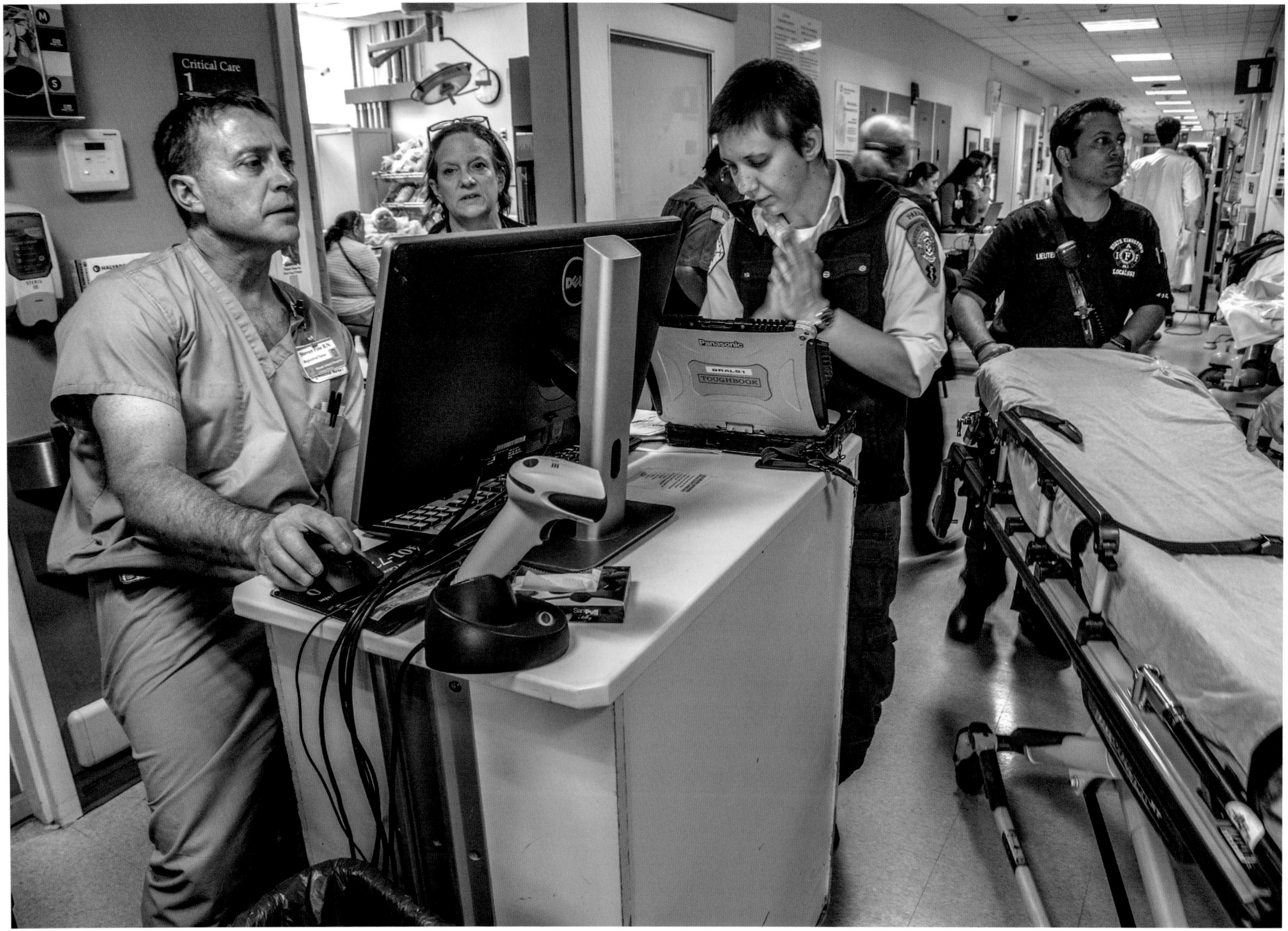
Critical Care
1
Panasonic
TOUGHBOOK

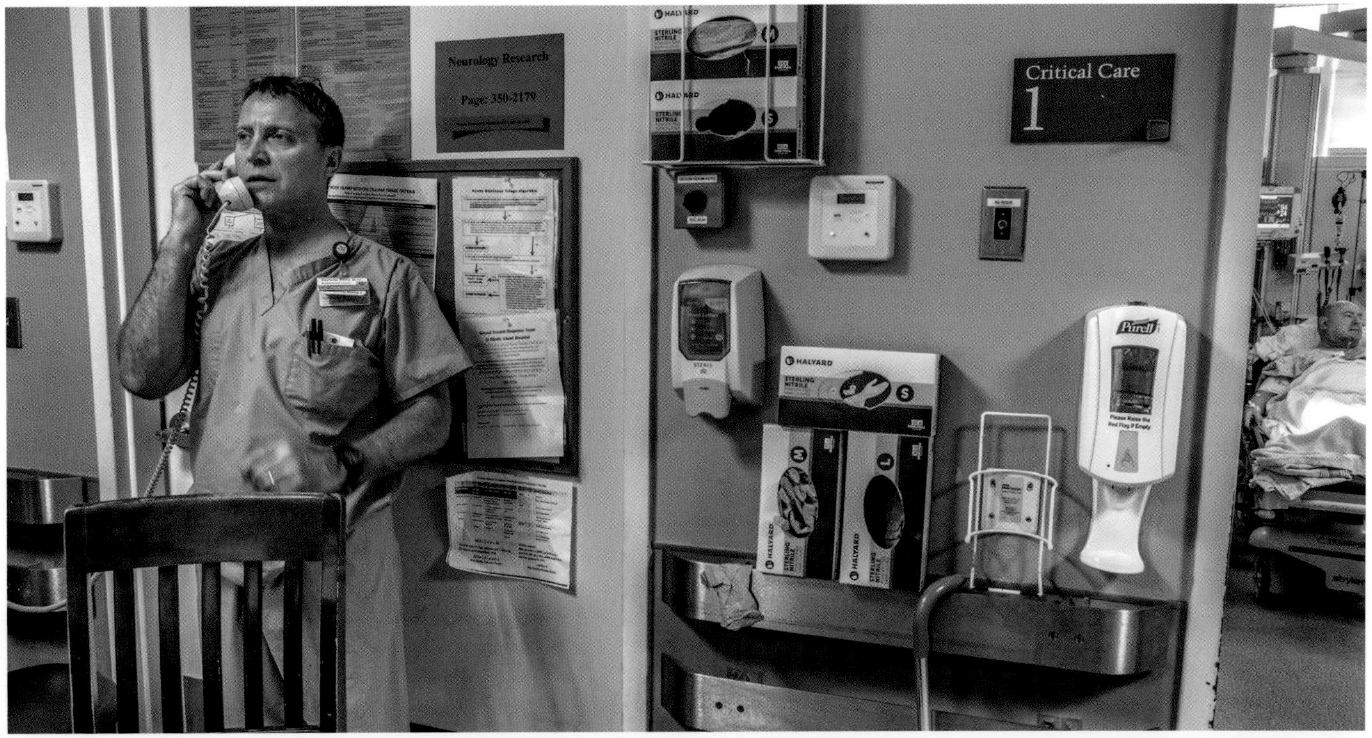

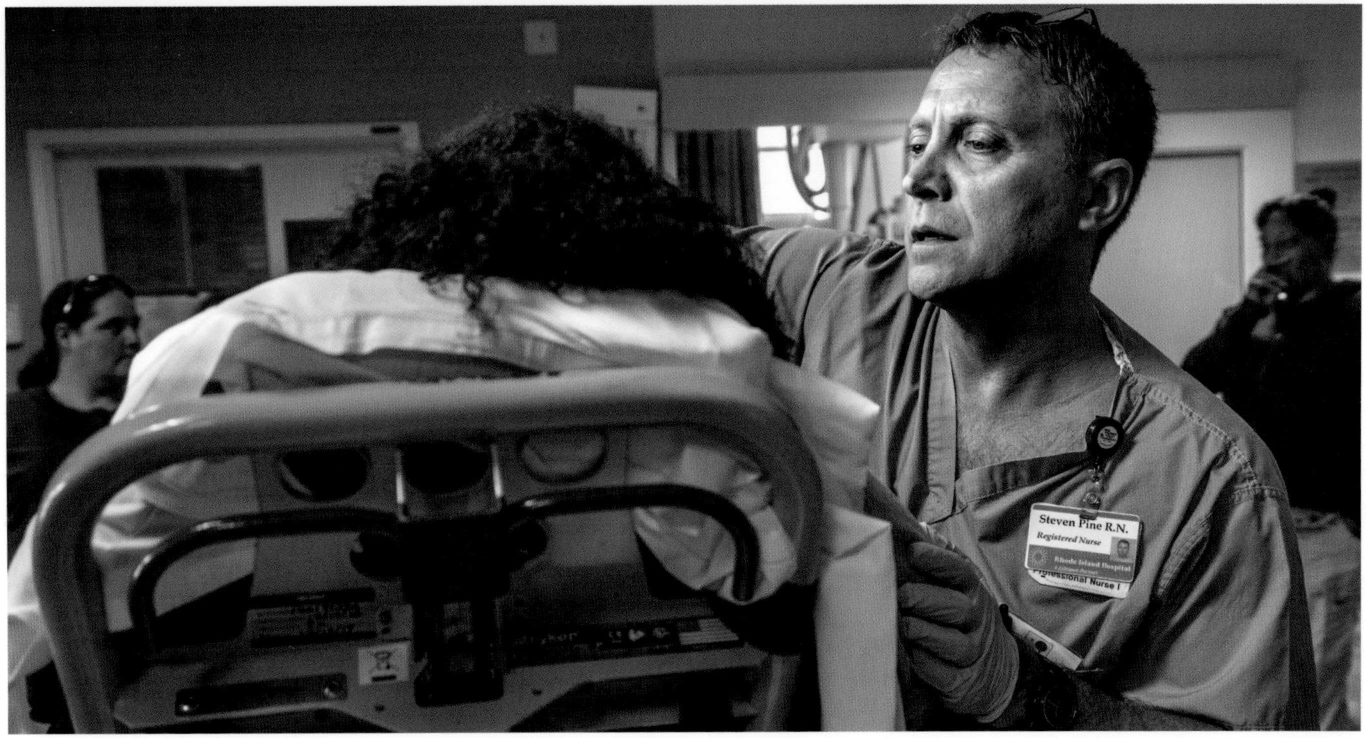

I was in a critical care room one day, and there was this suicidal patient; he was being watched by security. He was in his pajamas and yelling that he needed to go to the bathroom, so I volunteered to escort him. I kept one foot in the bathroom door and my other foot outside in the hall. He finished, but I thought it was taking him an awfully long time to wash his hands. When I opened the door, he turned around and was holding a knife to his own neck. It was a pretty big blade. He said, "I'm sick." I pretty much did what I had to do. I just knew people were going to get hurt, so I had to jump him. I pinned him against the sink and flicked the knife out of his hand. Security came around the back, and we escorted the patient back to triage.

Management, head of security, and a few of the other supervisors came down because they'd heard an employee had gotten stabbed. It took a few minutes before I realized they were talking about *me*. I was too busy filling out my report . . . I hadn't noticed I was bleeding all over the place.

The security guard and I received an award. In all the years I've been here, I'd never seen a nurse get anything like that — and there are a lot of nurses who do a lot of good things that get overlooked. There must have been fifteen guys in suits from New Jersey and Connecticut who came down to present the award. And they gave me a little bar, a little captain's bar.

So, if I decide I don't like nursing anymore, I can always get a job in hospital security. ✚

Hany Atallah, MD

Emergency Physician & Emergency Department Medical Director
Atlanta, Georgia

There are only two things I ever wanted to be — a doctor or a stunt car driver. I chose the first, but my wife will tell you I'm still trying to be the second.

When I interviewed for residency, the guy who would later become my advisor said, "Your grades are *okay*. Your board scores, *okay*. But, I've got to be honest with you . . . you don't really stand out on paper. Why should we take you?" I gave him a big speech about how I'd work harder than anyone else . . . come early and stay late . . . give it everything I had. But I also said, "I'm a big believer in family. I want to be on a first-name basis with the CEO of the hospital *and* the guy who mops the floor. We'll probably spend more time together than with our own families, so we need to take care of each other." Several years later, he came up to me and said, " Do you know why you got a spot here? It wasn't what you said about hard work. It was what you said about family."

When you do this job, you learn to read people very well. You know when there's something they're not telling you . . . you learn to recognize fear in a person's eyes. And you can sense when you need to go the extra mile. I give out my cell phone number fairly often — sometimes to reassure a patient and show them I care but sometimes because I think it's important to follow their progress.

You have to be committed to this place. My family gets it . . . I guess we're all workaholics to some extent. The kids understand how important my job is to me and respect the fact that Dad's not always available. I try to bring home some of the life lessons learned in the emergency department. It's good to be able to say, "Hey, here's an example of someone who made a very poor decision that's going to change the rest of his life. He's going to go to jail . . . his loved one is dead."

My kids are teenagers now, so they like the funny stories . . . especially the ones with *language*. So, I say, "Mr. Williams, wake up. Wake up! What's going on today, sir? Did you have too much to drink?" And the patient goes, "Fuck you, motherfucker . . . I'm going to beat shit out of you!"

One of the beautiful things in emergency medicine is the simplicity of its mission: *I will take care of you*. I don't care if you're the president of a Fortune 500 company or if you're homeless, I just want to help you, the person in front of me. But I still alternate between feelings of frustration and empathy. During a busy shift, it's easy to forget that every patient is a human being, not just a line on a spreadsheet. I try to put myself in their shoes. I mean, what would I do if I were homeless and needed to get out of the rain? I might make up a bogus excuse to get dry in the emergency department, too . . . see if I could get something to eat.

On the other hand, we can't solve the world's problems. At some point, we're going to have to send these people home. As an administrator, your attitude must be, "If they don't belong here, write them up and get them out." As a physician, your goal is to figure out what brought a patient in and what you can do to help. But which hat do I wear? Just because something is efficient doesn't make it kind. Where do I draw the line? That question tears me up a little bit. ✚

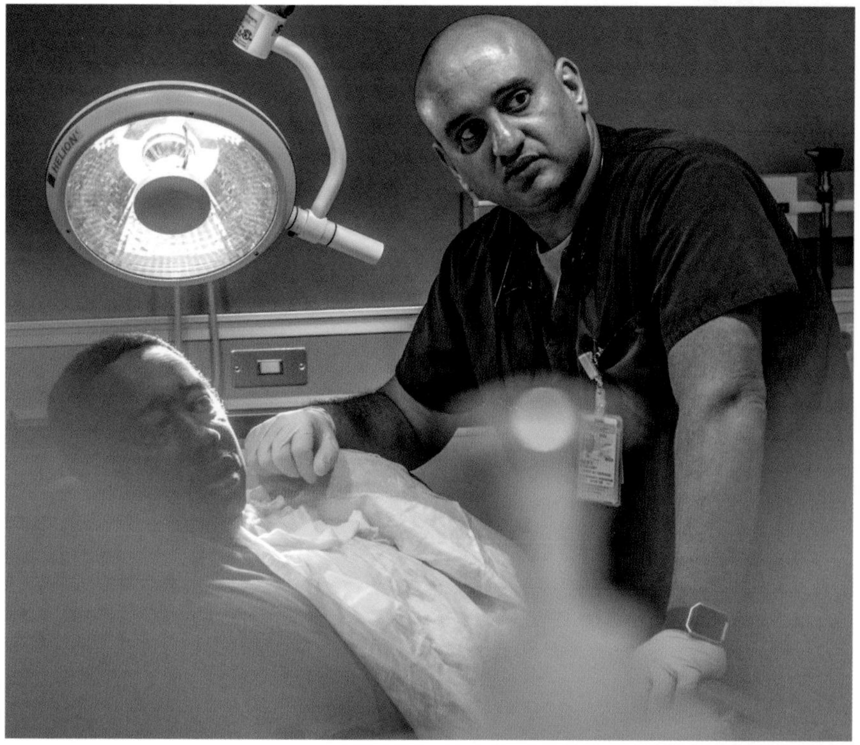

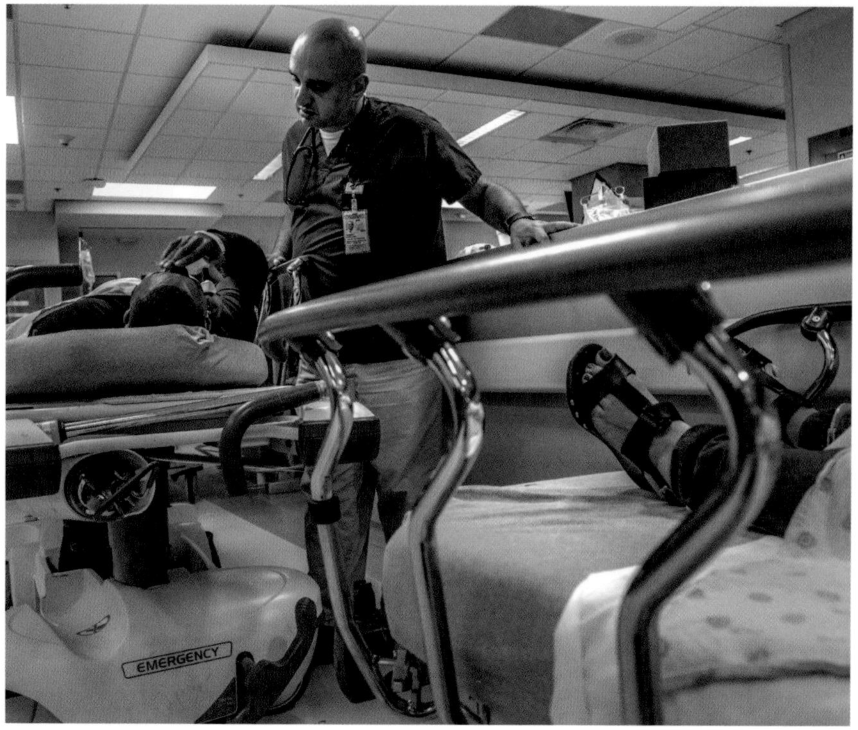

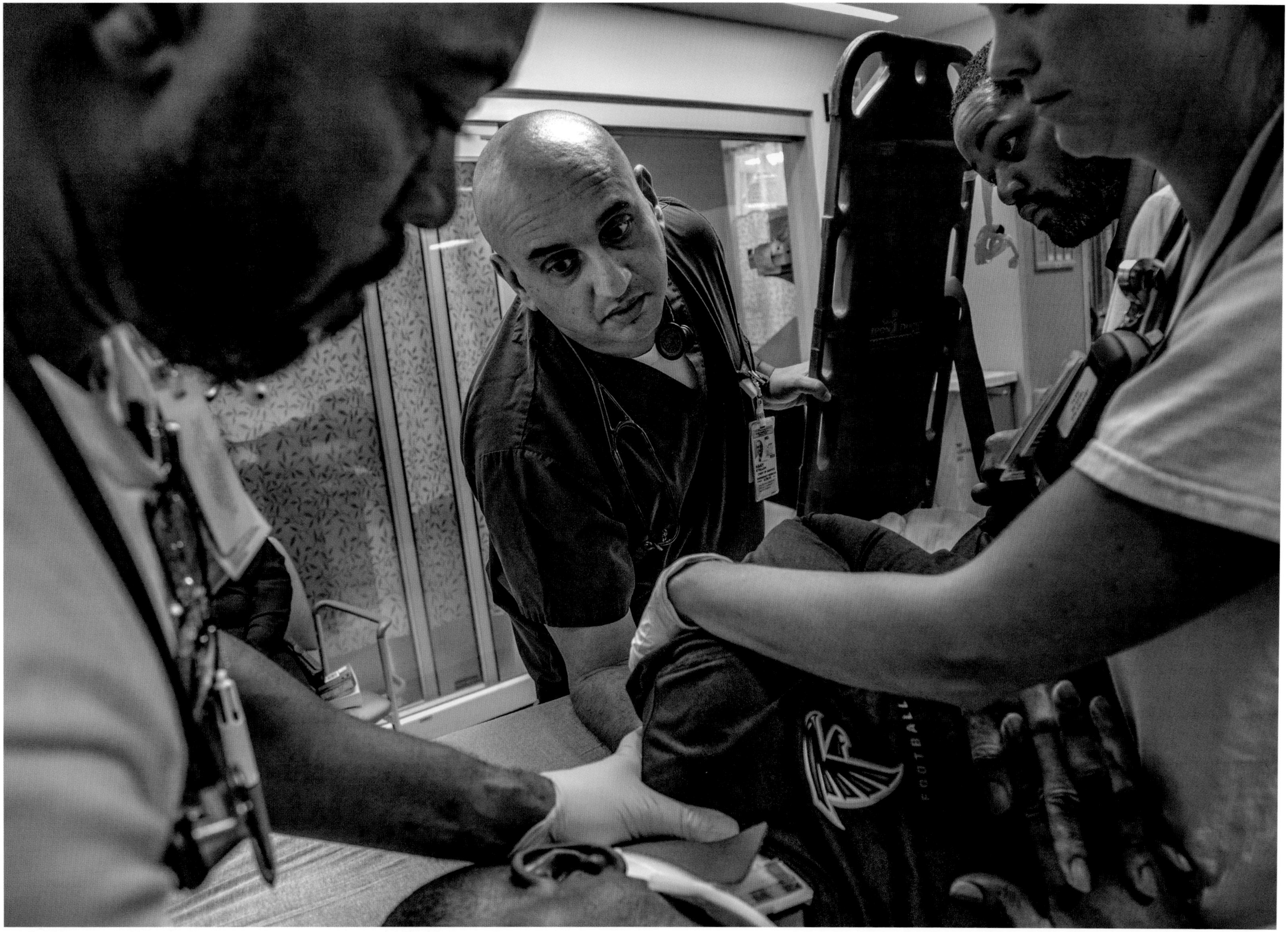
FOOTBALL

Erika Flores Uribe, MD

Emergency Medicine Resident
Los Angeles, California

When I was ten, my dad got shot. There was a lot of gang violence in south central LA, a lot of drive-by shootings. He was working a late shift and got caught in the crossfire. As a kid, I thought he was a superhero — nothing could hurt him — so it was strange to see him in the hospital, blood-soaked bandages covering his shoulders.

My parents immigrated here from Mexico and couldn't speak English, so they couldn't read my dad's discharge papers. I was only in fourth grade, but I had to function as their interpreter and advocate. Once he'd been released, we bought some big Q-tips at Rite Aid, so we could take care of his wounds at home. My dad was my first patient, I guess. I was his follow-up care — his primary care doctor.

I entered the fire academy when I was eighteen, the only female in a class of seventy-two cadets. I volunteered with the paramedics and was really drawn to the medical calls. One night we were transporting a patient who'd been shot in the head. When we got to the hospital, I looked around for a doctor but didn't see one at first. And then I realized, there she was — standing at the head of the bed. She just dominated the room. I think that was the first time in my life I'd ever seen a minority female physician. It was then I made the connection — I could be that person. I could be that doctor. Suddenly, a new world opened up for me.

My parents were very upset when I decided to pursue higher education. They thought it was a selfish thing to do. My dad would say, "Why are you wasting your time? You're going to do all this studying, only to get married and have kids. Then that's it! You're burning your eyelashes for no reason." American culture celebrates individual decisions, but my family functions more like a single unit. They still don't quite grasp why I'm doing what I'm doing, but they're getting closer.

I always loved school; it seemed fairer than real life. If you worked hard, you got rewarded. I got a congressional fellowship when I was in college and got to work on Capitol Hill. My parents came to this country as undocumented immigrants and there I was, walking through the halls of Congress. It was a surreal experience; I felt like I'd leapfrogged five generations in my own lifetime.

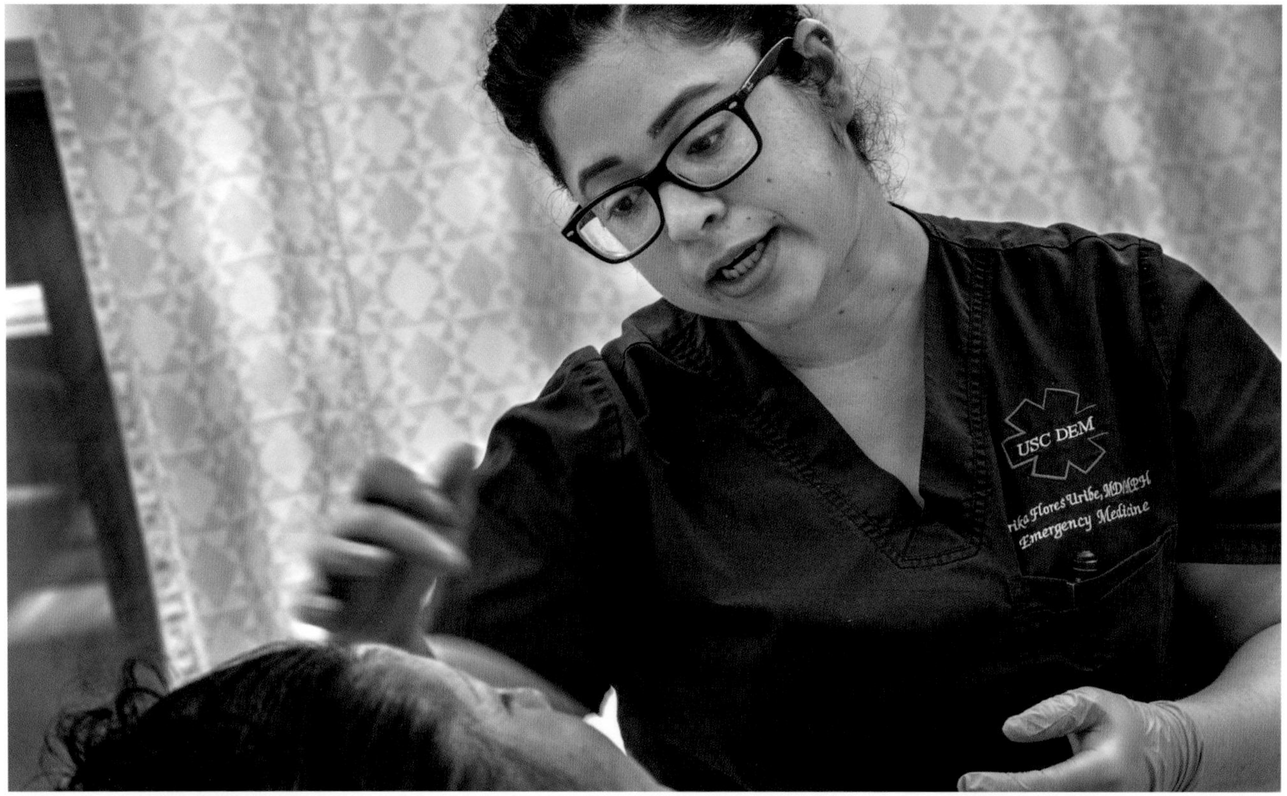

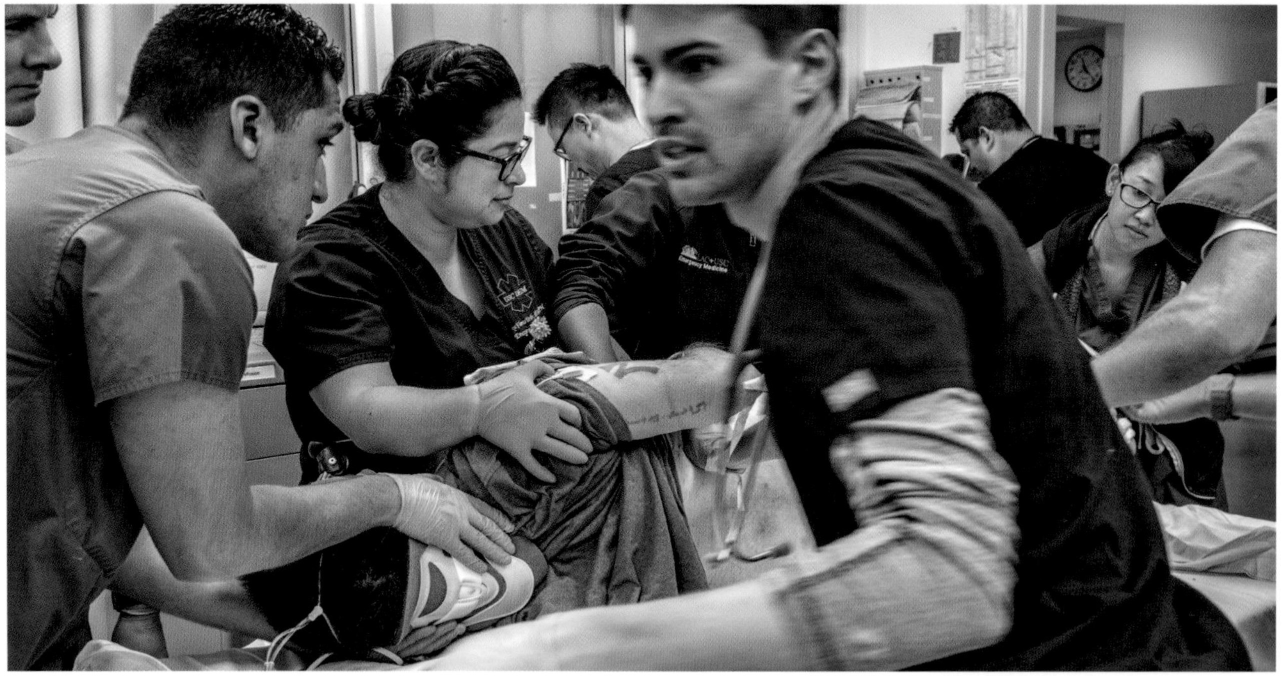

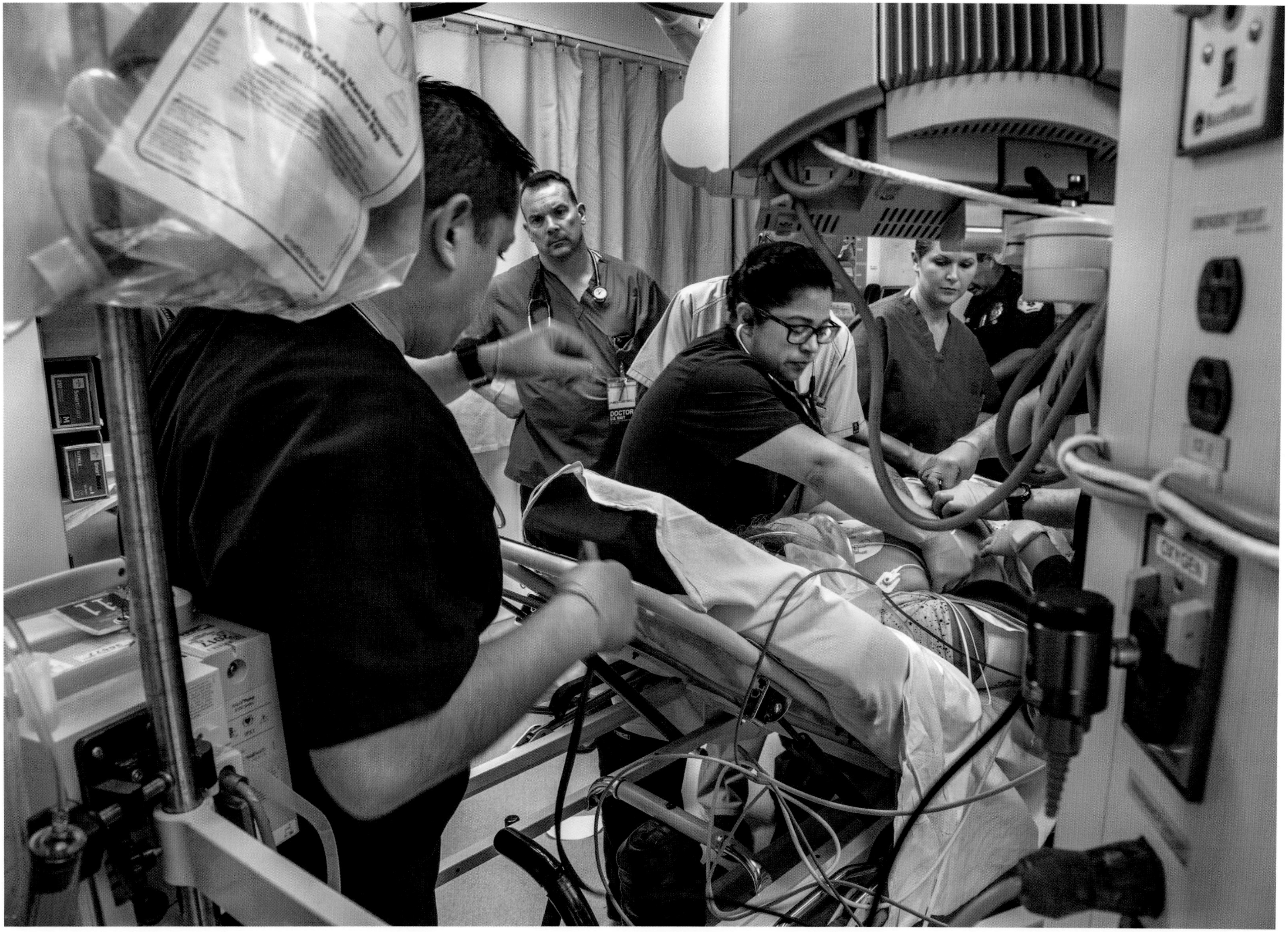
DOCTOR
OXYGEN

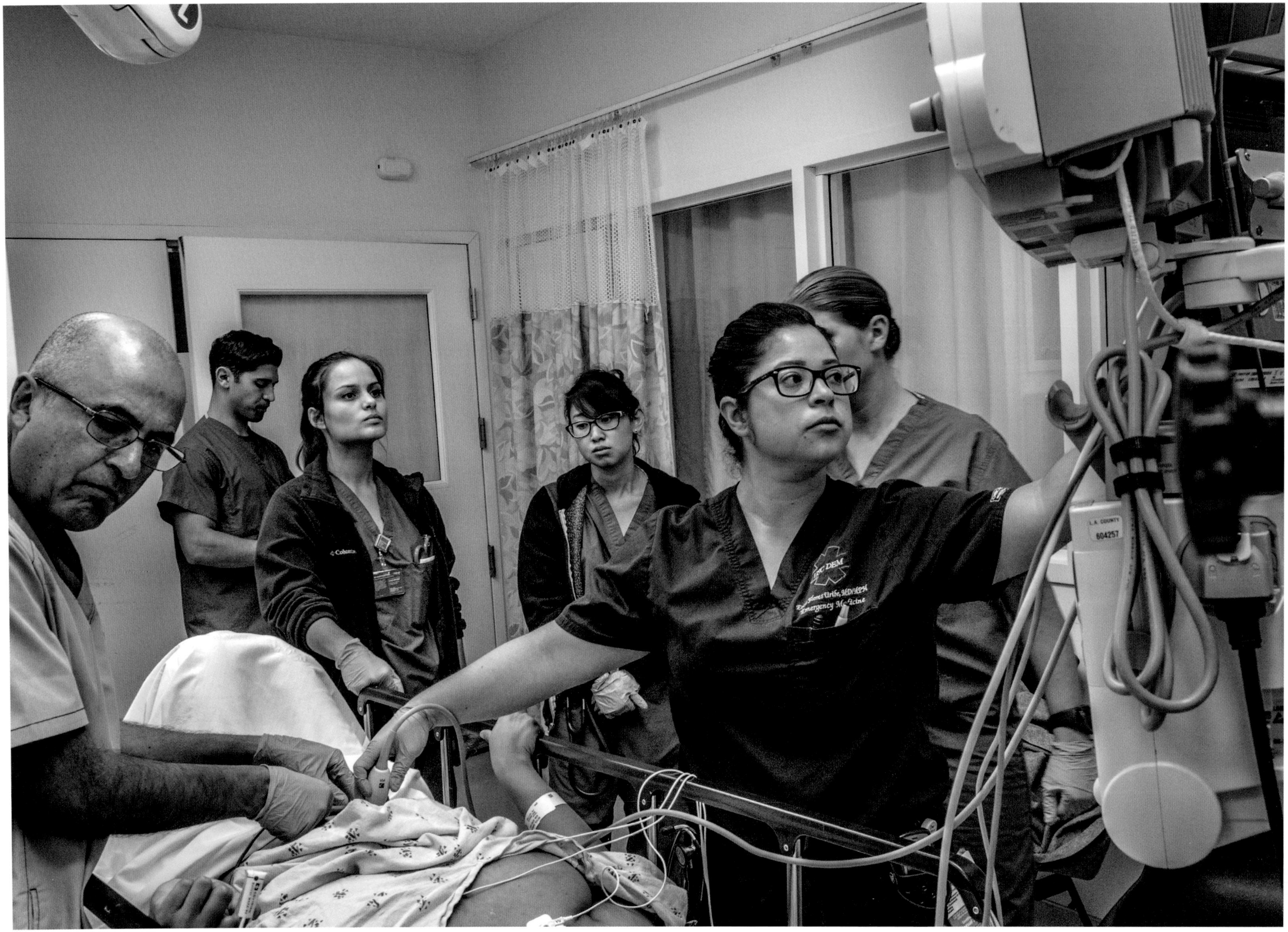
L.A. COUNTY
604257

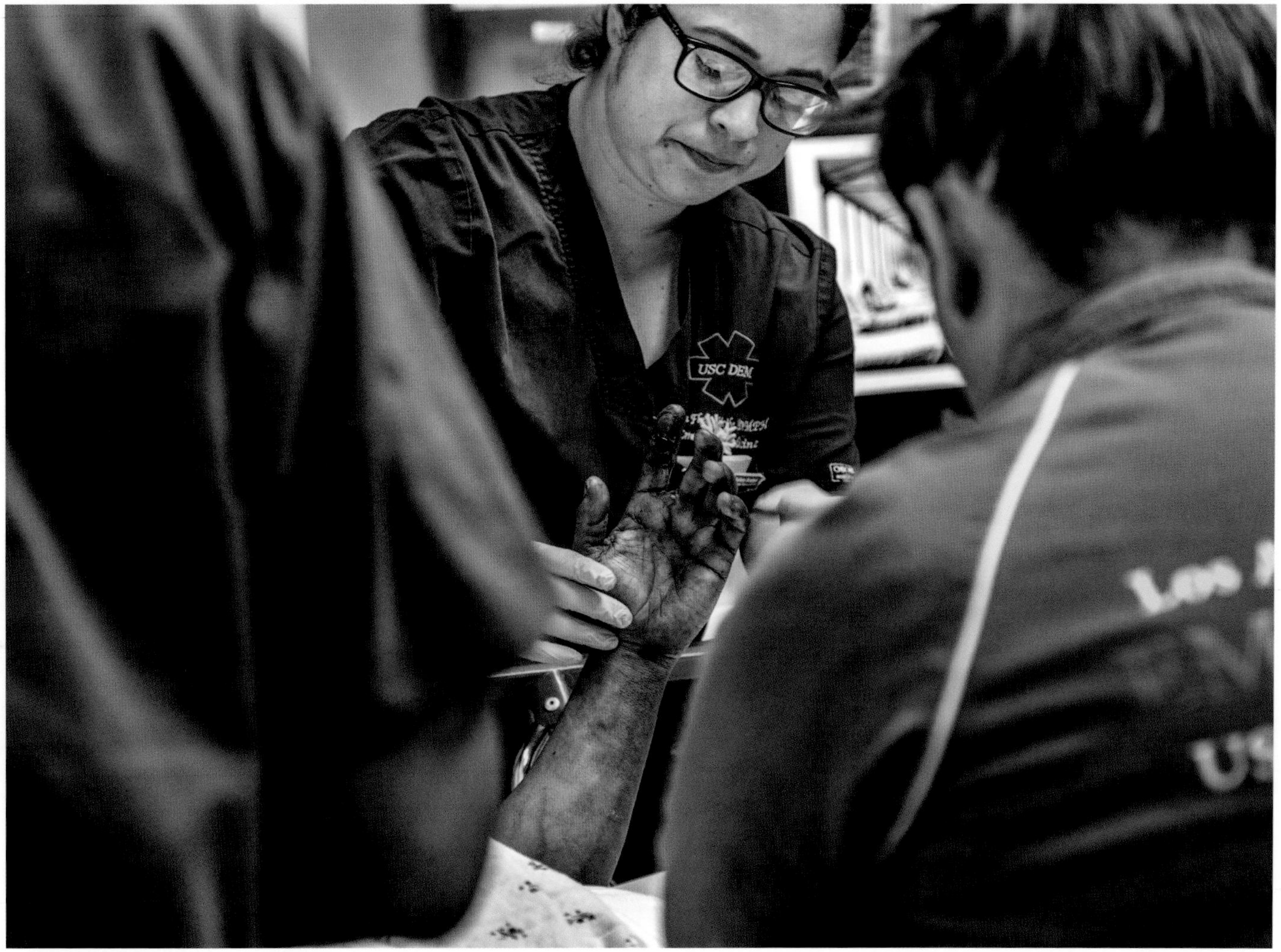

As much as I see myself as part of this community, I'm aware I'm also different. I don't have the same stresses, the same fear, many of my patients face. When I got into medicine, I envisioned being this great advocate for the patients of Los Angeles, and I assumed they would automatically respond with gratitude. Some do. But others are angry; they've been marginalized. I've been the reservoir for a lot of frustration expressed by people at the end of their rope.

I used to personalize those situations; they felt like failures. But I have learned how to put those expectations aside and just *listen*. There are voices everywhere that haven't been heard for many, many years. I can't always lessen their burdens, but I can treat them with dignity, be beside them in their most vulnerable moments, and acknowledge them as human beings. Emergency medicine is where I can be that type of doctor. ✚

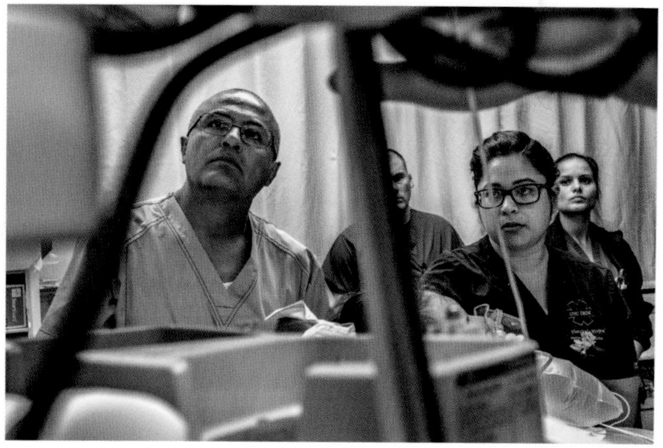

Edidiong Ikpe, MD

Emergency Physician
Atlanta, Georgia

My father called me his "tiger." My parents let us know that, as girls, my sisters and I could do anything; the sky was the limit. That freedom was unique, especially for a traditional Nigerian household.

Some patients make certain assumptions about me and my qualifications because I'm a black female. I'll occasionally have to let a patient know, "Hey, I've been doing this for this many years, and this is my professional opinion. . . ." But those situations don't necessarily offend me. If I'm dealing with a one-hundred-year-old southern white man, how can I hold it against him when he calls me "Honey" and tells me to bring him a blanket and asks me when his doctor will be in to see him? This is how he grew up . . . this is his world view. It is what it is.

The emergency department is like a snapshot of the community. We see all kinds. Patients who are angry . . . sometimes mentally ill . . . sometimes intoxicated or delirious. It's dangerous. But in medicine, there's this notion that the patient is always right. Doctors are expected to be superhuman — able to tolerate insults and even physical abuse.

Little old ladies — patients who look like they couldn't hurt a fly — can break your wrist. They'll kick, hit, spit. In any other environment, that person would be arrested or sued but we're expected to just take it. "Oh, they didn't mean it . . . they're in distress. . . ." But I think we must demand a certain level of respect; we can find better ways to protect each other and ourselves while maintaining compassion for our patients.

Atlanta is the capital of human sex trafficking. Sometimes I'll pick up on body cues that make the hairs on the back of my neck stand up. I'll just know something is wrong. Very wrong. I saw one young lady who was what we call a "frequent flier" — she had been here more than once. She couldn't have been more than twenty years old. The EMS workers had labeled her "combative," and I remember being a little annoyed by her behavior. We see so many patients who are intoxicated, you can make assumptions and it's very easy to become desensitized. But this patient was scared, hysterical, and *very* clear about not wanting a male provider. She said, "I cannot be held responsible for what I'll do if another man comes in this room!" But, when one of the female nurses or I would approach her, she'd calm down. She eventually told us she had been trafficked since she was twelve — sexually abused, passed around. She said she hated men — hated what they'd done to her. And then she pulled out a picture of her son and said, "*This* is the only man in my life that I love."

I had another patient — a man who came in with his girlfriend. I did not like their interaction. He was very rude to her, though not abusive in any physical way. Some weeks later, I heard he had killed her.

We see and hear a lot of terrible things. They may make me sad, but they don't break me. They don't break me. I try not to take any of the emotional baggage home. There, I can just be a wife, a mom. Within those four walls, I have permission to cry. I can be scared. I'm allowed to feel confused, overwhelmed. But at work, there's no room for that; a different persona is required.

But at home, I pray. I pray for my patients. I pray for myself. ✚

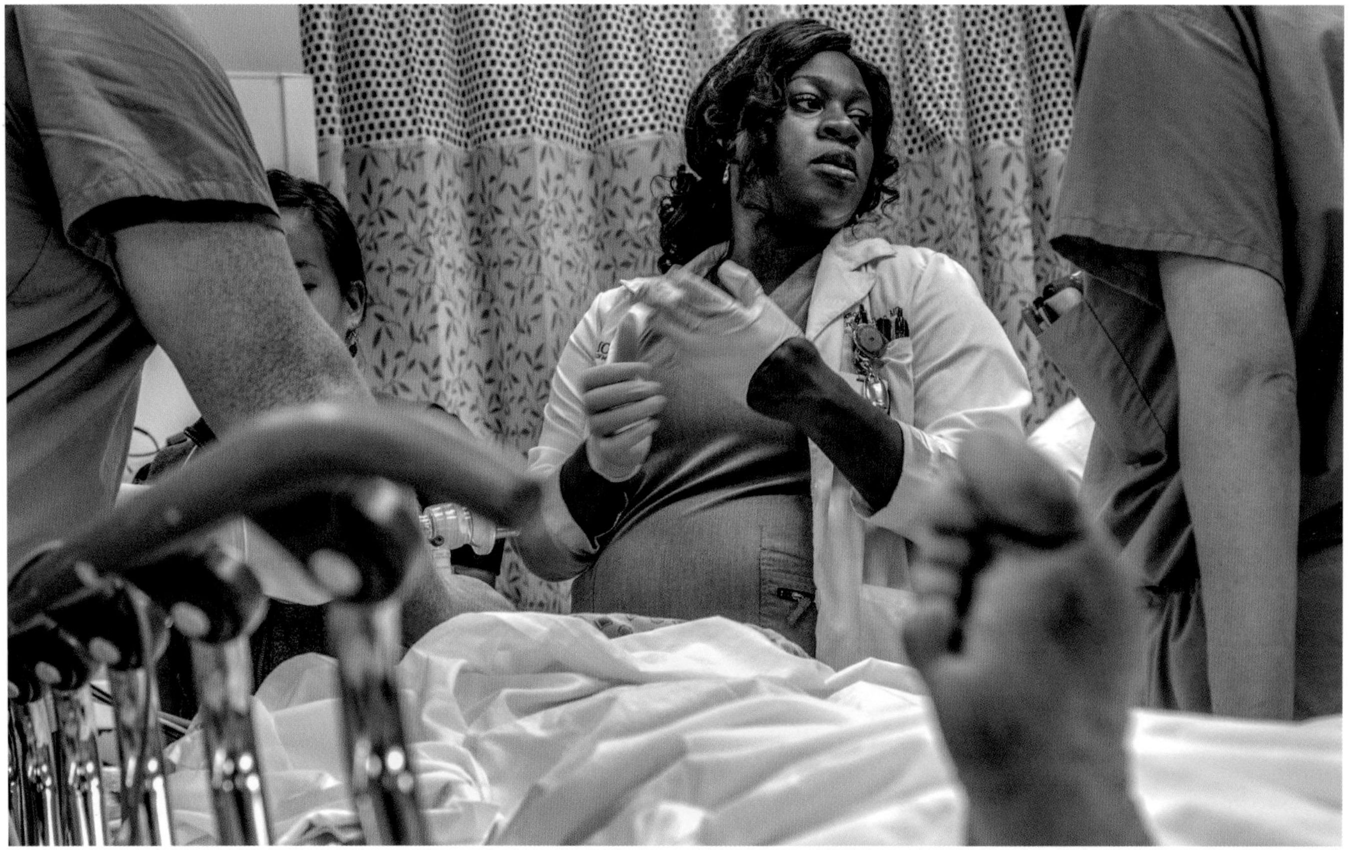

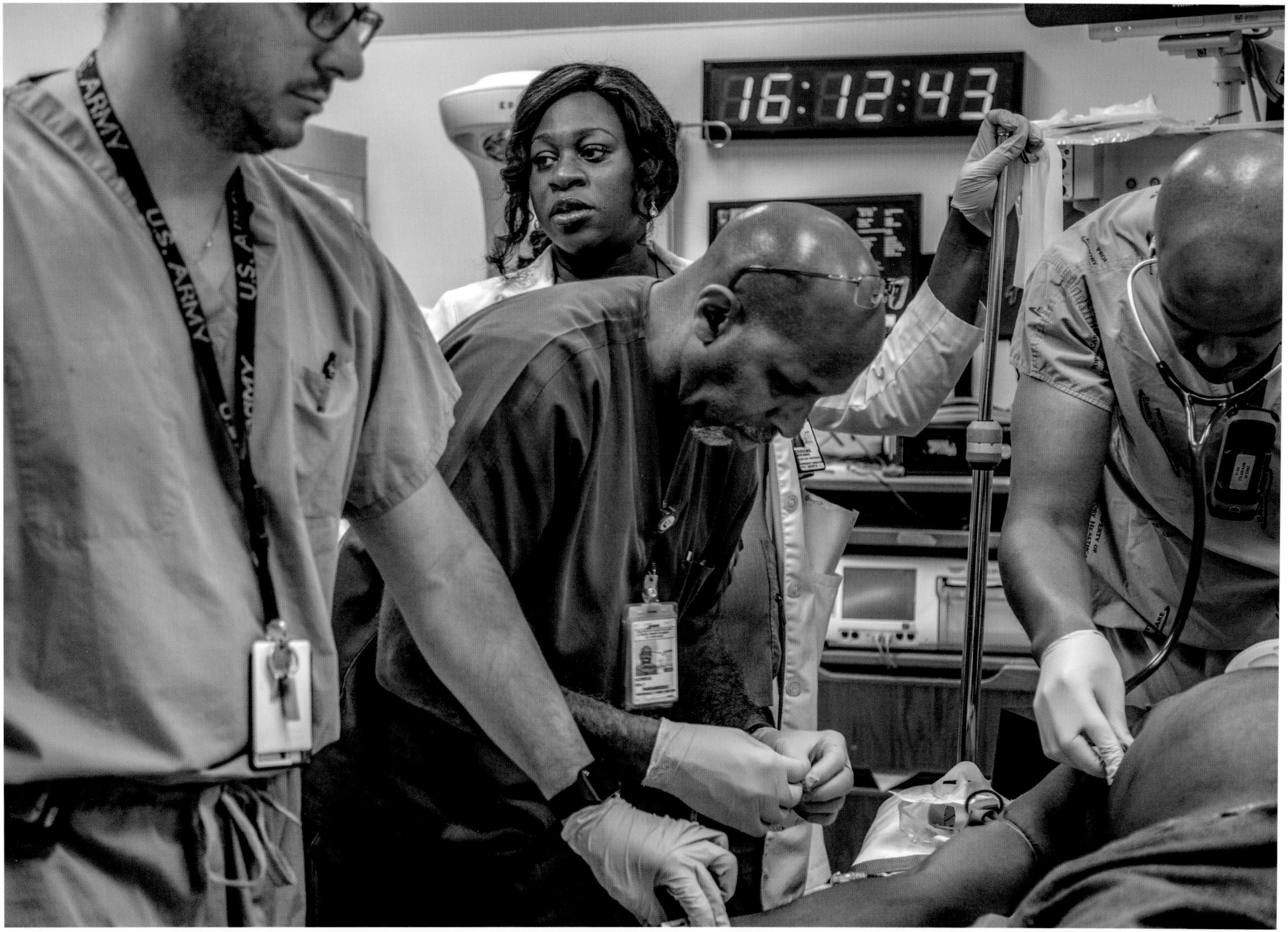
16:12:43
U.S. ARMY

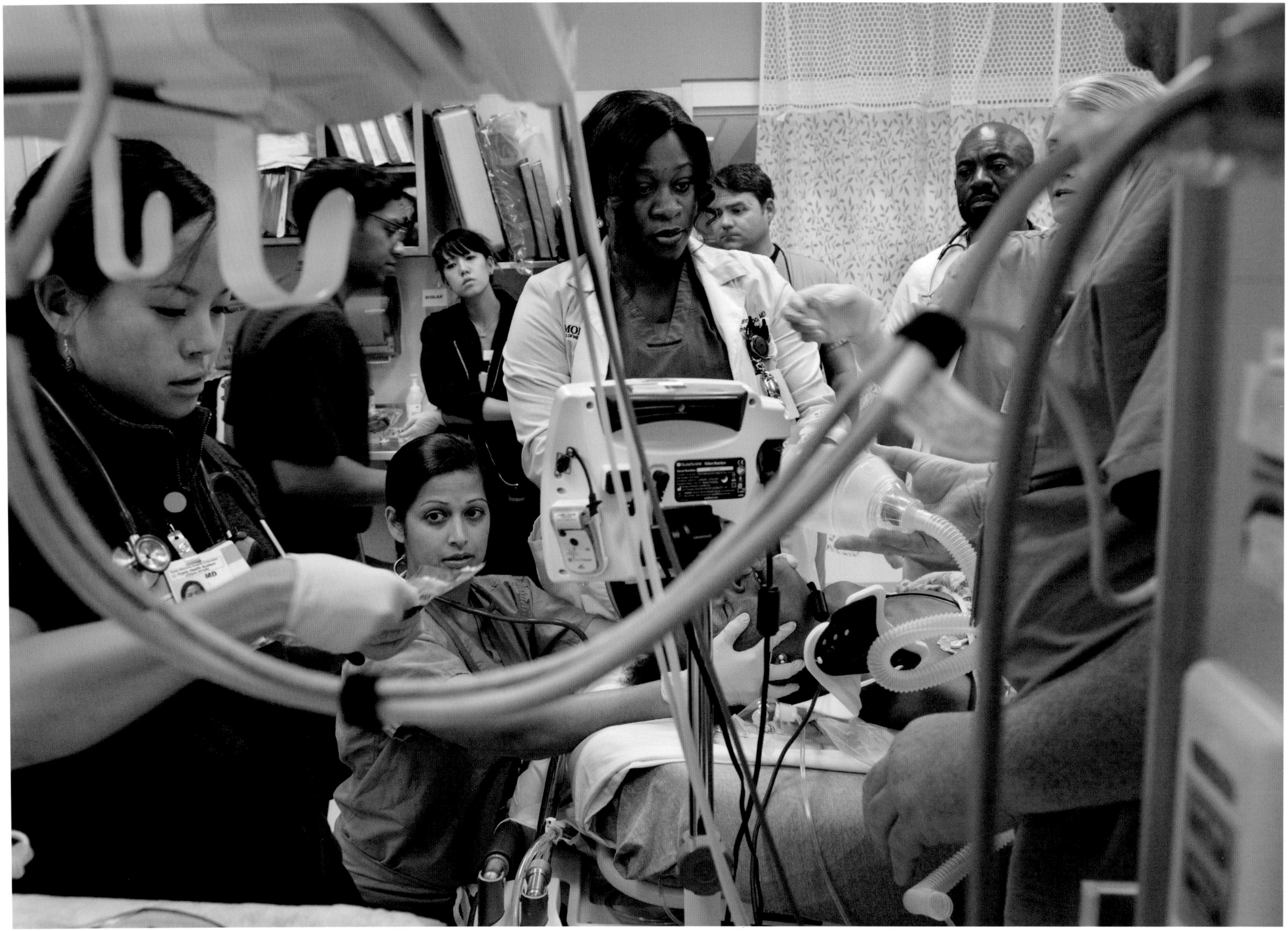

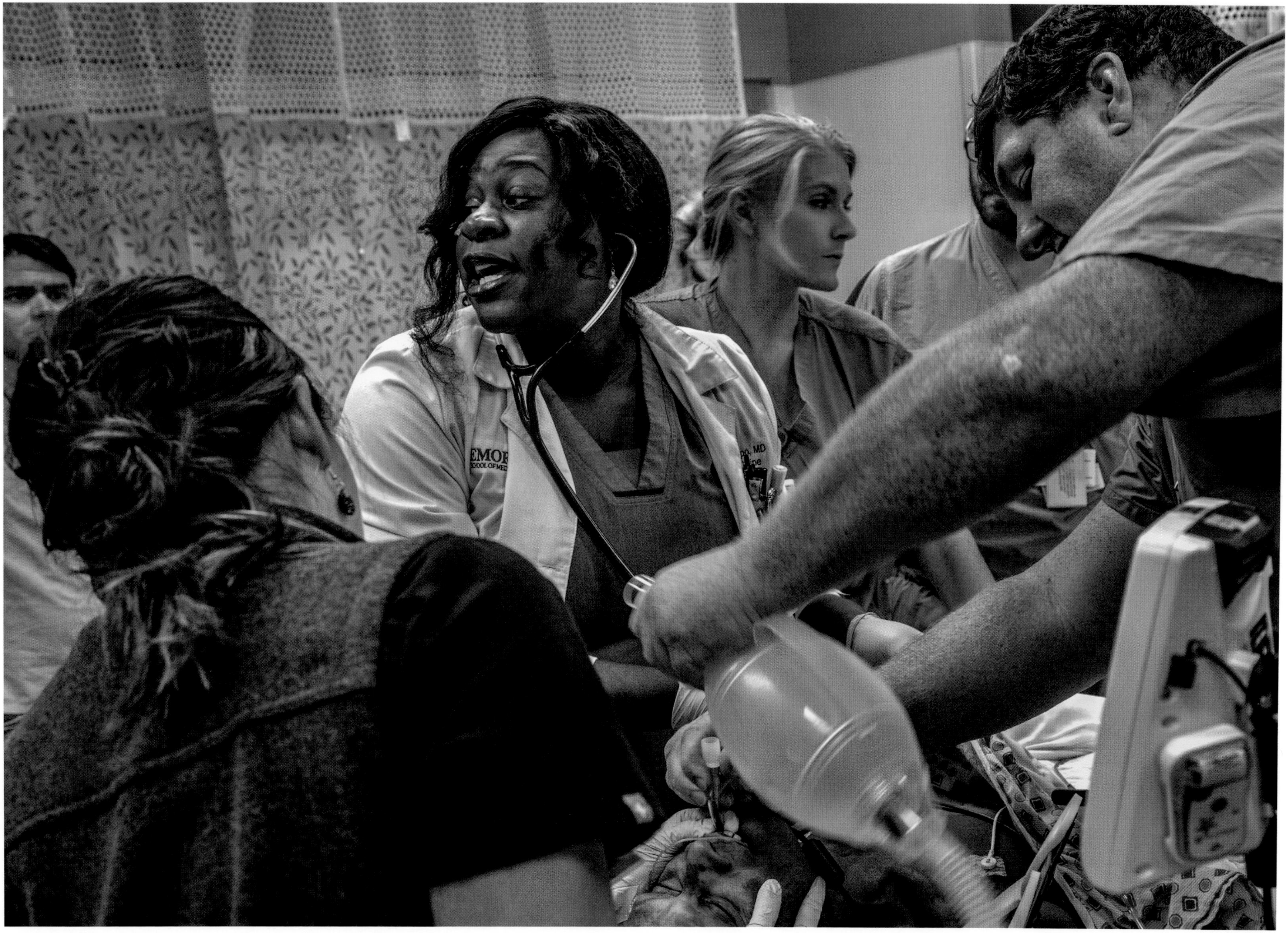

Richard Nowak, MD

Emergency Physician
Detroit, Michigan

If you could imagine any story — as bizarre as your mind could invent — it has happened to someone, somewhere and landed them in the ER. We used to keep a book called *Can You Top This?* We didn't have electronic medical records back then, so that's where we'd document the extremes . . . the crazy lab values . . . the wild stories. You just couldn't make this stuff up. One guy taped a bent quarter to one of the pages; it had been in the pocket of a woman who'd been shot. The bullet had hit the quarter.

We once had a patient come in after a sudden cardiac arrest . . . he'd collapsed at the plant where he worked. His wife shows up, and we have to break the news, " We're so sorry to tell you that his heart stopped beating and we were unable to resuscitate him. He's passed away." That's always the hardest thing ever. You look at the person's face and you know they're thinking, " Is this a joke? Are they lying?" And then, of course, here it comes . . . tremendous emotion, tears, and all the other stuff. She asks to see him, so we escort her to the room. But she takes one look at the patient and says, " That's not my husband." Walks out.

We're just standing there like idiots going, "Are you *sure*?" It turns out two people with the same name were employed by the factory. Somebody just called the wrong family. I bet she's still telling that story at parties to this day.

The ER is a different place than when I first started. Medicine, in general, has turned into a business, driven by third-party payers and the government. The problem is, we're not in the business of producing widgets. What we do is about human beings. You can't tell a patient, "Sorry, your life is going to be miserable . . . but, hey, I've got a bottom line to meet." How do you handle that? I'm not exactly sure.

I grew up in Canada, so when I first moved to Detroit I was struck by the level of drugs and violence. There'd be an incident and we'd get two or three people who'd been shot. I'd never seen those kinds of things before, so I'd think, "Oh, this is big! This story is going to be all over the 5 o'clock news." But the next day, I'd see a one-liner in the newspaper . . . buried on page fifteen . . . just a footnote. Why wasn't it on the front page?

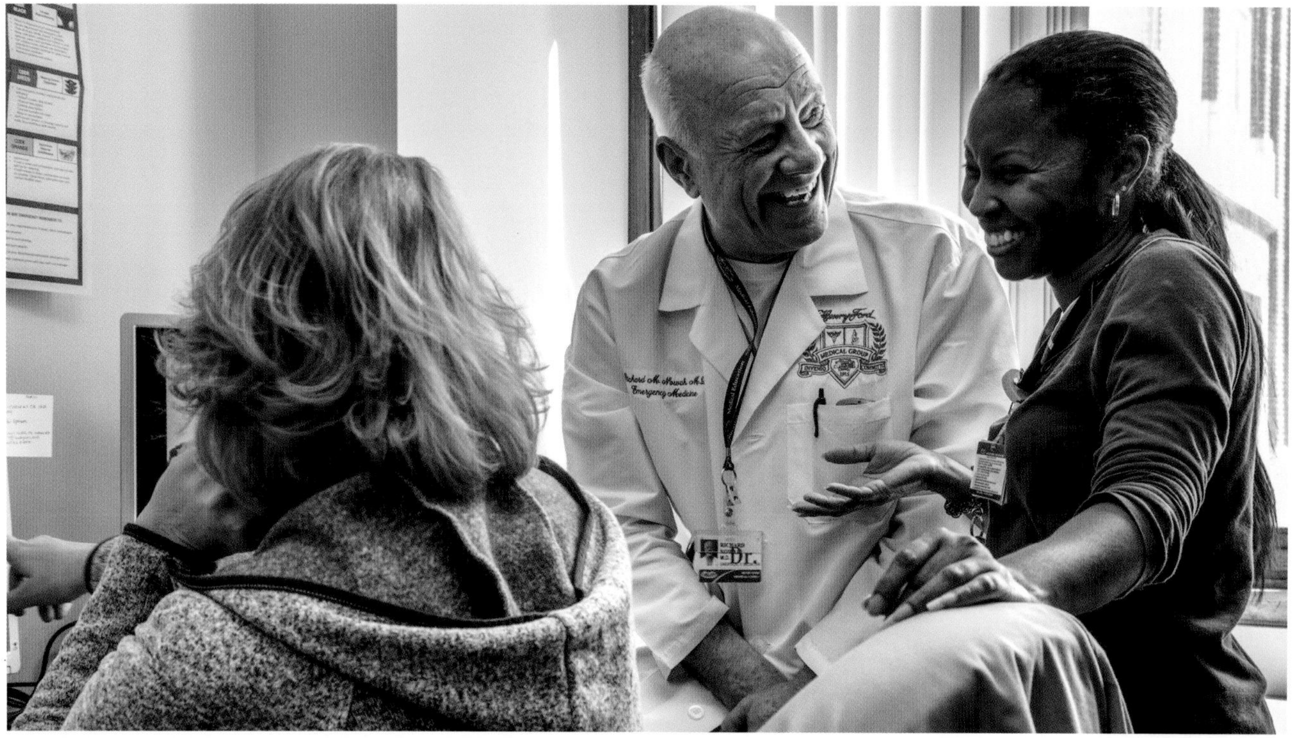

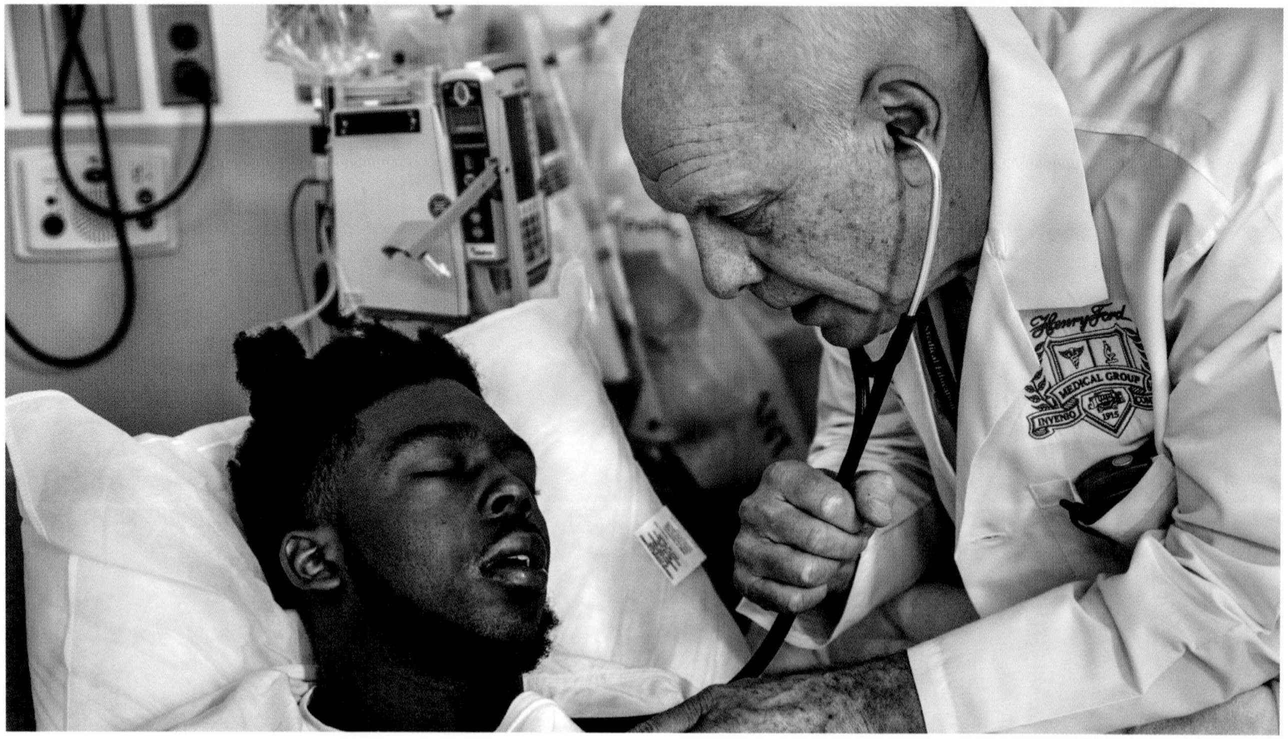

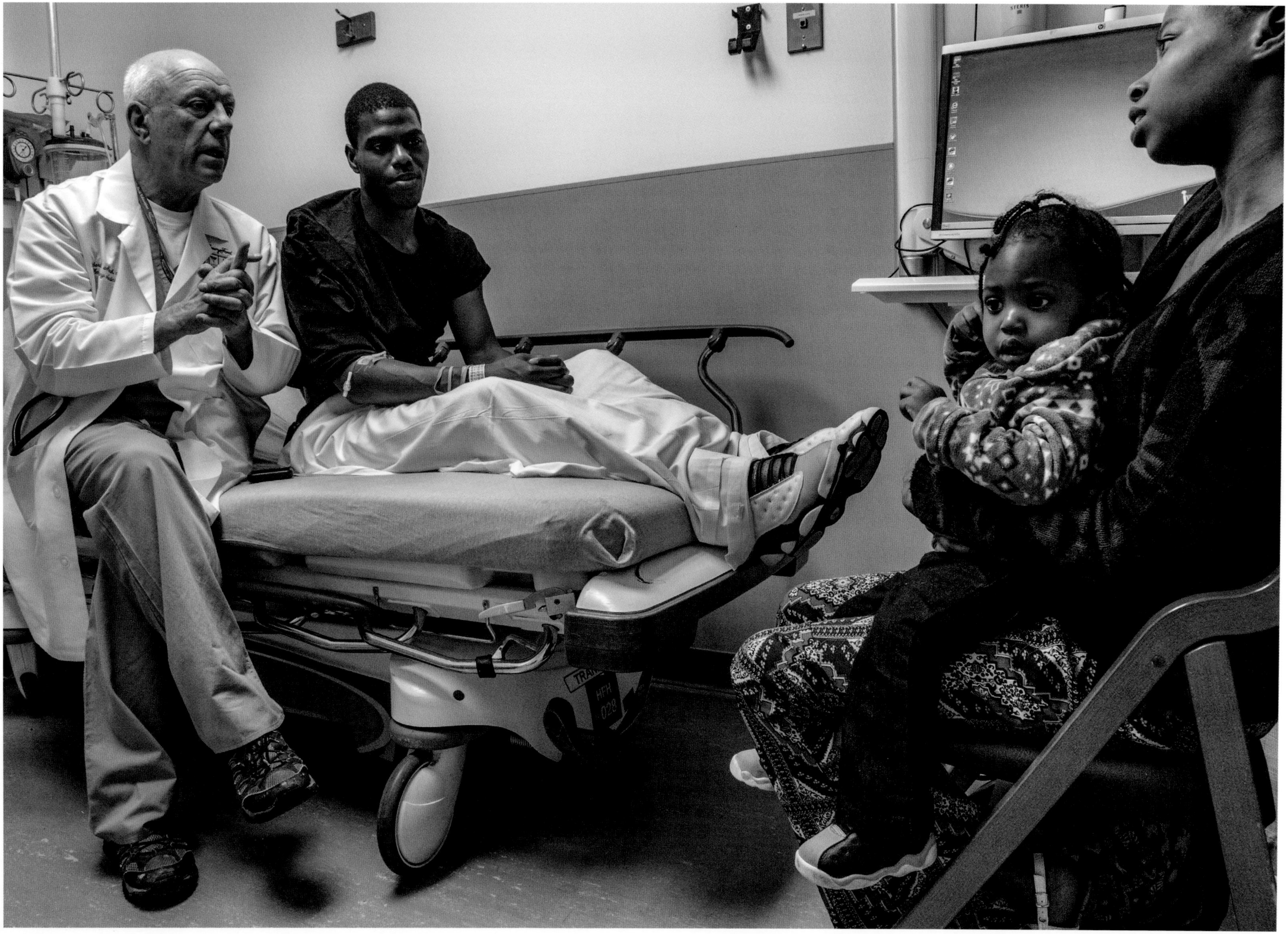

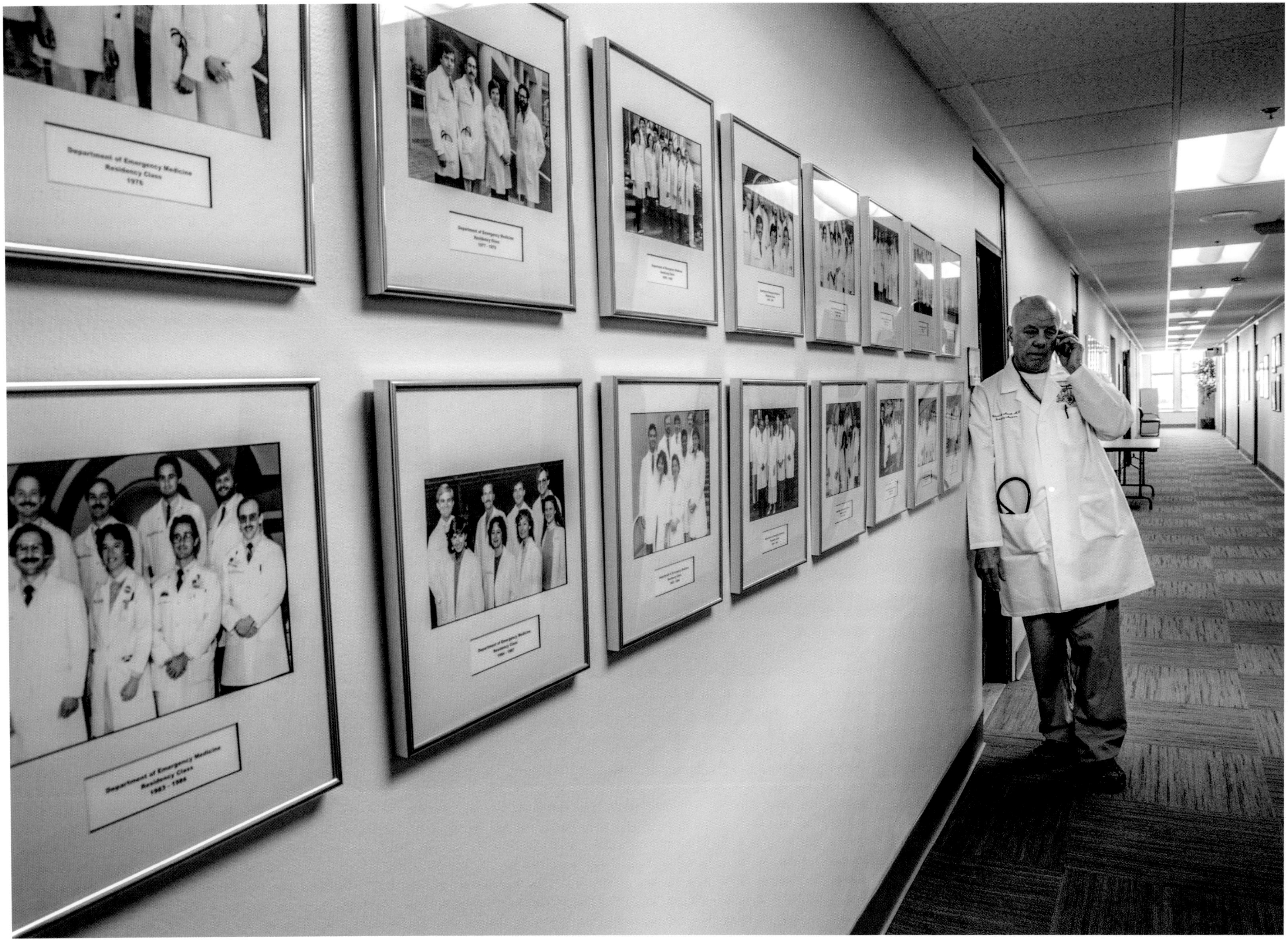
Department of Emergency Medicine
Residency Class
1975
Department of Emergency Medicine
Residency Class

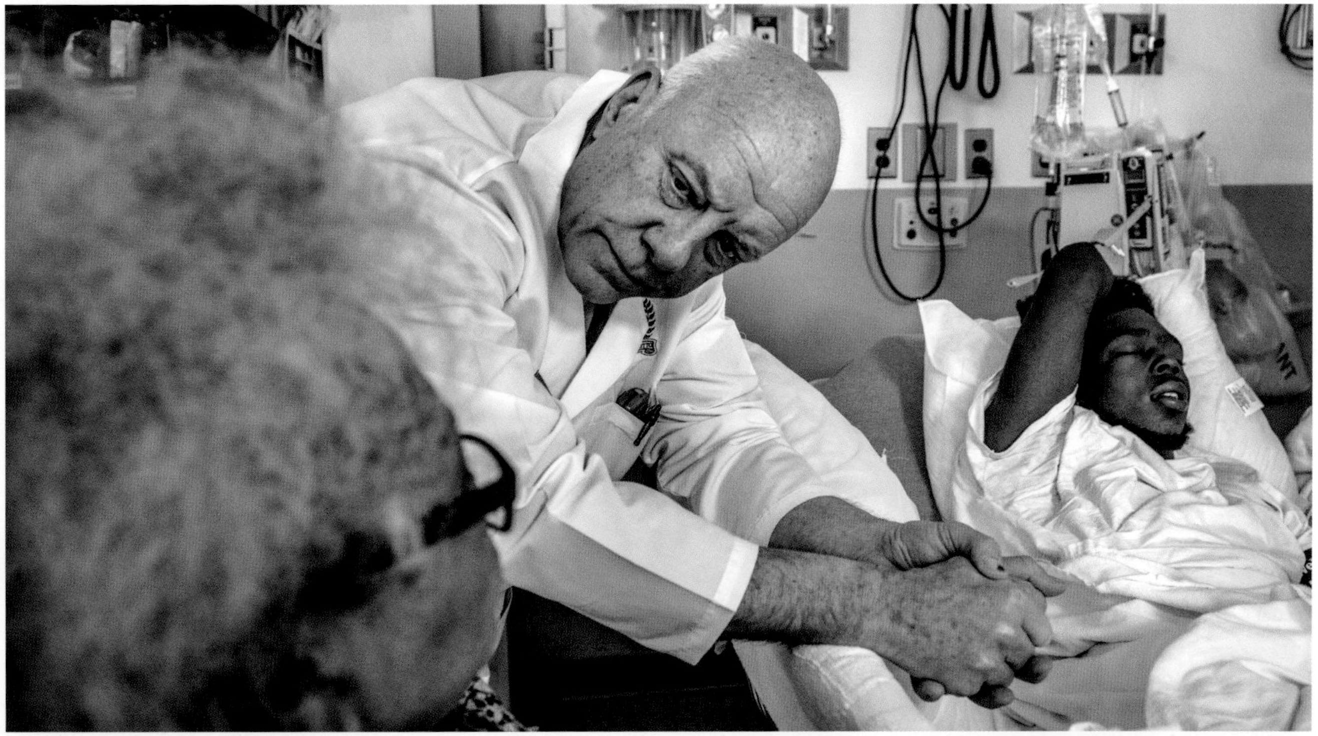

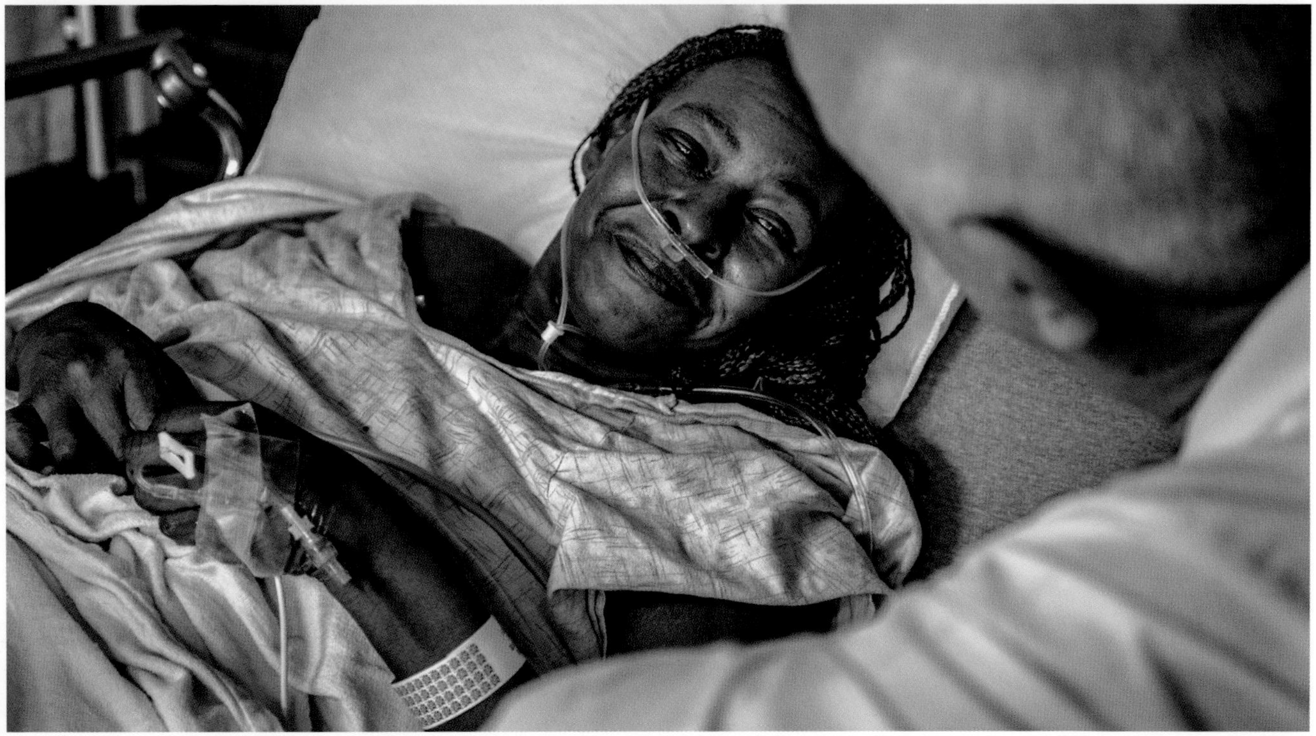

A patient's parents would tell me, almost nonchalantly, that their son had been doing drugs. In Toronto, that would've meant the kid was maybe smoking a little dope. Here, they'd be talking about IV heroin. The thing that struck me was this attitude of tolerance. I've always found that to be really sad . . . how a society can become so accepting of things that are so bad for it.

Canada subscribes to more European beliefs . . . its social systems operate with the assumption that government is good . . . we have a responsibility to help one another. But in the United States, individual rights are supreme. Americans are much less trustful of their government and much more protective of their own civil liberties. There's got to be a middle ground, but I'm not sure where it is. The whole thing is complicated as hell.

If you want to be successful in emergency medicine, you can't be arrogant. Most of us learn that very quickly. If you treat people with respect, most people will respond in kind. I remember reading an interview with David Bowie, and the reporter asked him about his accomplishments. He said, "You know, I'm not really that interested in the past. I'm more interested in the future." That's how I feel.

I mean, I've had a great career. It's been a riot. I hope people say nice things about me when I'm dead and gone. If they do, I think I'll rest peacefully. ✚

Rachel Bengtzen, MD

Emergency Physician & Sports Medicine Specialist
Portland, Oregon

Emergency physicians view the world with a biased perspective. We have a heightened awareness of all the things that can go wrong. We can be a bit superstitious about becoming patients ourselves — we'll even joke about it. But, no, I didn't think those conversations would ever hit so close to home.

Three years ago, we were expecting a daughter. It was, in the grand scheme of things, a very healthy pregnancy. I was a little past my due date and the baby was showing signs that were a little bit concerning, so my OB recommended we start the laboring process. Things seemed to be going fine, until I had two contractions that were just exponentially stronger than any I'd had before. Suddenly, the OB rapid response team came barreling into the room. The baby's heart rate had plummeted and wasn't rebounding, so they rushed me down the hall to the operating room for a crash C-section. Things improved, though, and my daughter was delivered — healthy, vibrant, and amazing. Everything seemed to be going well.

But about eight hours later, I lost consciousness. I awoke to a sea of blue scrubs and one white coat at the foot of my bed, and I heard someone say, "Order the transfusion!" At first, I thought, " Boy, these guys need to get out more. What's all the fuss? I feel fine . . . I'm thinking clearly. . . ." All of a sudden, I felt a searing pain as they placed the ultrasound probe. My eyes followed the cord back to the machine, and I could see that my belly was full of fluid. I had an intra-abdominal arterial bleed.

I was still trying to process the nuts and bolts of what was happening when I saw my husband's face. That's when I realized the stakes. I knew I was very sick, and *he* knew I was very sick. In those moments, everything I could potentially lose came clearly into focus. I'd cared for people with severe blood loss before. Even when we'd done everything right, we'd still lost patients who were less critically ill than I was. I really was on the razor's edge of a cardiac arrest.

In the operating room, they found three liters of blood in my abdomen. I received a massive transfusion, and they were able to locate the arterial bleed and reverse the coagulopathy. And here I am.

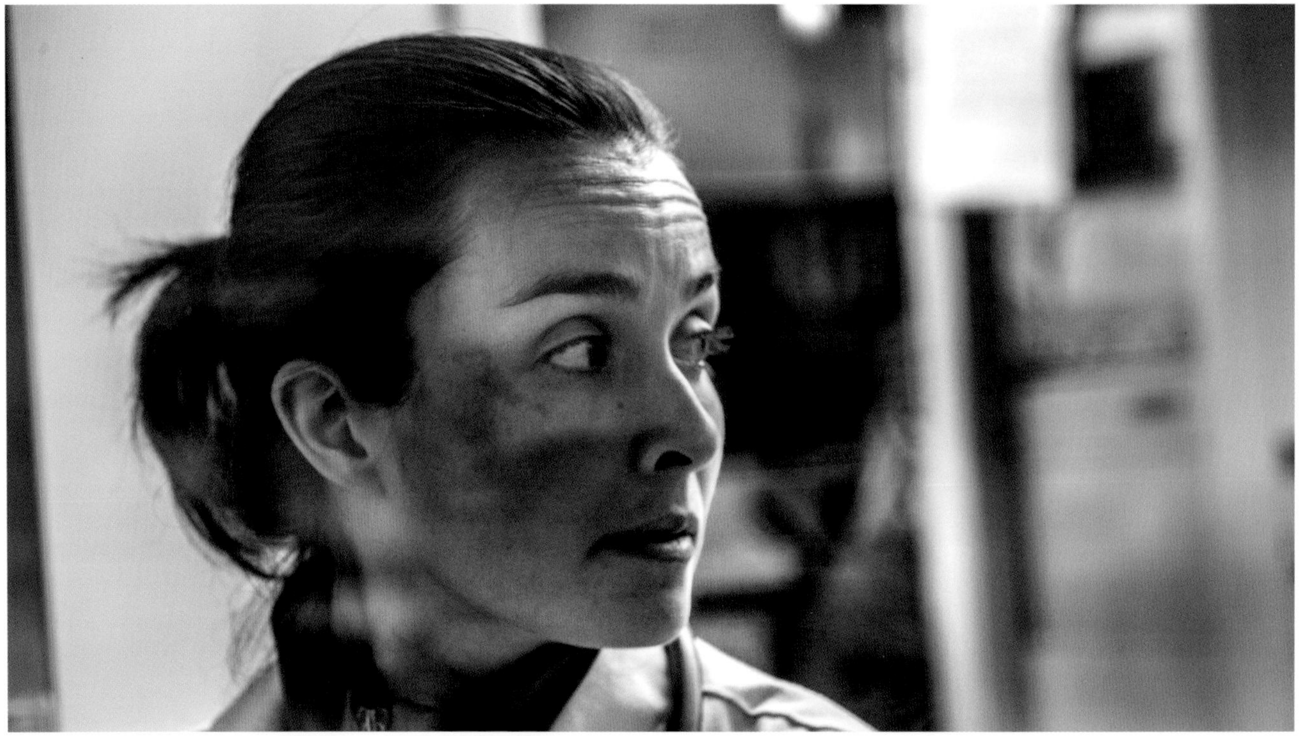

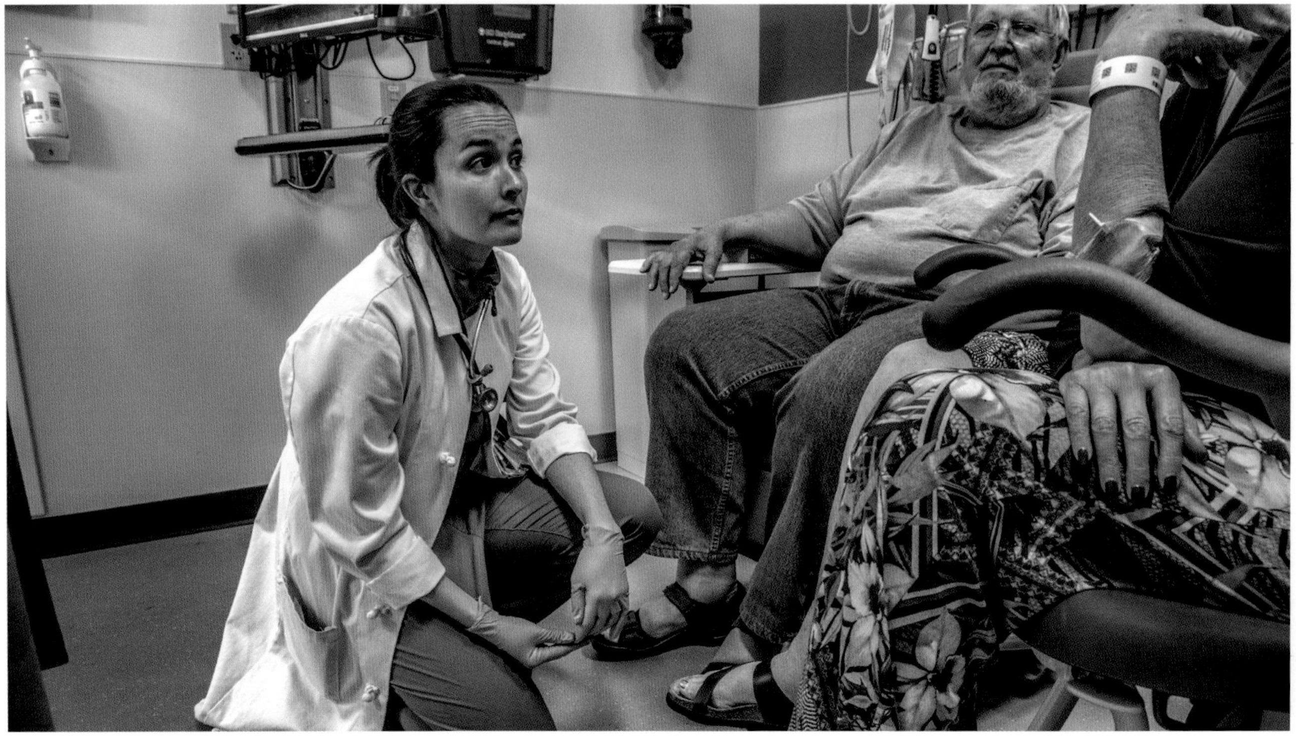

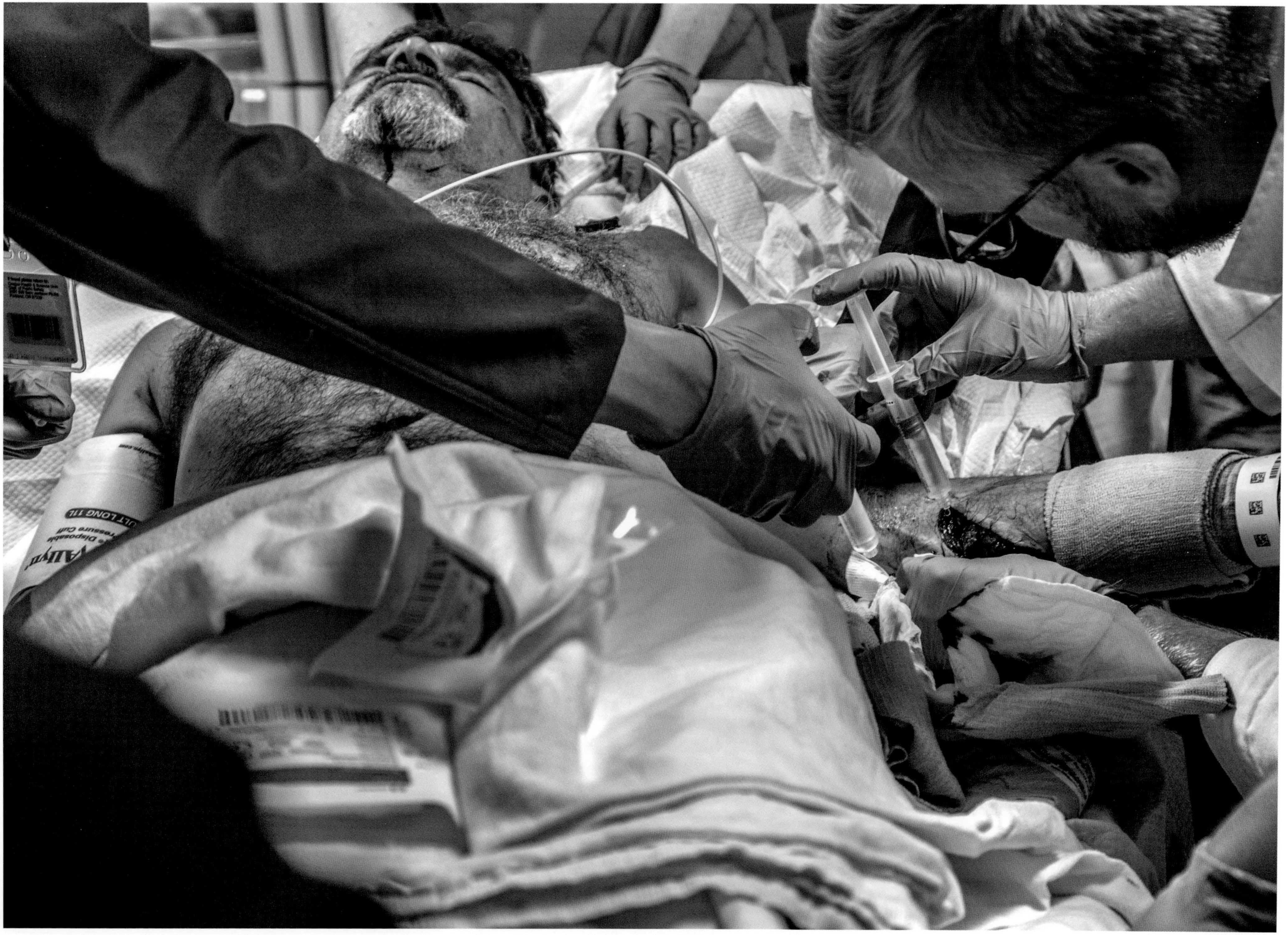

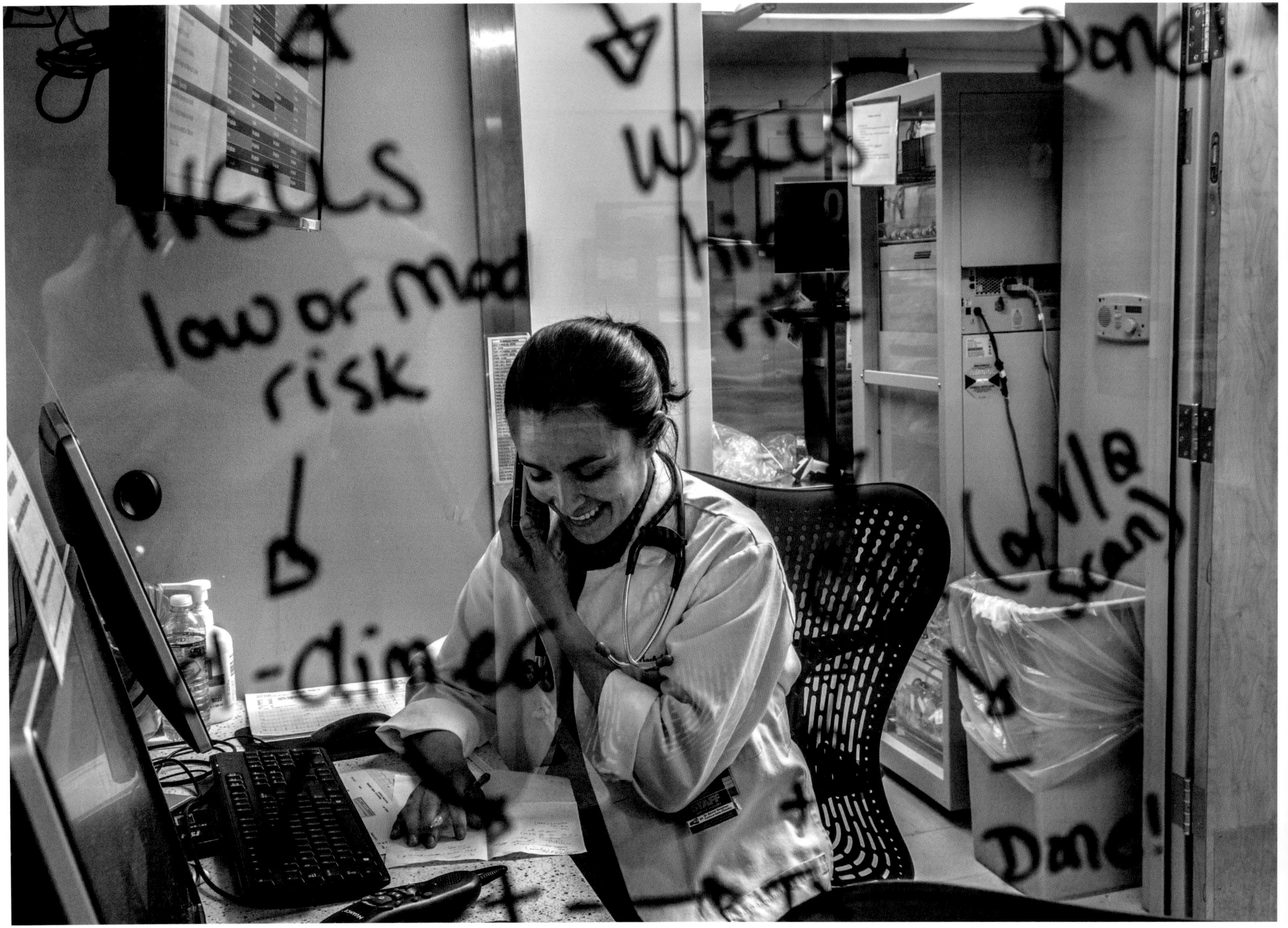
WELLS
low or mod
risk
WELLS
Done.
Done!

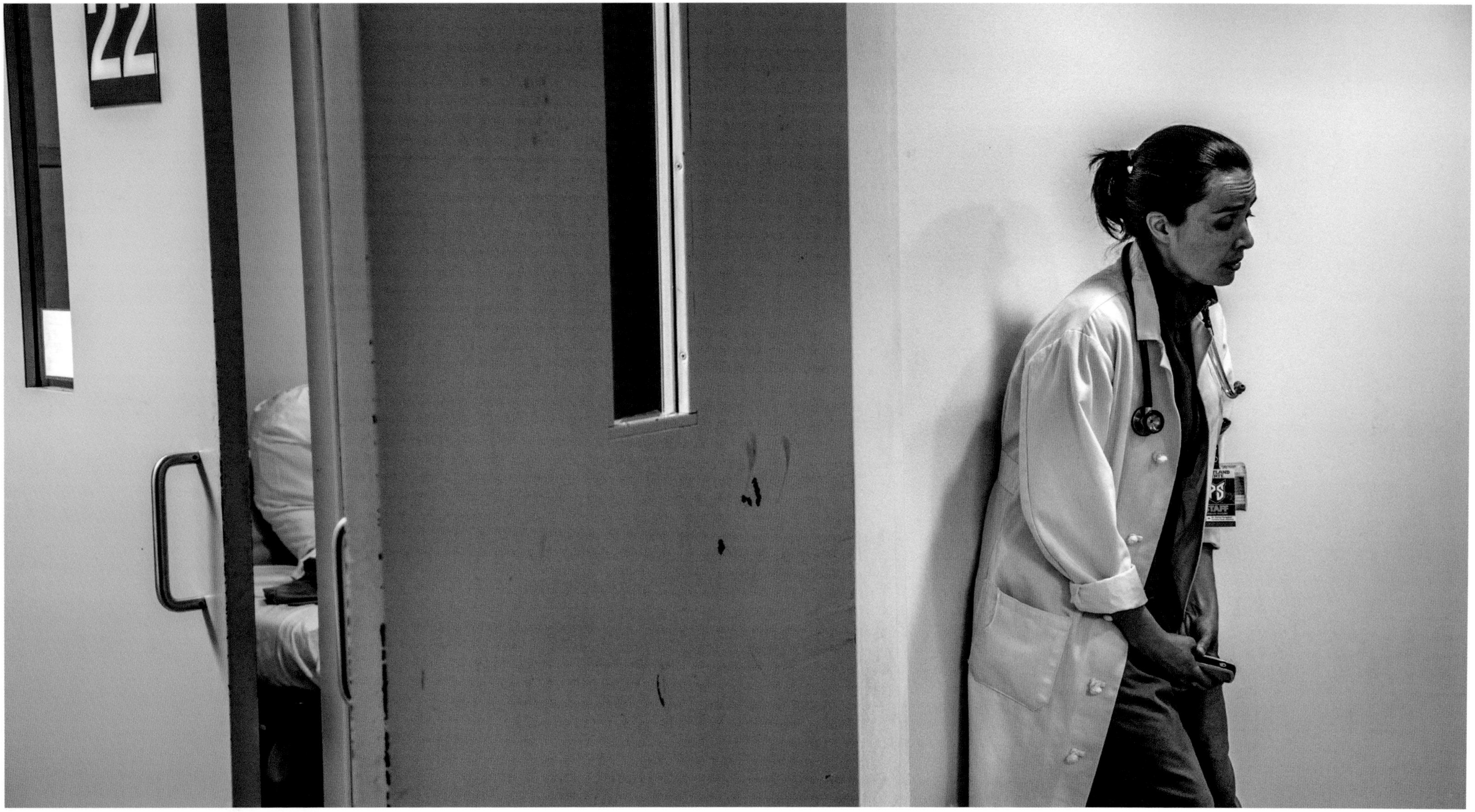

The recovery was very difficult; I had to take an extended maternity leave because I just physically couldn't do the work. As a former athlete, that was a new experience. Until then, I'm not sure I appreciated the kind of stamina required in the ED. I once heard the chess champion Garry Kasparov speak about the combination of intellect and physicality required to play the game. It reminded me of emergency medicine.

I've always been an empathetic person, so I really had to relearn how to keep a professional distance between myself and the patient — for the benefit of everyone involved. But when you live through a scare like mine, you truly learn the value of caring for someone in their most vulnerable moments.

During my ordeal, fourteen different people said, "We're going to take care of you." But there were two that mattered most: my own OB and a nurse I'd never met. The nurse had on the bouffant cap, the mask . . . I could only see her eyes. But I'll never forget the way she looked at me when she said those words — she meant them.

The whole experience has made me more proactive and present. I no longer put myself in a different category from my patients; I value my work at a higher level. I'm just fortunate to be back, to be able to do this. Being here is a gift. ✚

Steven Stack, MD

Emergency Physician & Former American Medical Association President
Lexington, Kentucky

I took on a paper route in grade school, which I inherited from another kid who'd made a mess of it. He would oversleep . . . deliver the papers wet . . . miss houses. None of the customers knew how much they owed or when he'd be by to collect payment. When I took things over, my dad told me I needed to run the route like a proper business, so I did. I'd get up at 5 am and wait for the delivery truck. I told people to call me directly if they had a problem. I converted everybody to a regular payment plan and figured out if I charged $1.60 a week, they would round it to $2.00 and I'd get a 40 cent tip every time. That experience taught me lessons about accountability I still carry with me. I learned the importance of fulfilling my commitments and how to take ownership of the quality of my work.

I've learned a lot from the hard-knock school of life. I was in Seattle for a medical forum and was headed to meet a friend for dinner one night. But I was staring down at my phone and missed a step on my way out of the hotel. In my defense, it was a very irregular step. In the hotel's defense, it was painted yellow. Anyway, I dove face first into a clay flowerpot and down into a well. I shattered my glasses . . . cut my eye . . . tore my jacket . . . my face was covered in dirt and blood.

When I got to the hospital, I explained I was an emergency physician and — in fact — was the president of the American Medical Association. I went through this whole thing about how I was scheduled to give a speech on electronic health records at that very hospital the next day. Unimpressed, they told me to take a seat. Just like that, I was in the club. There we were . . . a homeless person sleeping on the bench next to me . . . a schizophrenic woman scooting around in a wheelchair, looking for a ride. I sat there for two hours, bleeding through my gauze.

And that's what I love about emergency medicine — it's the great equalizer. You think you're awesome, huh? If you need a reality check, just walk into any hospital in the United States. And I don't mean that as a criticism — it's just the nature of the beast. In this business, we take care of people on a first-come, first-served basis and according to the urgency of their medical needs. It doesn't matter if you're rich or you're poor . . . no one cares where you work. When you're there, you are a patient. Vulnerable. Mortal.

People talk a lot about the American Dream, but for most it really is the American Fallacy. We generally operate within a caste system; where you're born is probably where you'll stay. That's not to say we should naively dole out "equal allotments" at every turn; however, it's very difficult to make the situation better if you don't call a spade a spade. The reality is this country offers very little in the way of social mobility, but we continue to foster this rugged, individualistic Marlboro Man mythology: *just pull yourself up by your own bootstraps*.

I like to think of myself as a moderate . . . that is to say I'm very pragmatic. Franklin Delano Roosevelt said, "The test of our progress is not whether we add more to the abundance of those who have much; it is whether we provide enough for those who have too little." And I believe that. It is in our enlightened self-interest to raise the tide for as many as we can.

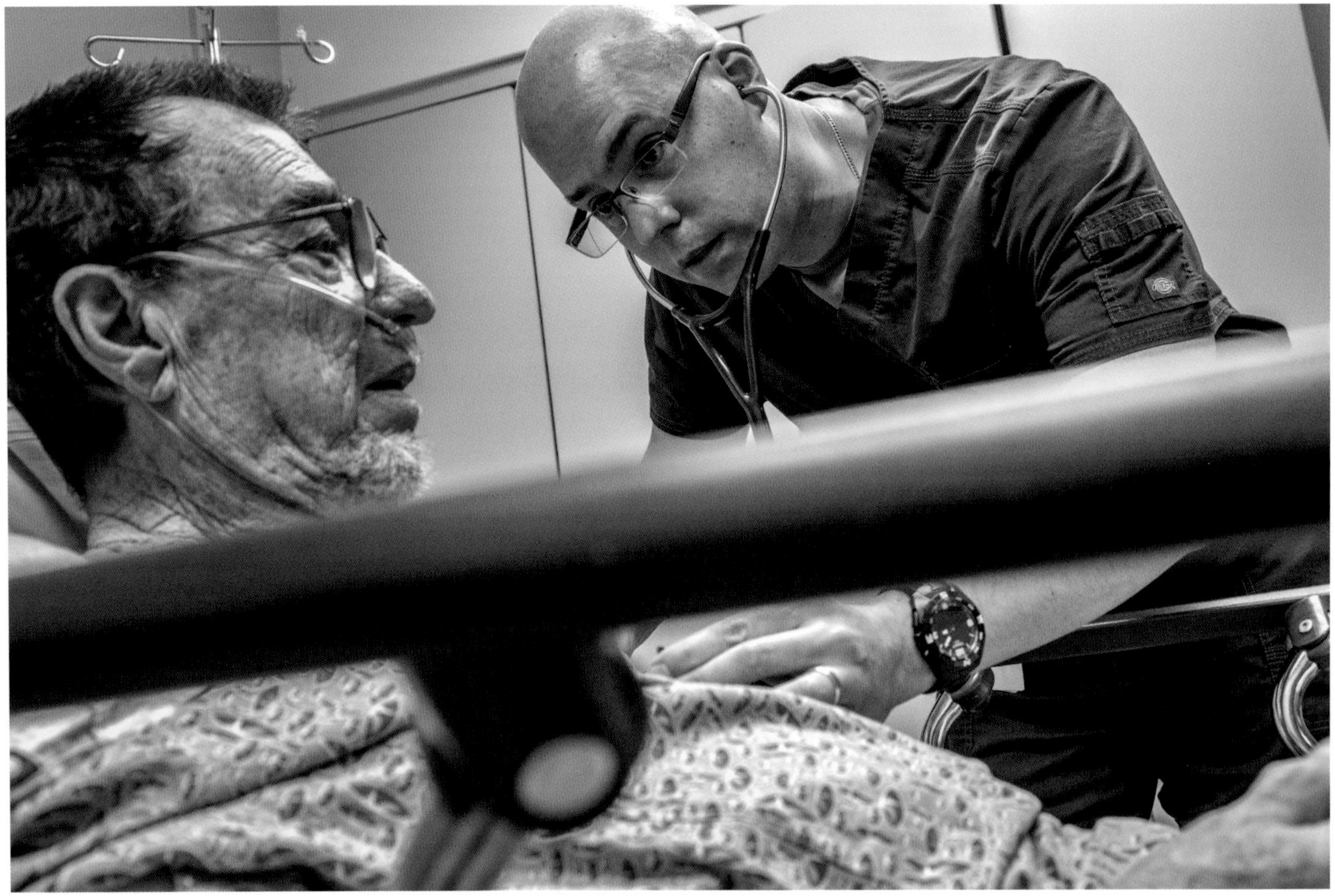

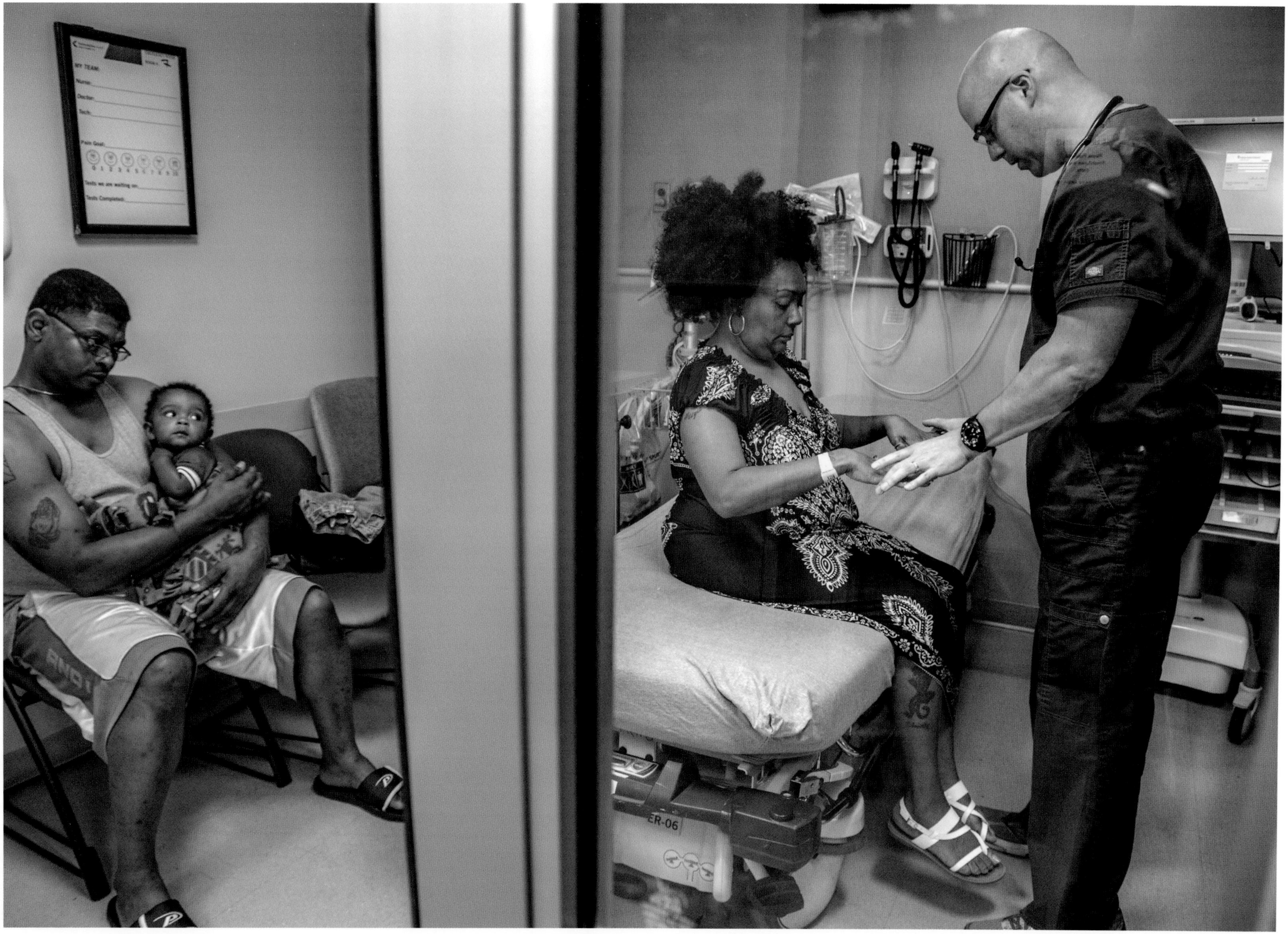
MY TEAM:
Name:
Doctor:
Tech:
Pain Goal:
Tests we are waiting on...
Tests Completed:
ER-06

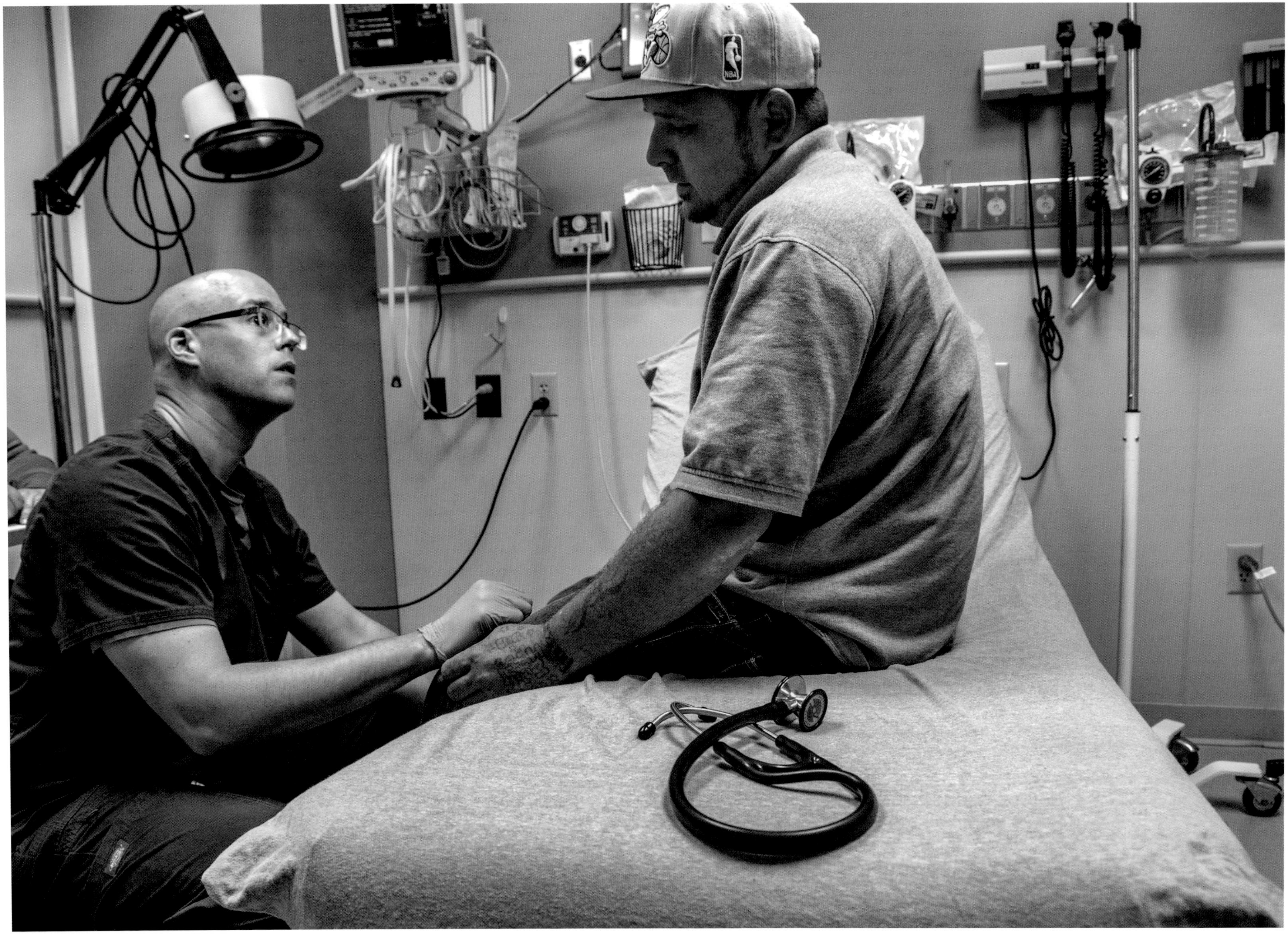
NBA

We sustain a system that is arguably one of the most inefficient on the planet. We're the richest country in the world, yet one in seven Americans must rely upon the charity of others to pay their bills. While it's true some of them may not care, there are many more who do . . . but we've given them virtually no path forward. I mean, what are you supposed to do when a thirty-day supply of medication costs $380 and it's more than your take-home pay? The political debates . . . the massive network of funding streams . . . the media spin . . . they all obscure the fundamental issue at hand: every single one of us has a need for health care. Why can't we create a system that isn't entangled in all this other stuff?

When you don't take the time to ask the right questions . . . when you prejudge people . . . you stop learning. That's true in emergency medicine *and* in regular life. People who lock themselves inalterably to rigid moral views probably have a peace I lack, but that security isn't worth the trade-off. You simply lose too much of what it means to be human when you presume you know right . . . and everybody else does not. ✚

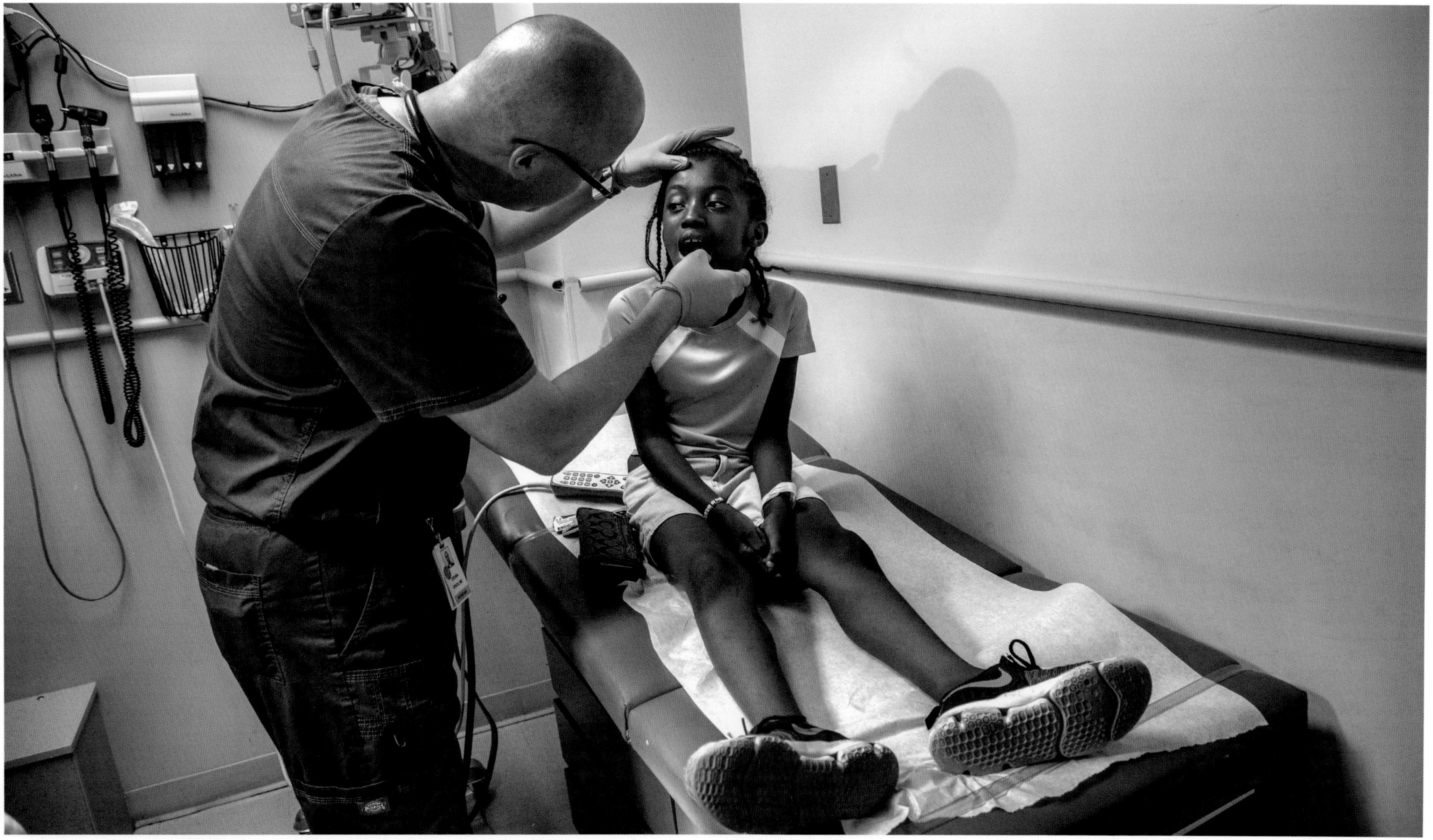

Brian Anderson, CFRN

Flight Nurse
Anchorage, Alaska

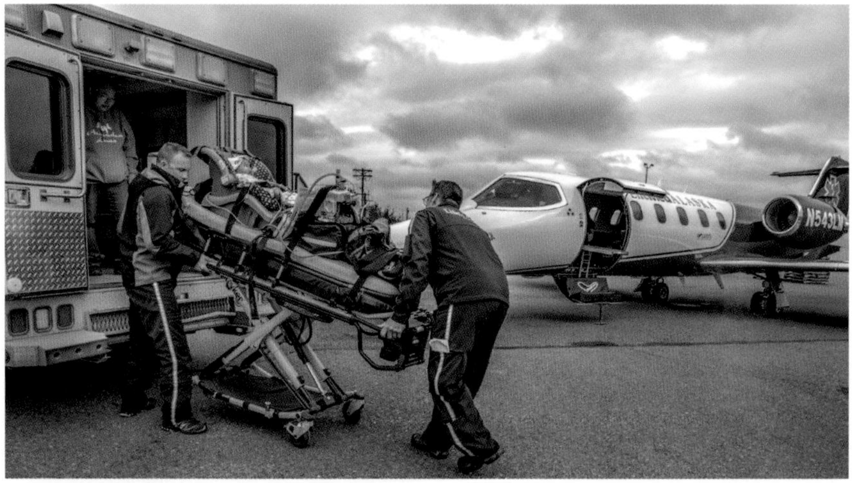

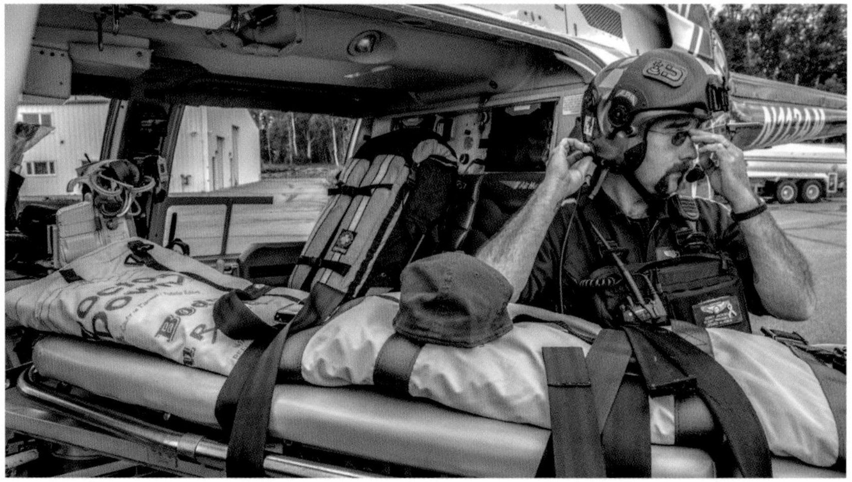

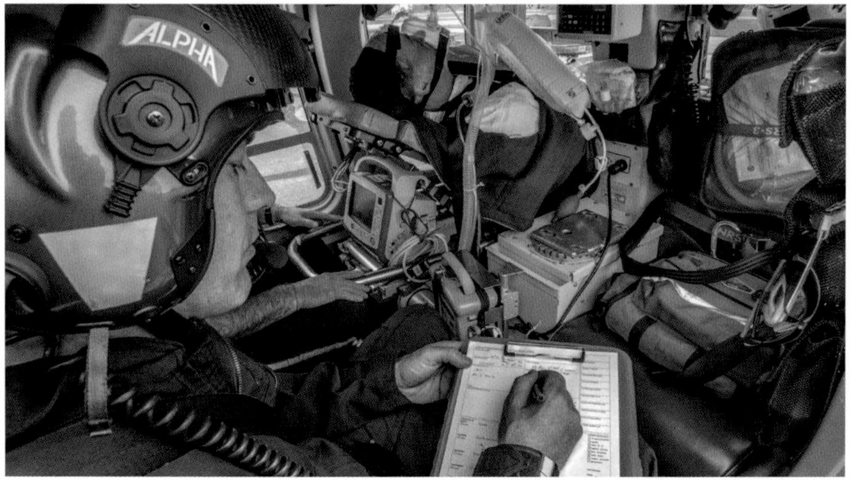

There was only one other man in my nursing class. The stigma was still alive and well in 1997 . . . people thought the work was all about fluffing pillows, stroking hands, and braiding patients' hair. I guess public perception got to me, too. I was embarrassed to admit I was in nursing school. I would just keep it vague . . . tell people I was in a "medical program." Since then, emergency medicine has undergone some big role reversals. We're seeing more and more female physicians and paramedics . . . several of our helicopter pilots are women. It's a reminder to teach my five daughters they can do anything and everything a man can do.

Alaska can be a hostile, dangerous environment. We work as a team and put a great deal of trust in our pilots and their ability to forecast the weather, which can change in a split second. You never know what you're going to get out here, and we've seen a lot . . . a *lot*.

We got a call about a bear mauling a couple of years ago. They're not uncommon, so my partner and I weren't worried . . . figured it was all going to be a big nothing. So, we land and I start walking toward the patient. His face is covered with a hooded jacket, but as I get closer, I can see one white eyeball floating in a red mass. His whole face had been degloved and was just hanging there . . . his ear and nose had been ripped off . . . bubbling holes every time he took a breath. It truly startled me, and I thought, "Ohhhhhh, shit. . . ." But I must've actually said it aloud because the guy turned to me and said, "It's okay, son. Don't freak out." When he talked, the skin on his face went *brrrr* . . . it just jiggled.

We put his ear in a bag of ice water, and when we got to the hospital, the patient told the plastic surgeon he wanted it sewn on backwards. We all just laughed, but he was serious. He said, "I want to hear those damn things coming up behind me next time." We learned later he had a bear tooth lodged in his butt. He said he was going to leave it there . . . a way to remember the bear. Nobody argued with him, of course.

We've got so much wilderness . . . sometimes the only way you can respond is by helicopter. I remember landing on a glacier to rescue a guy who'd fallen 120 feet into a crevasse. He'd just left his tent to use the bathroom. But . . . when you're on that kind of terrain, you're not at liberty to walk wherever you please. In situations like that, we put ourselves as close to the patient as we safely can, but we sometimes have to trek a mile or more.

We travel with a pilot and a two-person medical crew, so our resources are limited. Our aircraft are small, so we work in very tight spaces and don't get to travel with a lot of extra equipment. I remember flying over the water one evening with a pregnant patient in labor. The plane was just bouncing her all over the place . . . she'd literally come up off the stretcher two to three inches every time we hit an air pocket. I got out of my seat belt to comfort her, which I shouldn't have done, and got thrown into a ceiling vent. It hurt, but I kept going about my business until she looked at me with these really big eyes and said, "You're bleeding!" I'd cut my scalp pretty badly, but I just wiped the blood off my face and went about my night. I feel the scar every time I comb my hair.

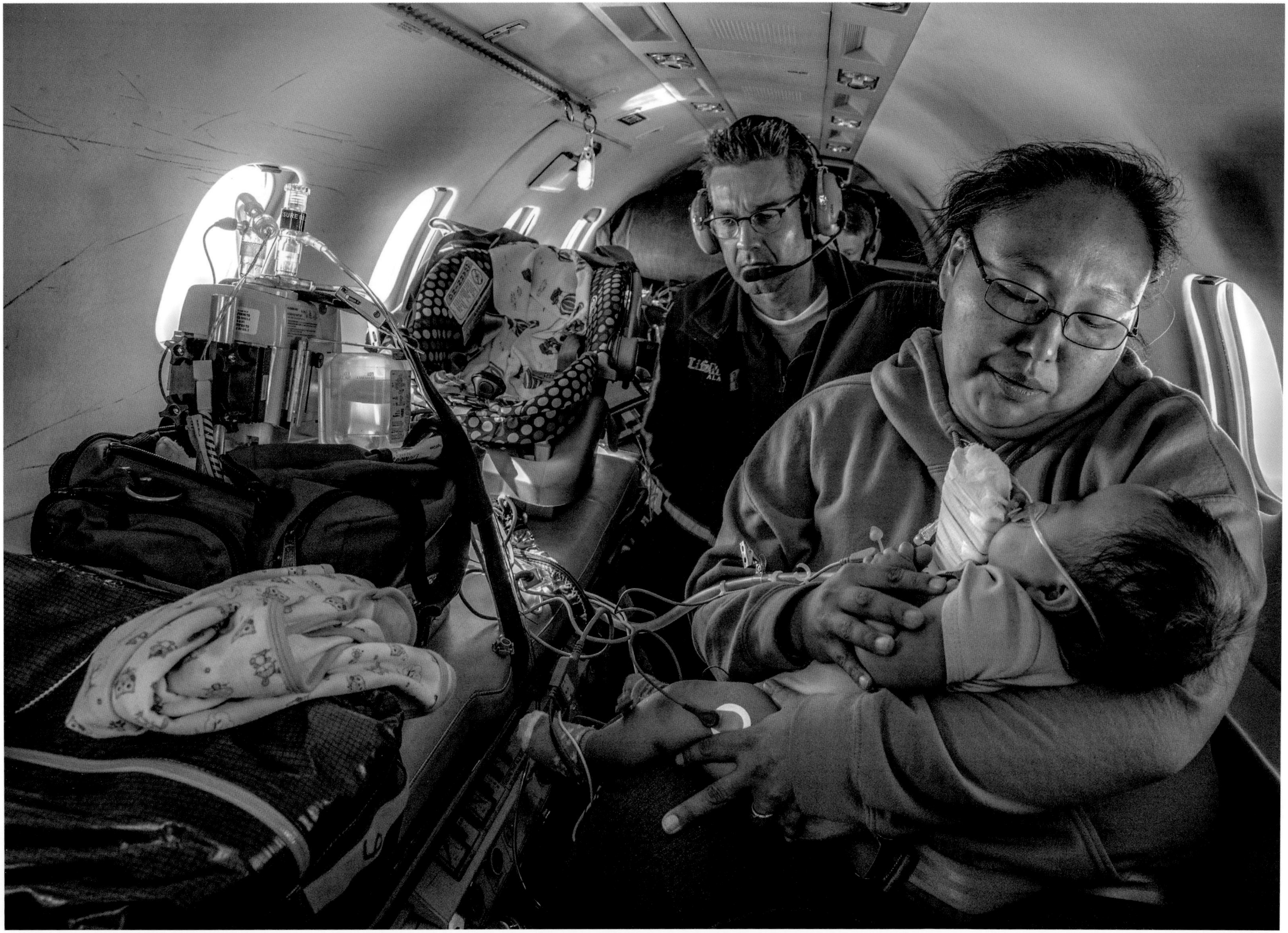

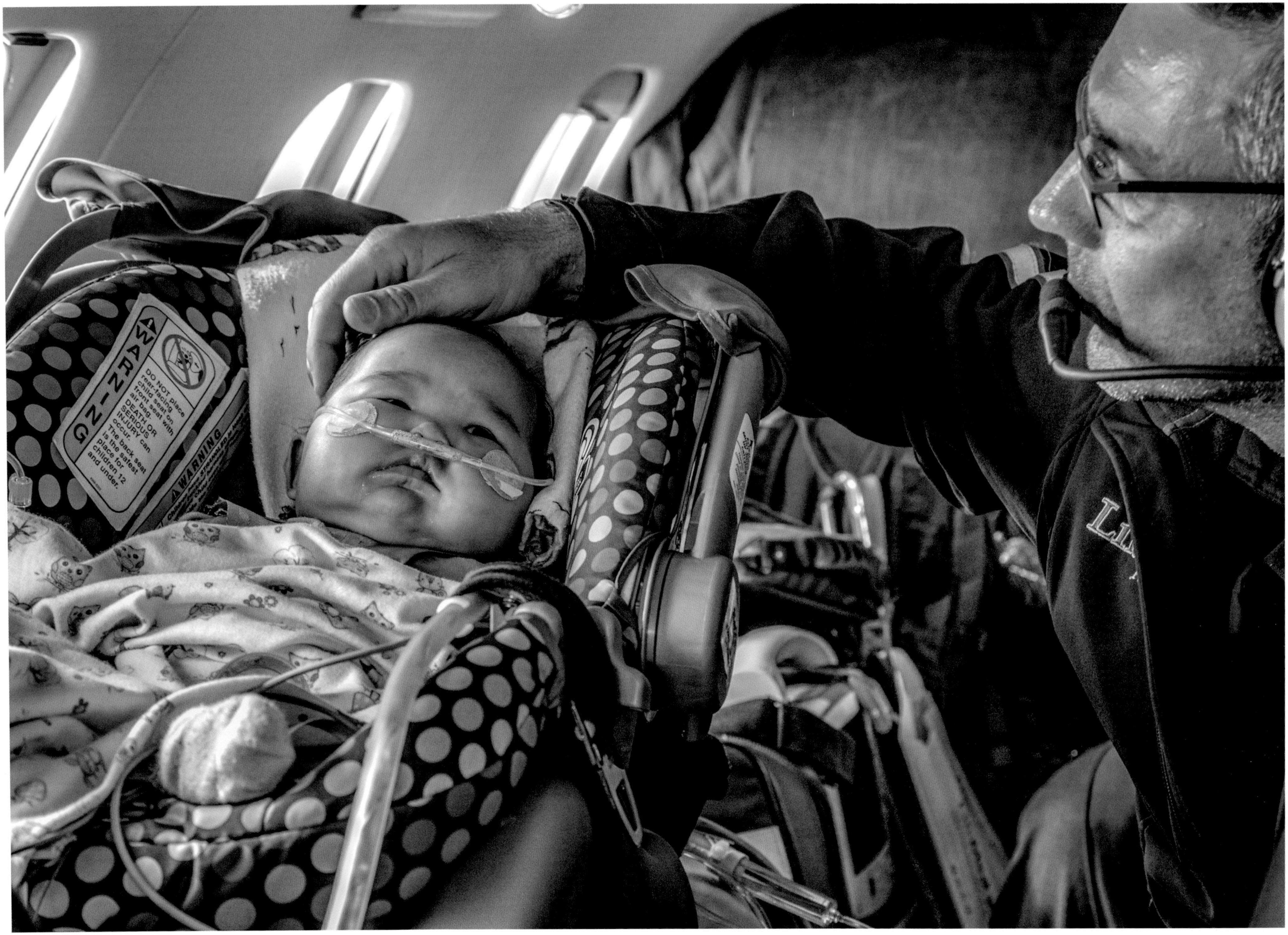
WARNING
DO NOT place rear-facing child seat on front seat with air bag. DEATH OR SERIOUS INJURY can occur. The back seat is the safest place for children 12 and under.
WARNING

I'll admit it's pretty cool to step off that aircraft and walk to a scene — it makes you feel like a hero. But that's not why I do the work . . . I do it for the autonomy. Although we practice within a scope, we have the freedom to think for ourselves. There's more than one way to skin a cat (or treat a patient), and we get to exercise our knowledge and creativity every single day — at 31,000 feet.

In this line of work, we always hope for the worst. We want the ugly stuff . . . that's just the nature of our personalities. But there's nothing better than knowing a patient lived because you were there. You land . . . and you do something good. ✚

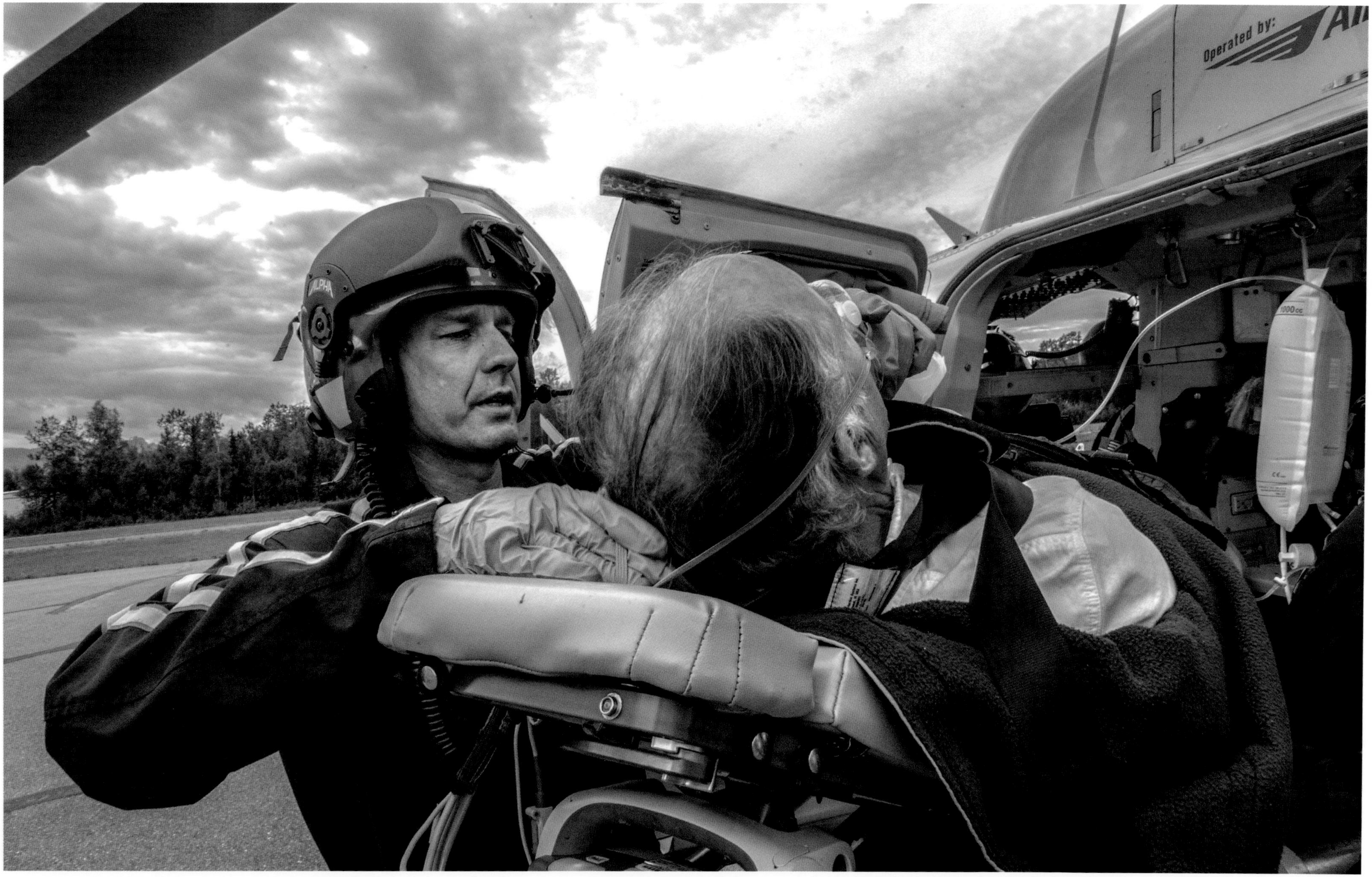

Mohamed Umar, PA

Military Physician Assistant
San Antonio, Texas

I was born in Cambodia after my family fled Vietnam. Eventually, the Khmer Rouge forced us into the countryside, where we were placed into a refugee camp. My father and I were the only ones who survived; the rest of my family members starved to death. My sister was the last one to die. She was very weak and asked me to help her, but I was cooking and said I was busy. She walked by herself to the edge of the hut, and the next thing I heard was a thump. She fell right there and died.

Things I cannot fix I tend to push to the side . . . but every time I think about my sister, the emotion comes flooding back. I cannot do anything now . . . I have to compartmentalize her. She's gone.

At the end of the war, I was sent to live with my uncle in a camp at the border of Cambodia and Thailand. We were given the choice of immigrating to Malaysia, France, or America. My uncle had a friend with a contact in America, so it seemed like a sensible choice. We landed in San Francisco in January of 1982. It took me a couple of days to get used to the smell . . . it was just different. The weather was cold, and I only had shorts. My English was terrible. It was tough.

I went back to Cambodia in 1990. A cousin of mine was very sick — with cholera, I think. I can still see the eyes of his mom, begging me to help . . . and I couldn't. I understood then that with a little knowledge of medicine, I could've done something. It was a strong motivator for me.

I joined the US Army in 1992, but it was a difficult decision. When I was in Cambodia, I'd encountered a whole lot of dead people who had been executed. It left a bad taste in my mouth for soldiers. But the experience has been much different than I expected. I'm Asian. I'm Muslim. But no one in the military looks at me any differently than they would if I were Christian or Jewish. We like each other.

I'd never had the financial means for medical school, but when I learned more about being an army PA, it sounded very attractive to me. The yearning to be a physician has never gone away, but I'm lucky in that I get to see a full range of patients: trauma, stroke, heart attack, and sepsis. When you're a PA, you have a lot of autonomy . . . but when you don't know something, you have to have the humility to seek additional help. That's where the line is drawn.

I ask God every day to bless me with the wisdom, knowledge, and skill to take care of patients safely and efficiently. Growing up as an orphan, you yearn for the kindness of others. And now that I'm an adult, I can give that. ✚

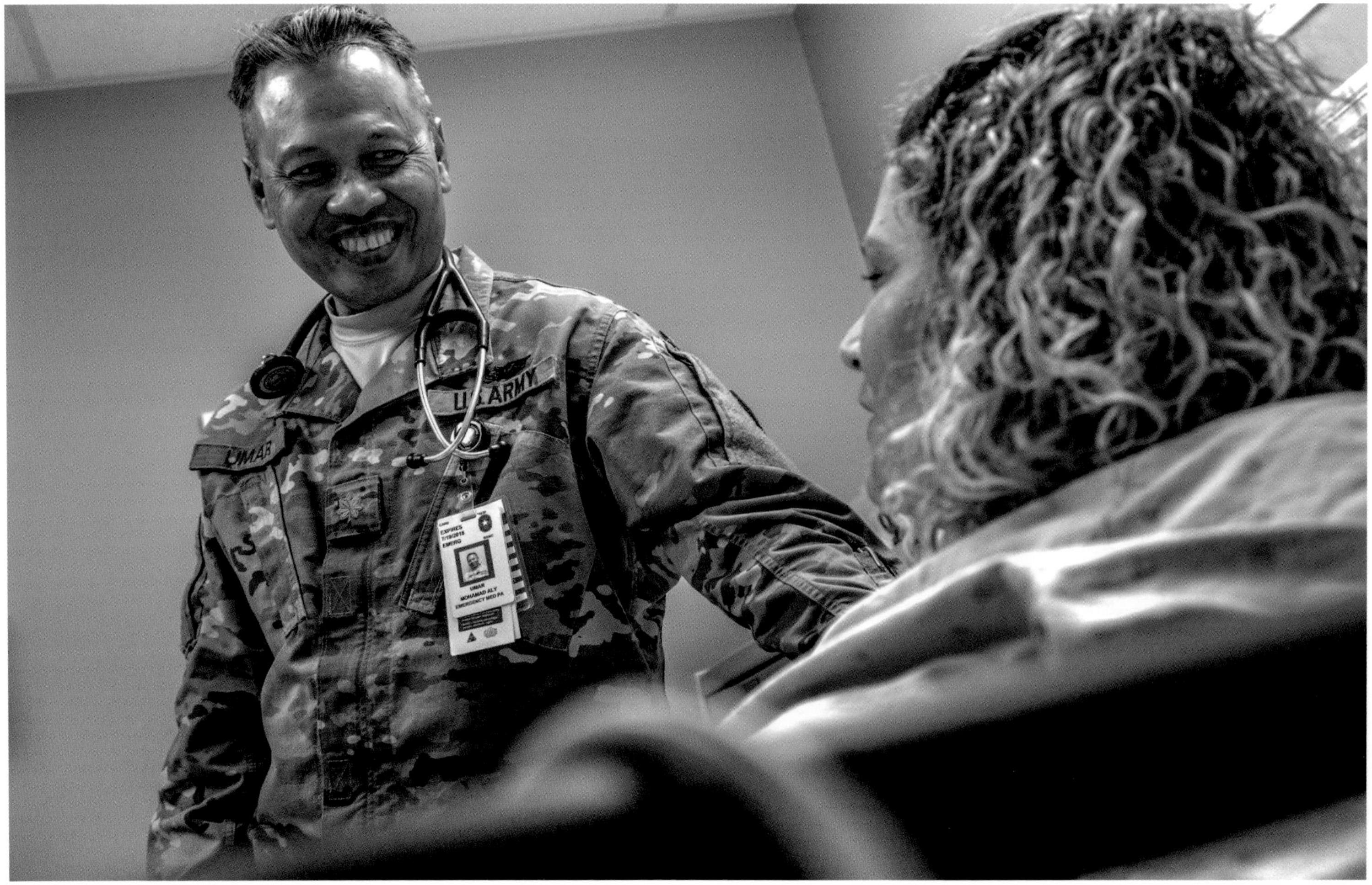

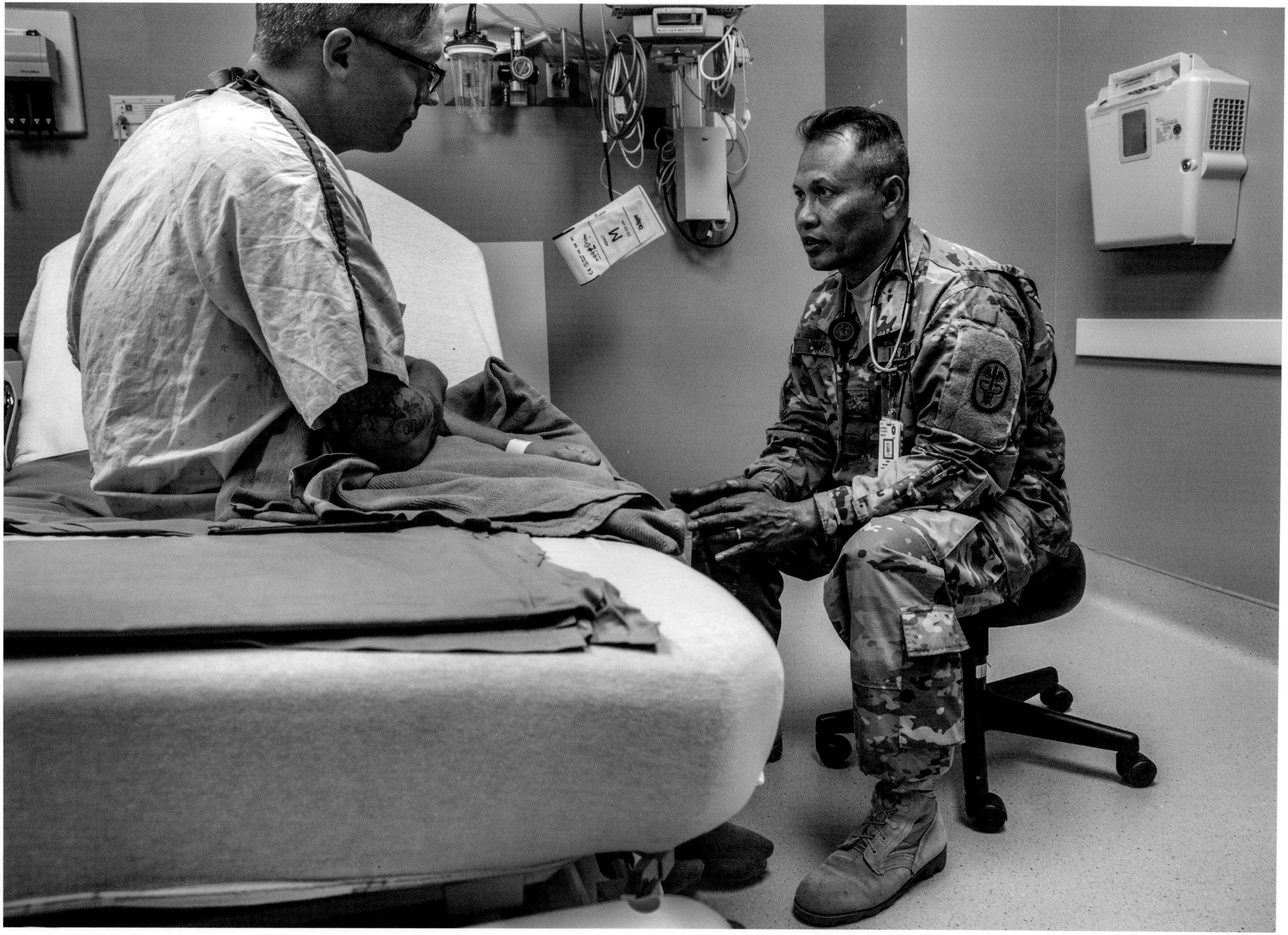

Mohamed Umar, PA

Katie Bakes, MD

Emergency Physician
Denver, Colorado

I totally recommend almost dying. Not dying but *almost* dying. I developed swimming-induced pulmonary edema during an open-water swim at the Chatfield Reservoir and came very close to not making it. I started out with a breaststroke and all of a sudden I was 250 yards out and couldn't breathe. I was yelling for help, but nobody was there. I remember thinking, "This is how I die." I felt the presence of God.

I yelled one last time . . . it's all I had in me . . . and a guy jumped in and got me to shore. I didn't know it at the time, but I have a genetic condition that can cause the vessels in your arms and legs to clamp down in certain situations. The phenomenon shifts the blood into your chest, and you just drown in it. I lost half my blood volume through my lungs and spent a few days in the ICU. I was an obnoxious patient . . . signed out on the third day against medical advice. I was really traumatized and couldn't stop crying for the first few days. But then I had this "aha" moment . . . I was just so happy to be alive. I've always been a searching person, but that experience really brought me to the next level. It left me with a lot of gratitude — and very few fears.

Our society — and medicine in particular — is so focused on outcomes. But the truth is, the story ends the same way for all of us. I mean, what's it all about if not the experiences in between? Partly because of my faith, life feels palpably transient. I believe what really matters is how you handle *moments*. You show kindness. You connect with people. You don't leave without them knowing you care.

I started becoming cynical at one point during residency. I think it really is a natural human response to the situations emergency physicians face, but it scared me. I fought against the feeling, though, and consciously worked to maintain my empathy. Every time I went into a patient's room, I would tell myself, " This is about them . . . somebody loves them and they love somebody . . . I'm just going to focus on the person in front of me." I did that for a year until I didn't have to do it anymore.

People are so interesting. I think that is what sustains me in medicine. The reasons a patient is in the ED are complex. I'm talking about the circumstances that go beyond "I drank too much" or "I got shot." There's something mystifying about people . . . their hopes and dreams . . . their accomplishments . . . their expectations . . . the things that make them human.

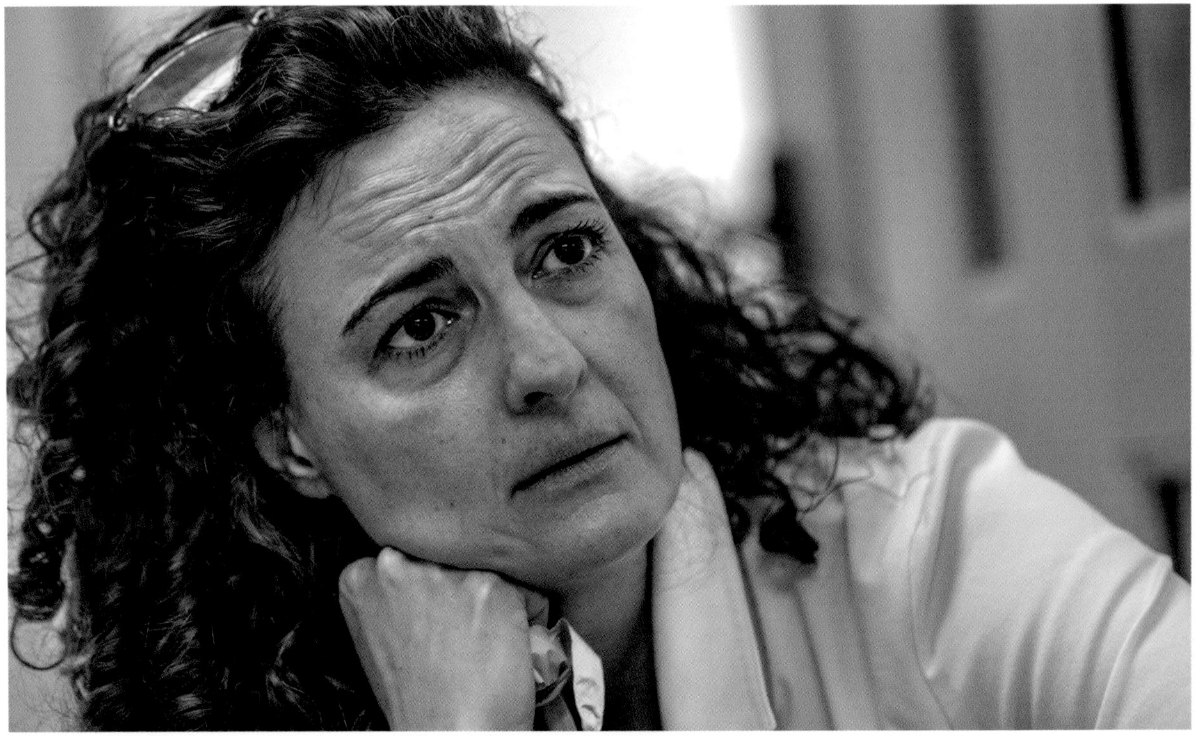

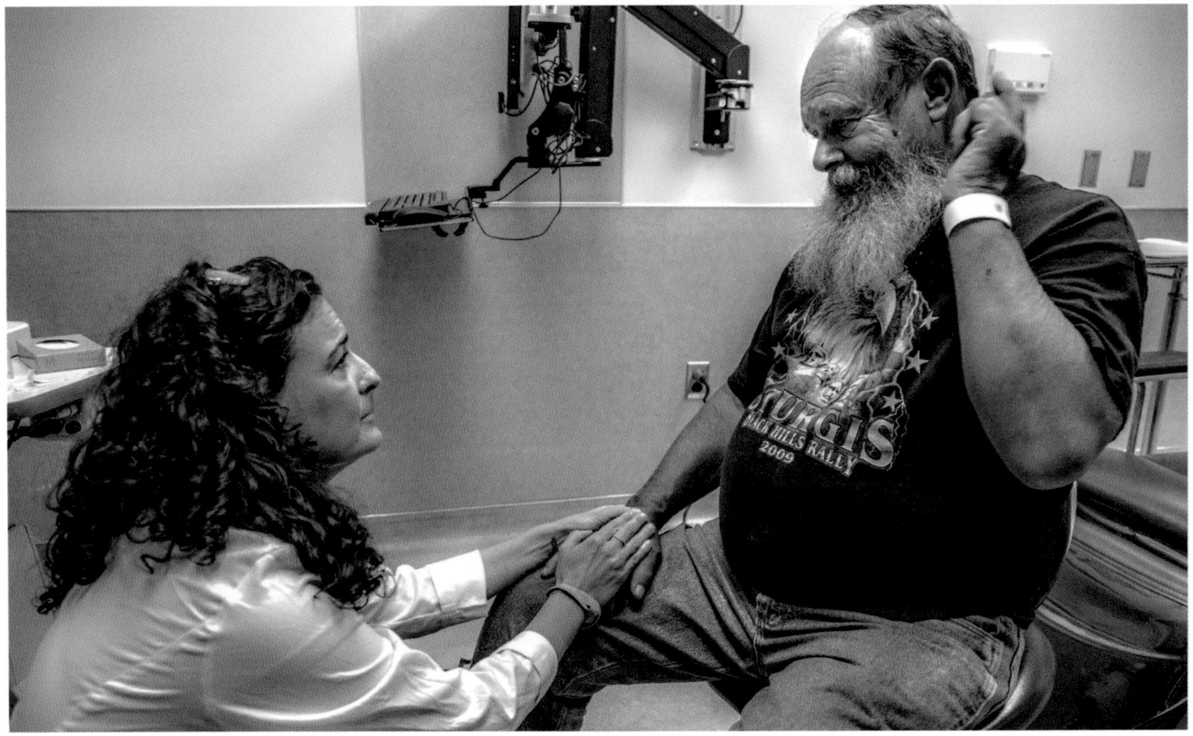

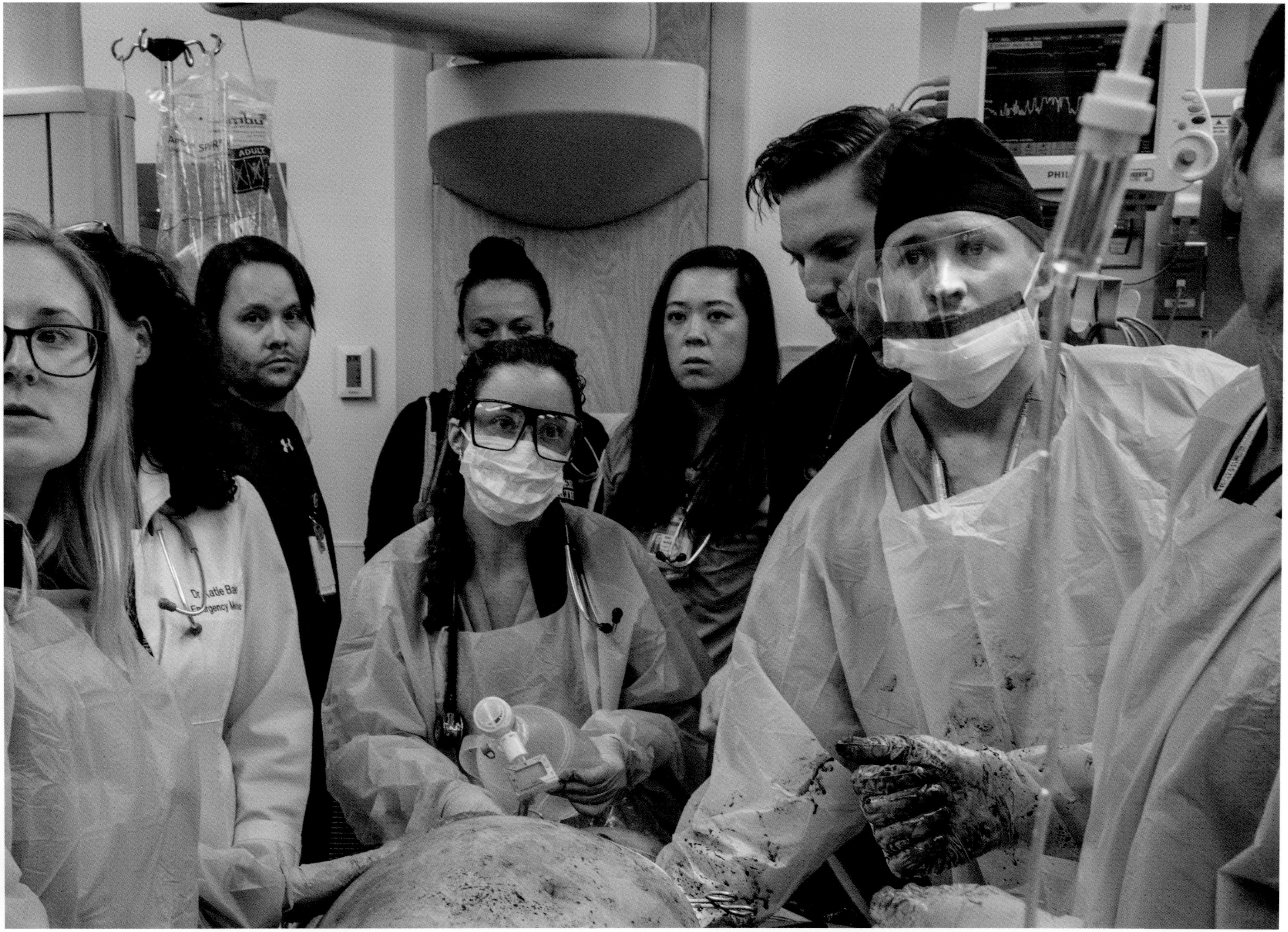
ADULT

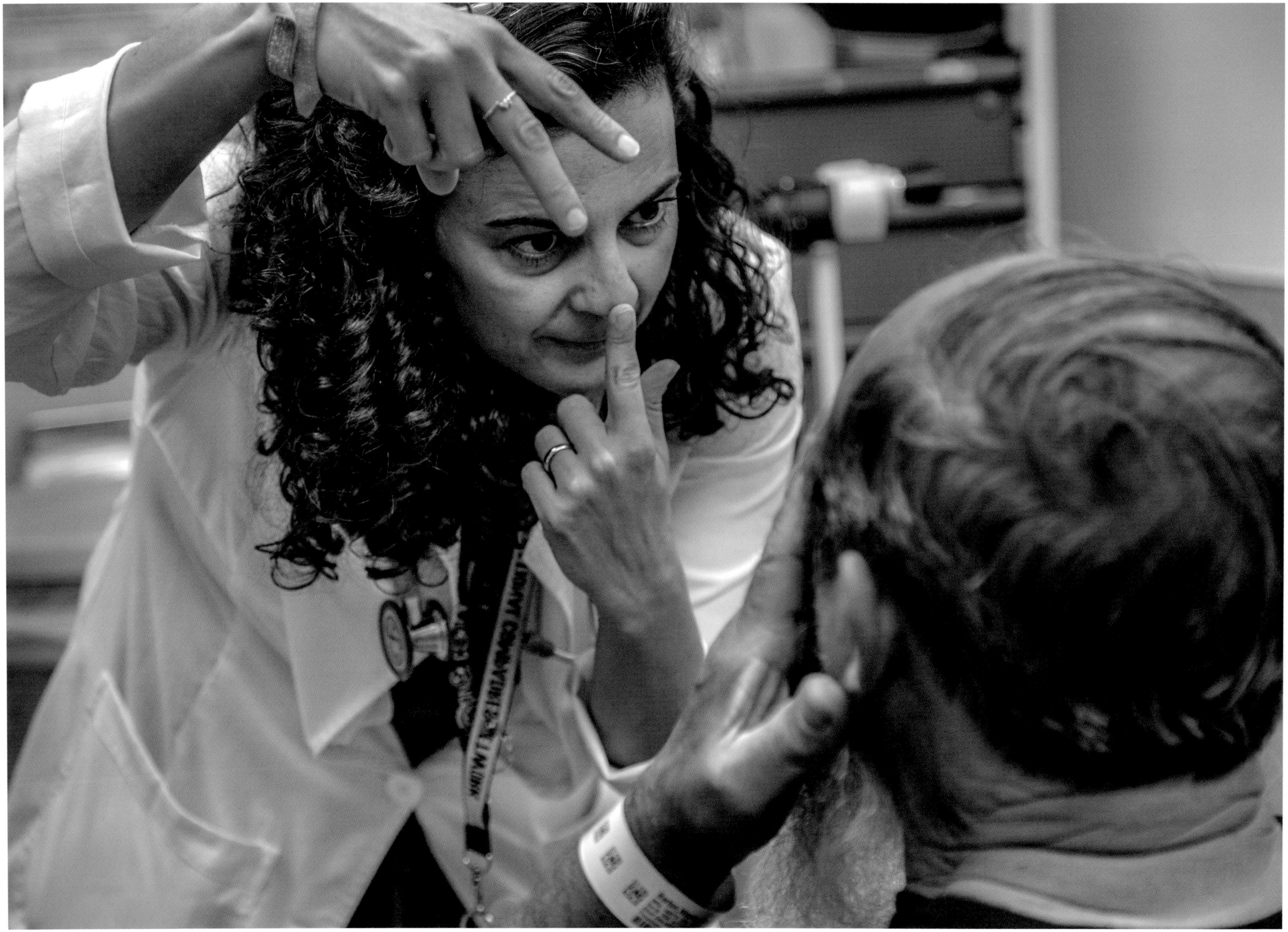

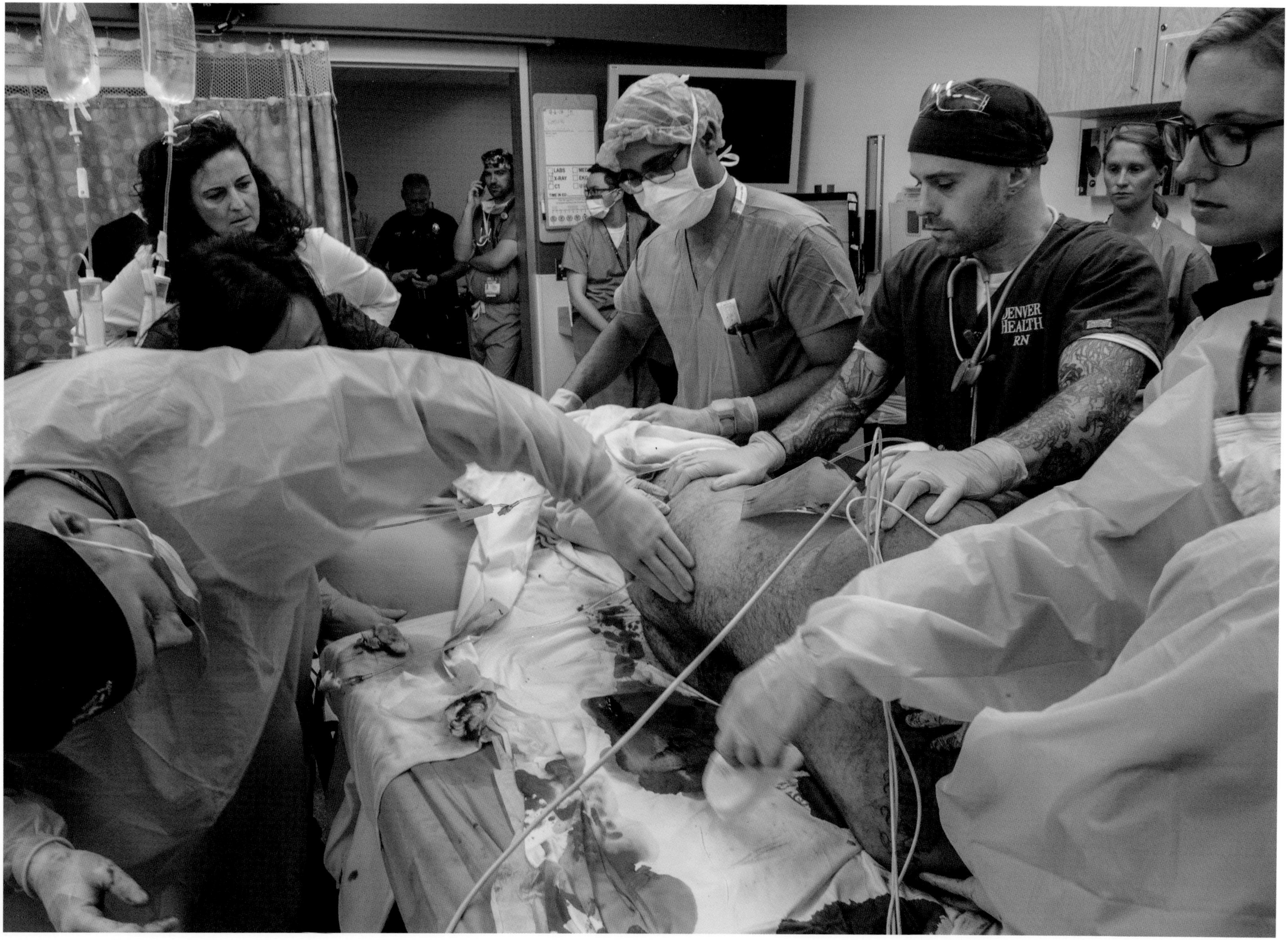
DENVER HEALTH
RN

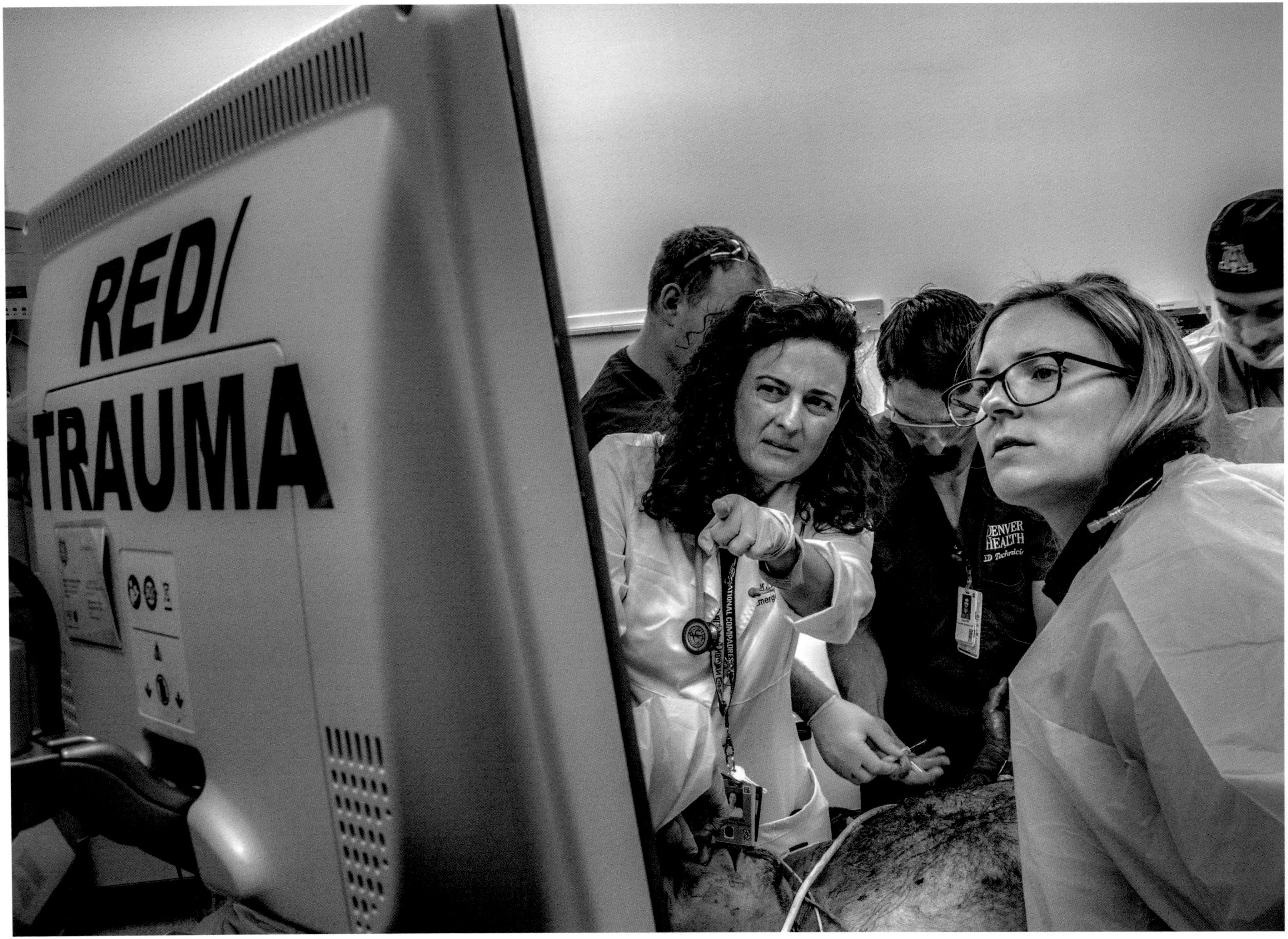
RED/
TRAUMA
DENVER
HEALTH

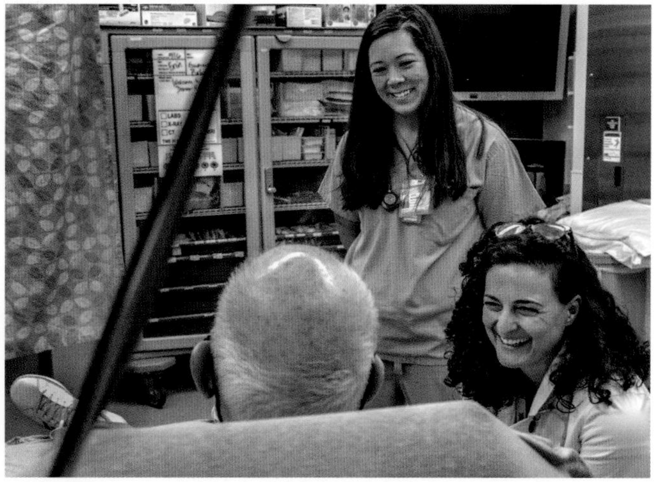

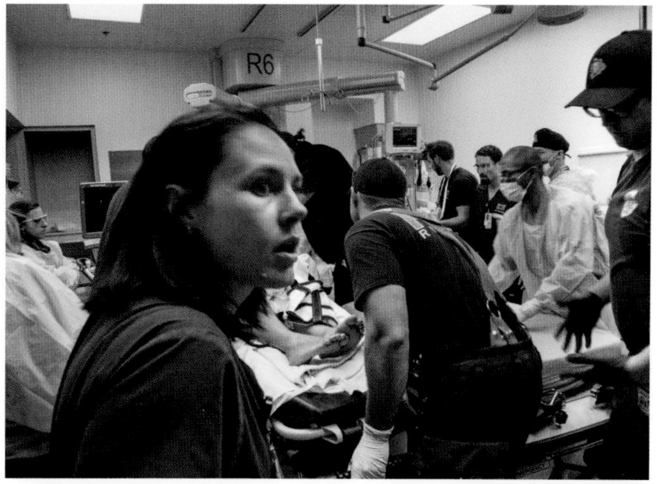

After I had my second baby, I went through a bad depression. I was obsessive . . . I compulsively worried . . . I couldn't sleep. It got to a point where I didn't want to live. That was my wake-up call. I'm open about that experience because I think one of the keys to providing (and receiving) help is destigmatizing this stuff. Depression is an illness — like hypertension — not some indication that a person is *less than*. I've seen how patients open up when I talk about what I went through. We all fear being judged, but the only way to dispel the shame is push it into the light.

Most physicians have been high-achieving "A" students who are used to succeeding in life. Being up front with weakness is not one of the things that got them to where they are. But I'd like to see that change. I believe vulnerability is the key to power. ✚

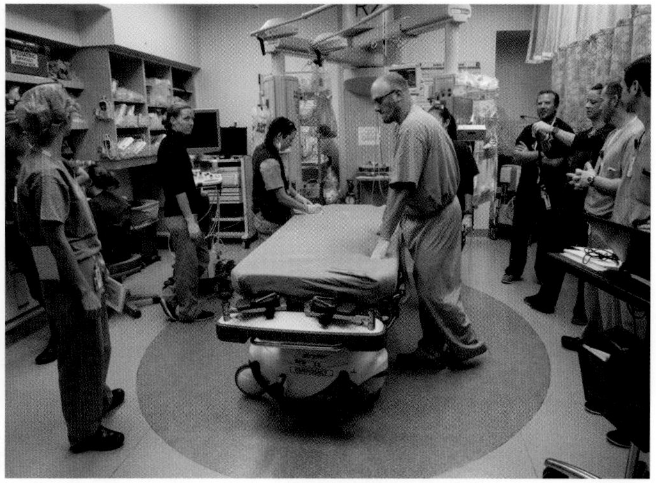

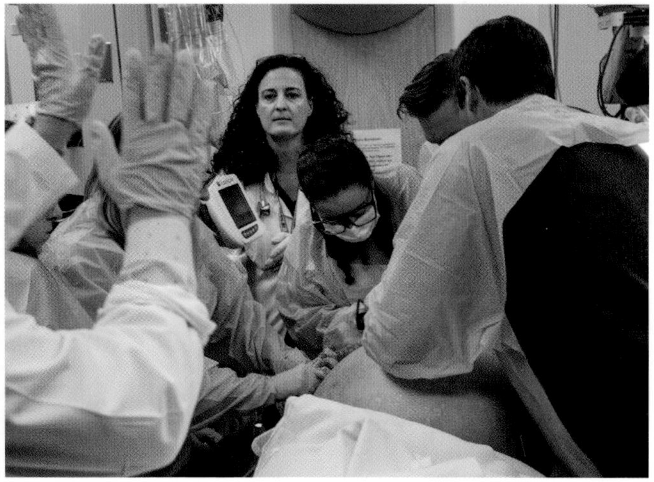

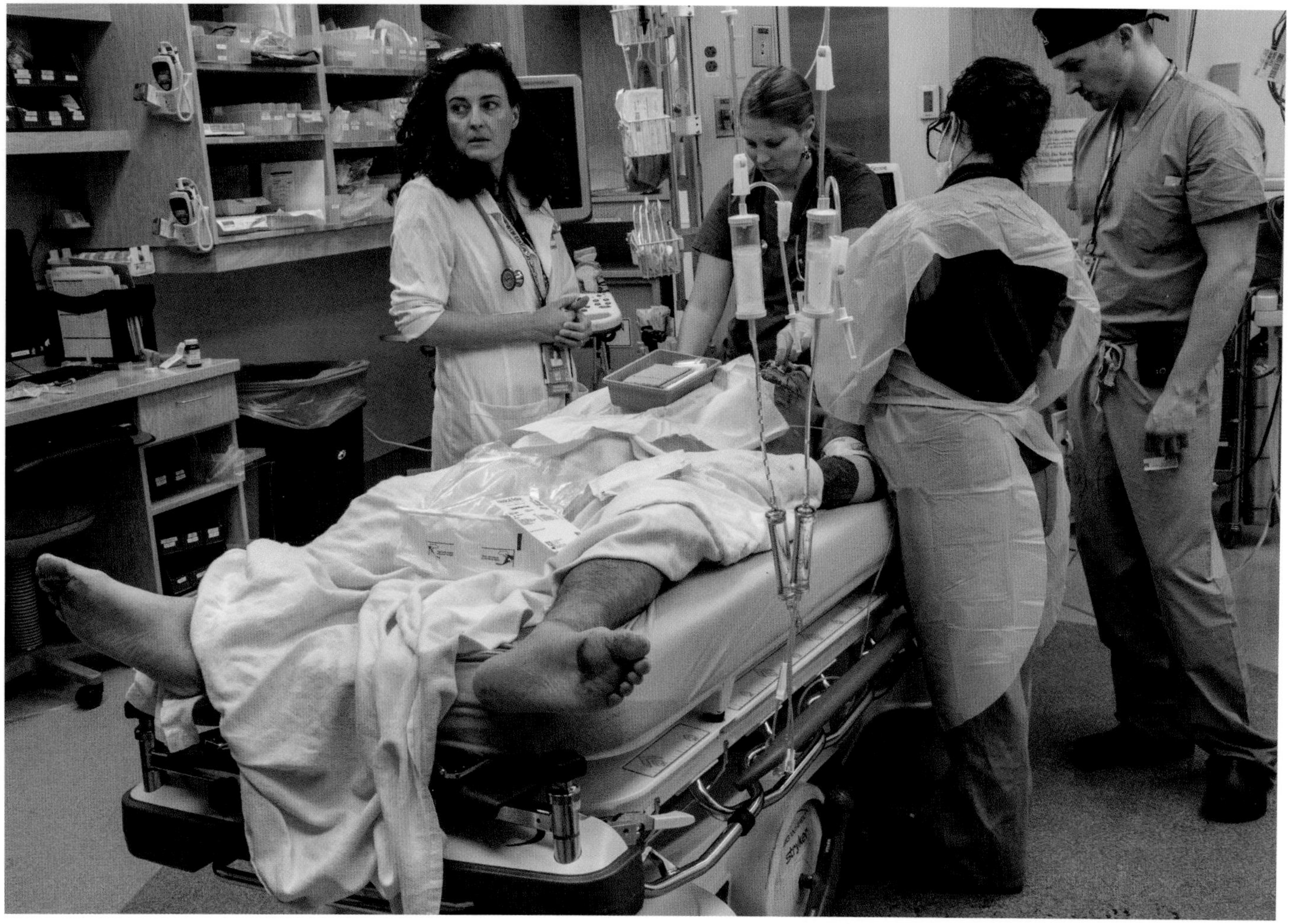

Nadia Pearson, DO

Military Pediatric Emergency Physician
San Antonio, Texas

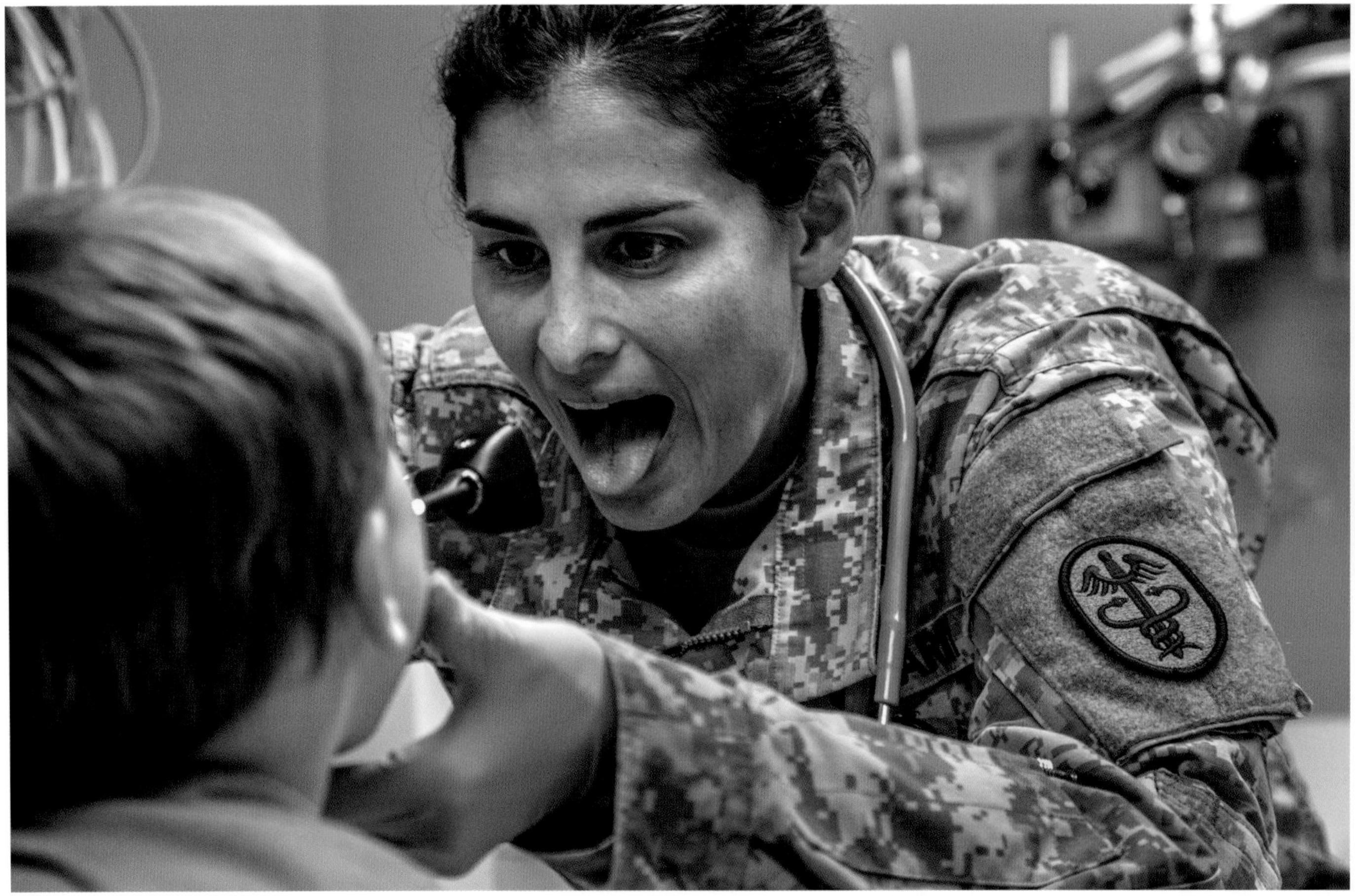

Everything changed for me on September 11, 2001. I had just enlisted in the US Army and had started my first year of med school. Suddenly, we were at war; I had no idea what to expect. I knew how to wear my uniform and I knew how to salute, but that was about it. I hadn't even been through basic training.

I was clueless about the military when I signed up. The recruiters were like, "Hey, do you want a free education? Come to — ." It was mainly a financial decision. They said they'd pay for my schooling and give me a stipend. I thought it sounded fabulous, so I signed on the dotted line.

My first deployment was to Iraq in 2007, about a fifteen-minute flight from Baghdad. We treated the usual — car accidents, gunshot wounds, IED and mine explosions, that kind of stuff. But a lot of our patients were victims of retaliation. It was the good guys versus the bad guys. People in the Middle East like their tea, so there was never a shortage of boiling water around. It was a popular weapon; we saw a lot of burns.

I suppose being in the army is a lot like being in the ER — you're in a combat zone either way. We see the worst of the worst, things regular people can't even fathom. Any kind of sensory experience you can think of — it's ours on a daily basis. We have to have that camaraderie; otherwise, we'd probably go crazy. I think emergency medicine is one of those fields where you actually feel like a "real" physician. You're in the ER — the epicenter of the hospital.

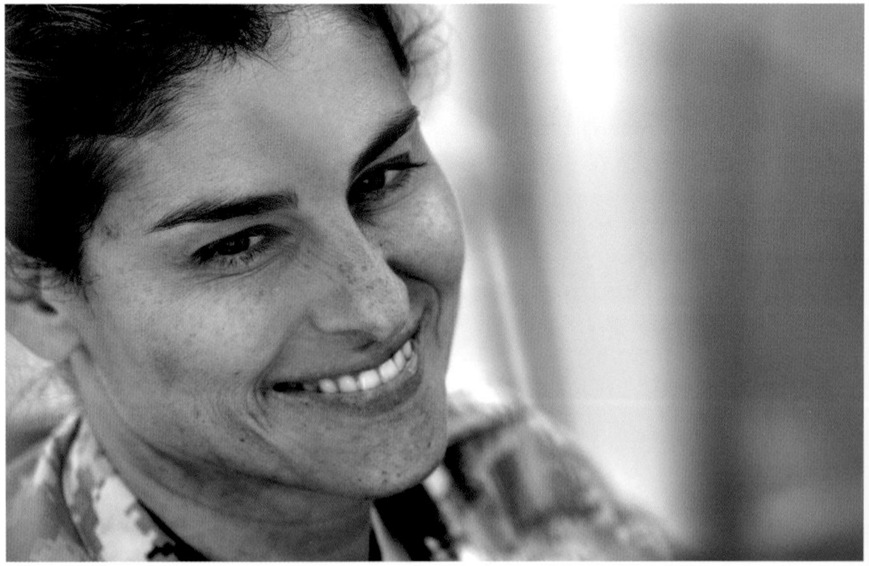

I started thinking about getting into the field when I was in college; I did some summer coursework in EMS. My first experience with CPR involved doing chest compressions on a patient who'd just eaten a bowl of SpaghettiOs. I forgot to bring the suction equipment . . . lesson learned. I wore his dinner for the rest of the night. Unfortunately, the gentleman did not survive the experience. I did.

I love taking care of all patients, but there's something special about taking care of soldiers. It has been very satisfying — an honor, really. I wear the same uniform they do, but I don't walk in their shoes. They're putting their lives on the line in a way I've never had to. So, when I'm out in public and somebody says, "Thank you for your service," I always do a double take.

I have friends from medical school; we're collegial. But your military friends . . . they're in a different league. These are friends for life; these are people who'd take a bullet for you. The bond you share . . . it's just different . . . you can't explain the feeling. ✚

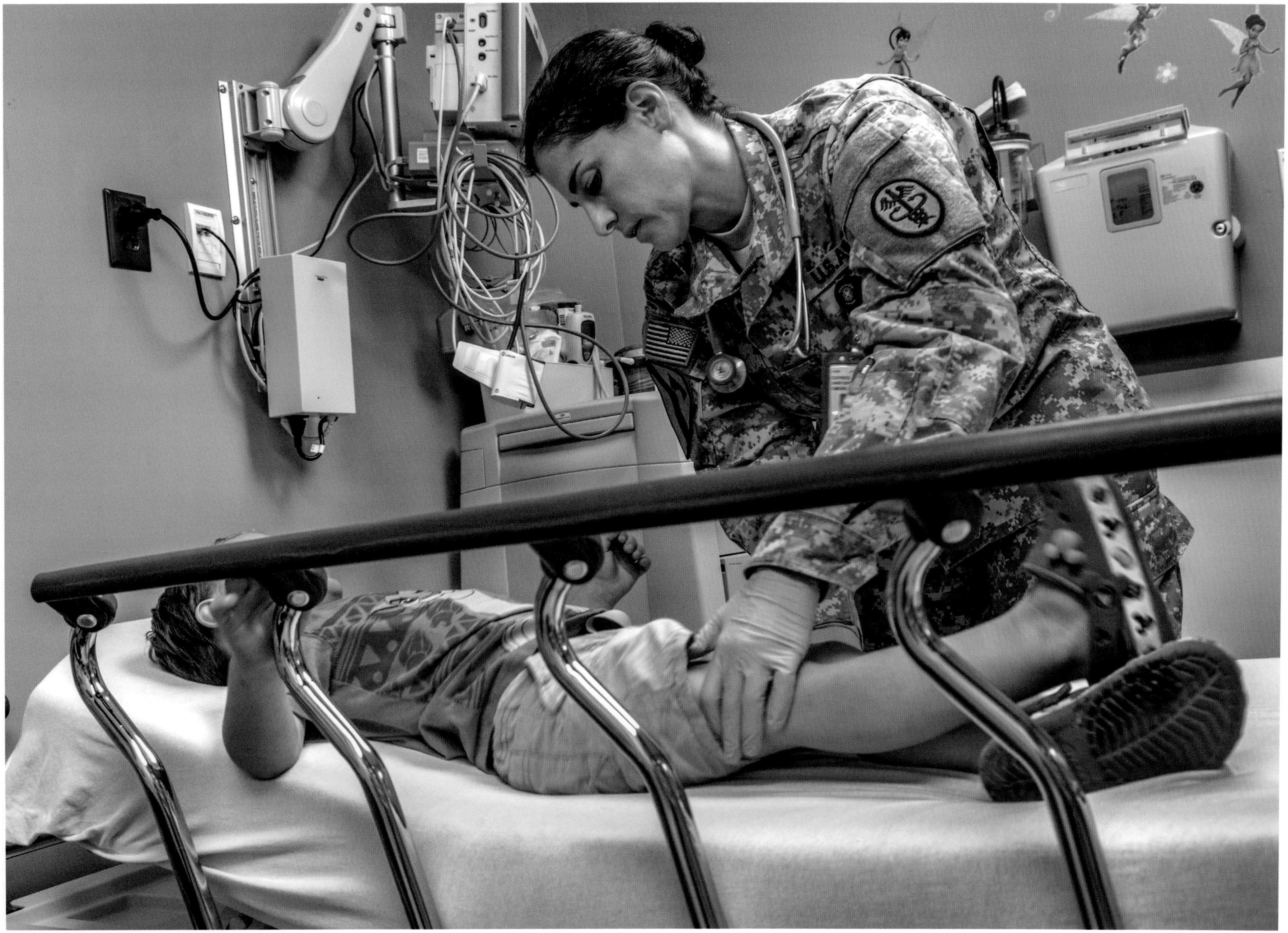

Nadia Pearson, DO

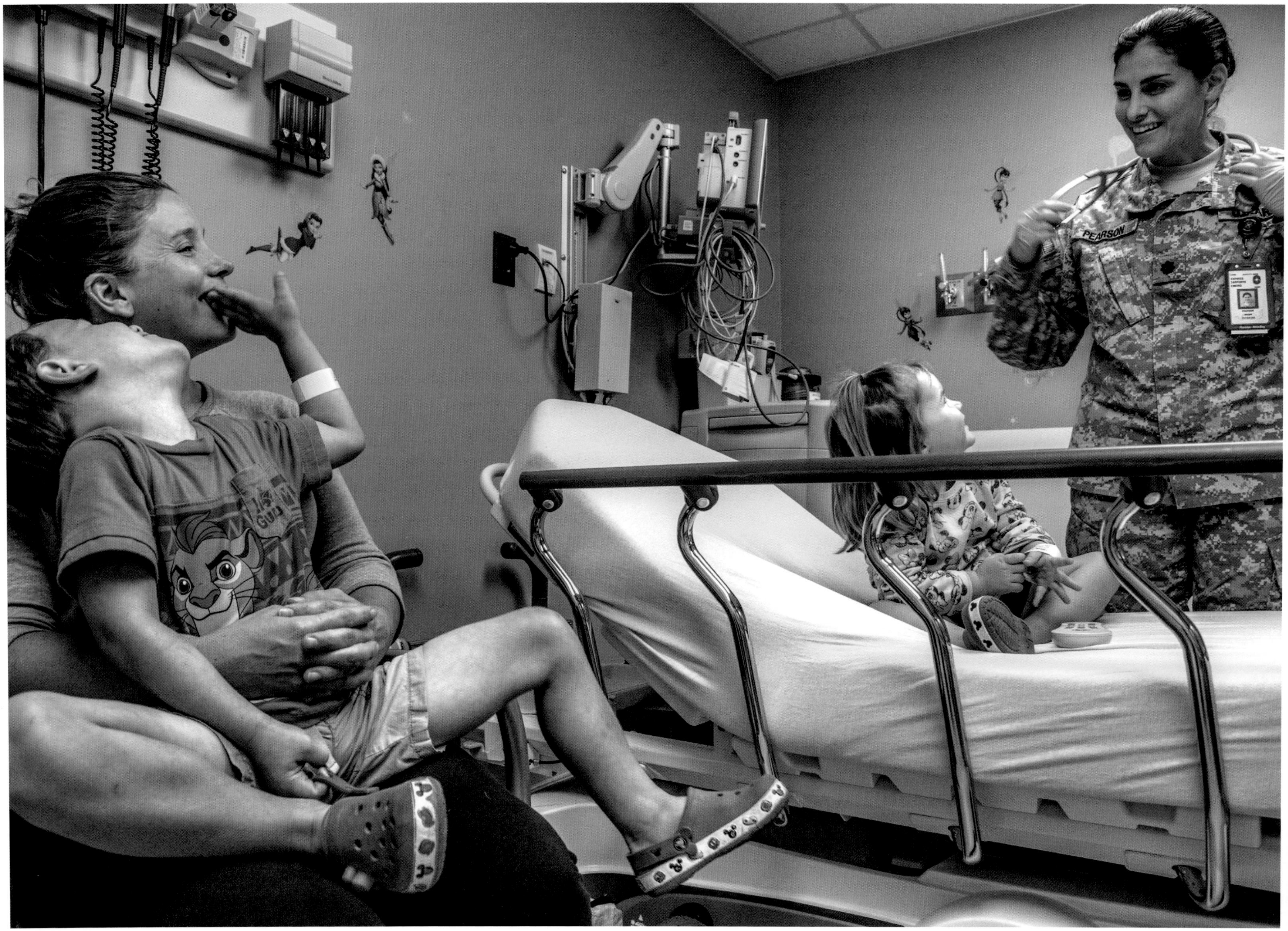
PEARSON

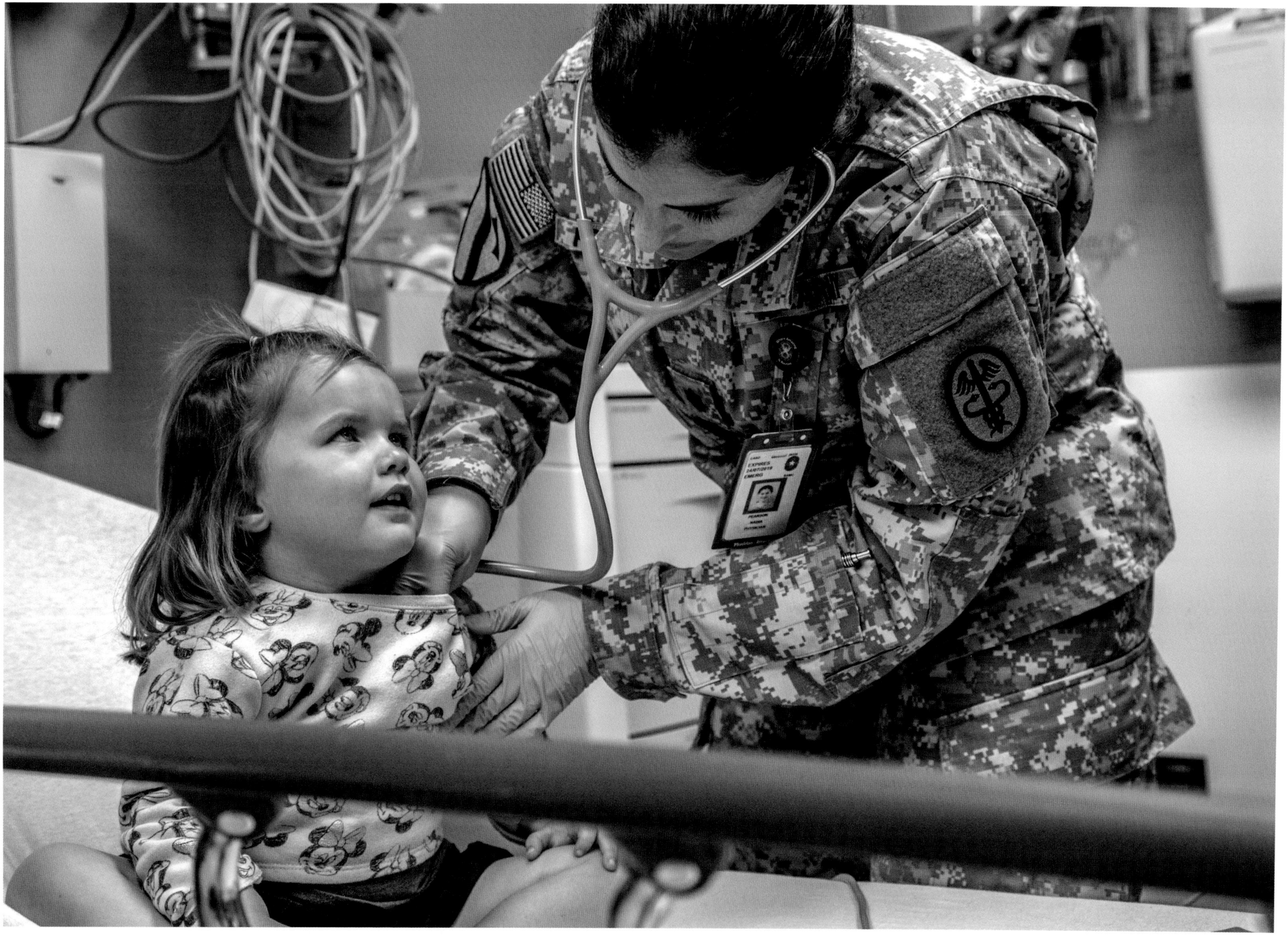

Nadia Pearson, DO

Christopher Celentano, MD

Emergency Physician & Disaster Medicine Specialist
Los Angeles, California

The guy who's working that fourteen-bed emergency department overnight with no backup is the real hero of emergency medicine. My dad was an old ED pit doc back in the day. He would work twenty-four-hour shifts three or four times a week . . . see ninety-six patients in a single shift. I couldn't do that. As I was growing up, his lifestyle didn't seem that appealing. I wanted to be an astronaut. But — as happens to us all — once I did an emergency department rotation, I was hooked.

I eventually fell into a niche of a niche. In response to tragedies like Hurricane Katrina and 9/11, the US government developed a national preparedness program to help hospitals manage disasters. Now I run an EMS resource center — one of only fourteen in the country — that specializes in mass casualty response. I guess my area of specialization functions a lot like an insurance policy. You may never need us, but we'll rise to the occasion if and when you do.

Back in 1963, a dam broke in the Baldwin Hills area of Los Angeles. The flooding destroyed 277 homes and killed five people. My dad heard about it as he was driving home and went to the site. He said there were firefighters and police officers at the site but no medical responders — he was the only one. There were no policies or plans in place, so he just started calling people to help — right there on the spot — and tried to do whatever he could to secure resources and pharmaceuticals.

Compare that response to the way we do things now — they're night and day. EMS has completely evolved. We have a medic alert center ready to triage victims and distribute them evenly to area hospitals, so no one center gets inundated. We have quick access to pre-deployed equipment and supplies. We've organized community allies, who understand the role they will play in the event of a disaster. We've got things under control.

Although mass casualty disasters are few and far between, one could argue that every day is a disaster in the emergency department. So, when I'm teaching and residents ask what kinds of illnesses or injuries they should focus on, my answer is, "The bread-and-butter. The heart attacks, car accidents, and gunshot wounds — the stuff you see all the time."

The first year our team provided aid for the LA Marathon, we had two patients who were elite runners — professional athletes — the kind who travel with a whole posse of trainers and handlers. One of them didn't win — she came in second in a tight race — and you wouldn't believe the drama. She had the whole diva thing going . . . collapsed as she went through the finish line . . . the whole entourage swooped in. It was pure theater.

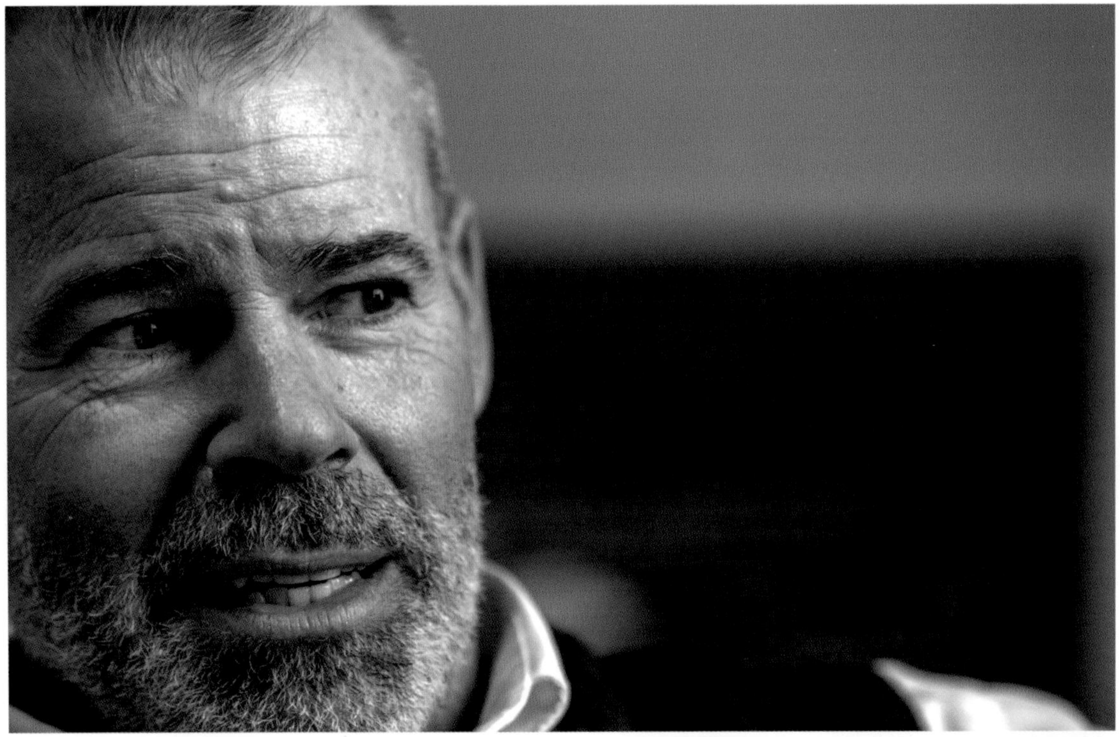

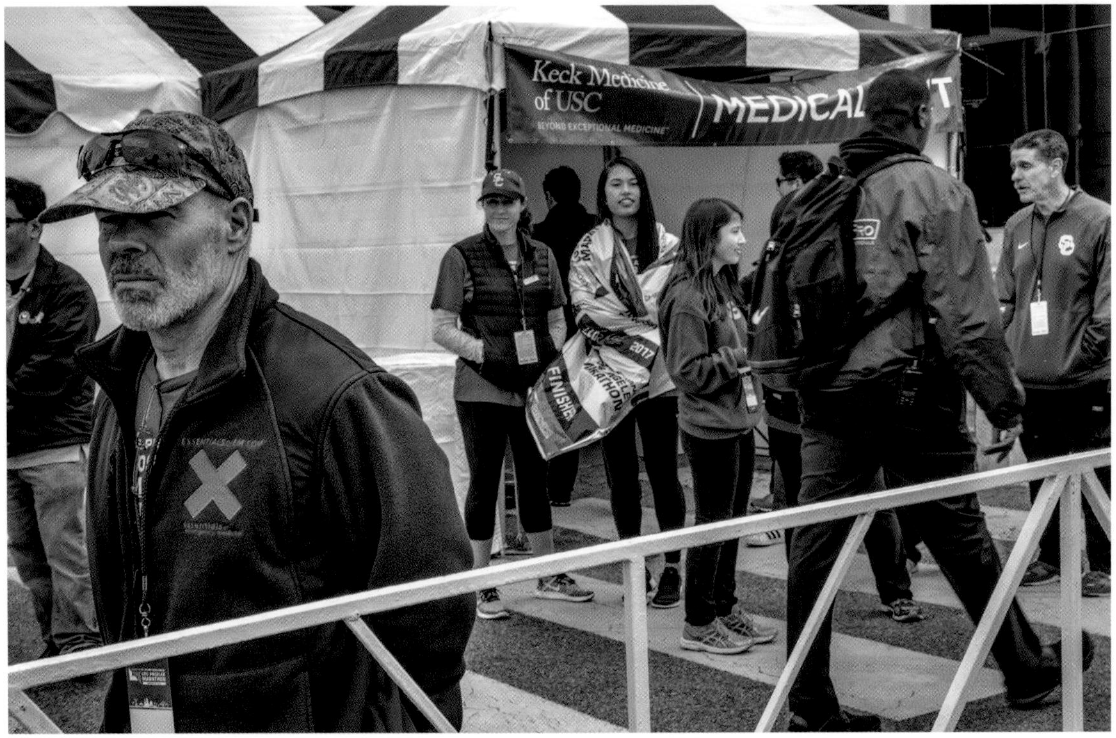

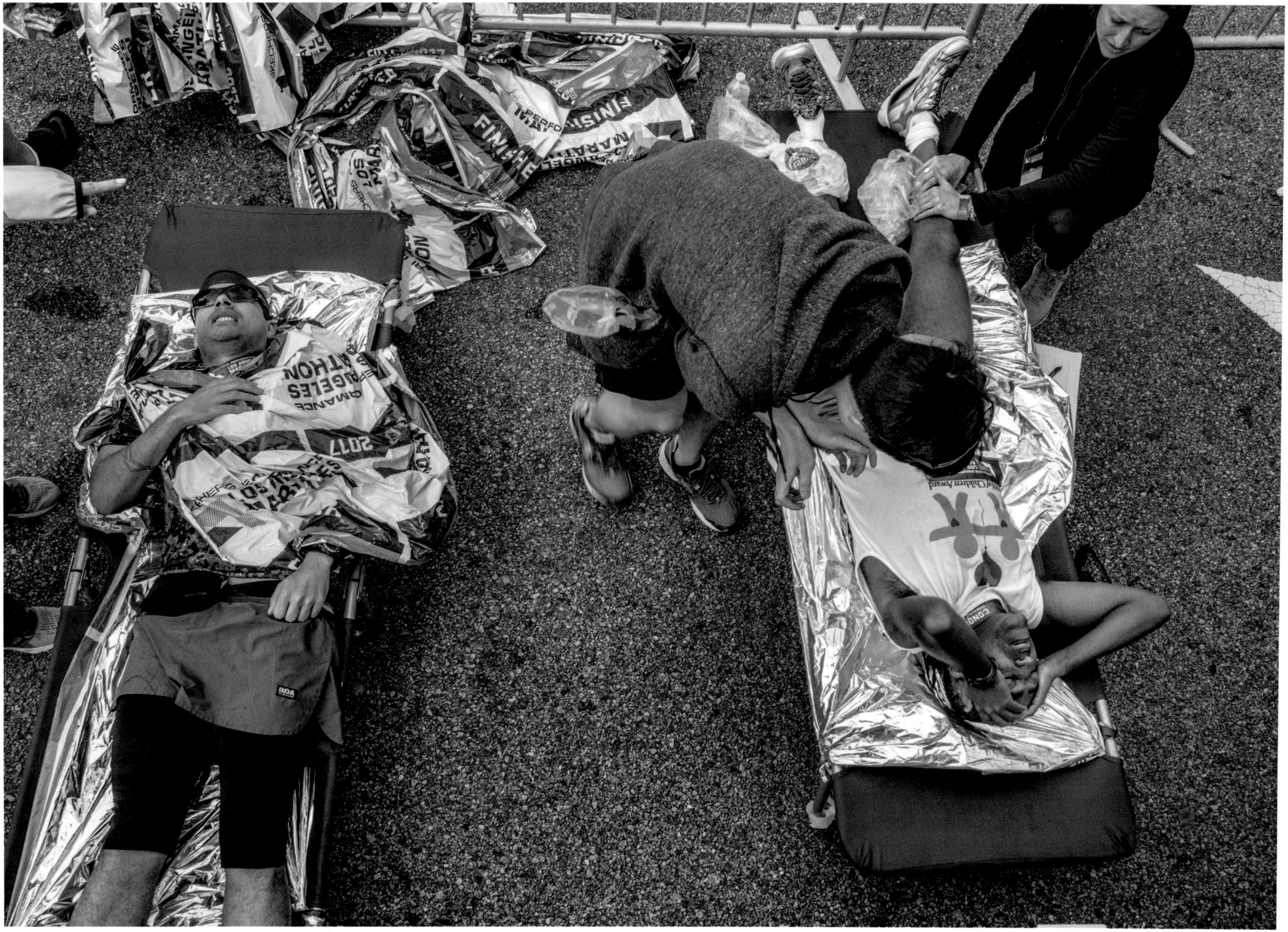
2017

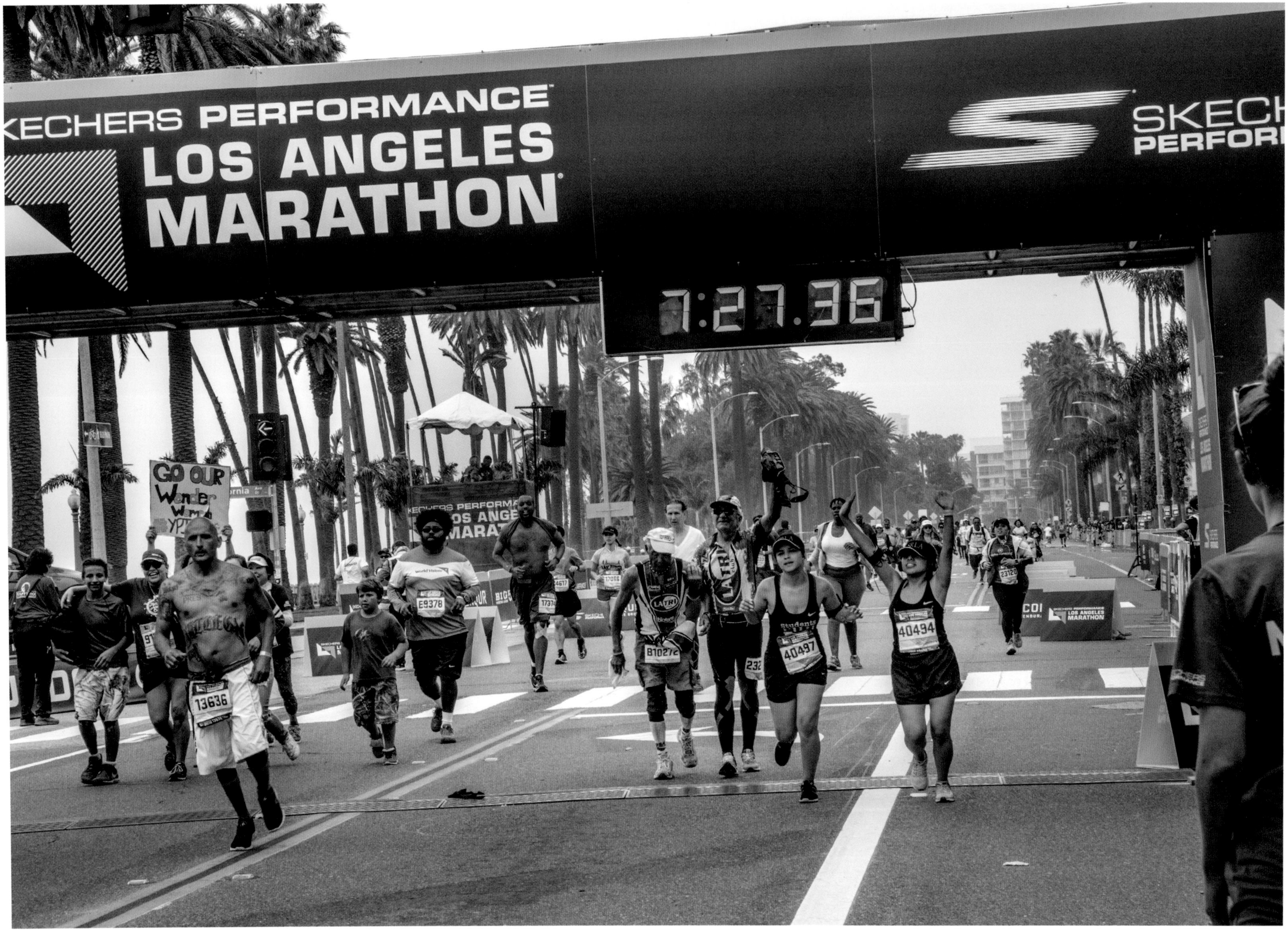
KECHERS PERFORMANCE
LOS ANGELES
MARATHON
7:27:36
GO OUR
Wonder
13636
E9378
B10272
40497
40494
23120

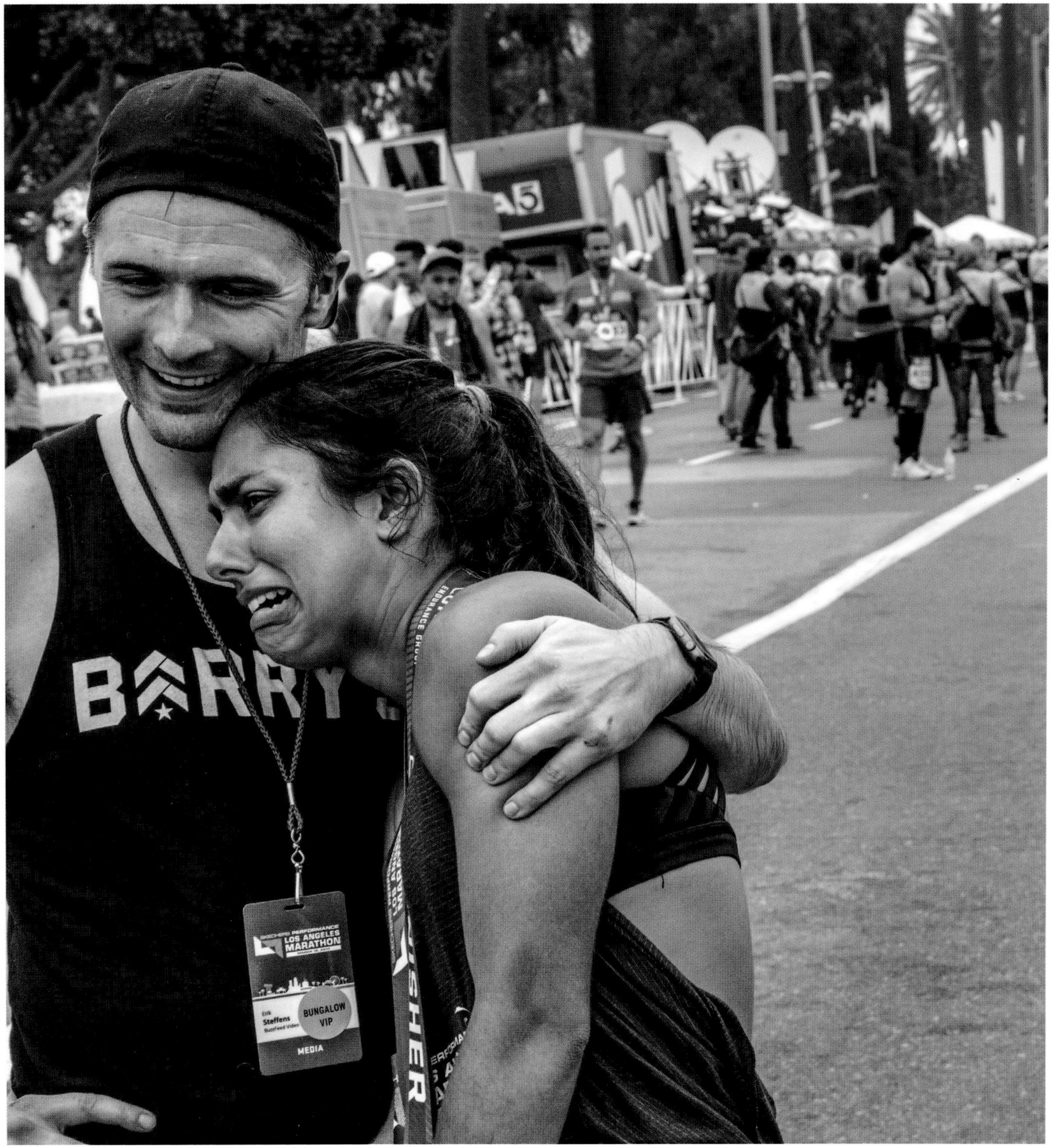

It's amusing when you contrast a scene like that to the *real* life and death situations we see in this business. Not long ago, I heard a sobering story by an emergency manager in Joplin, Missouri, which was devastated by a massive tornado in 2011. The town only had two hospitals within 150 miles. The storm leveled one and damaged a good portion of the other. Joplin is a small town, so everyone there knew or was related to one of the 160-plus people killed. He talked about a nurse whose home was totally leveled by the tornado — just gone. But even though she knew she'd lost it all . . . even though she was separated from her family . . . she stayed at work that day. She stayed to take care of patients. Now *that's* a real disaster. Those are real heroes. ✚

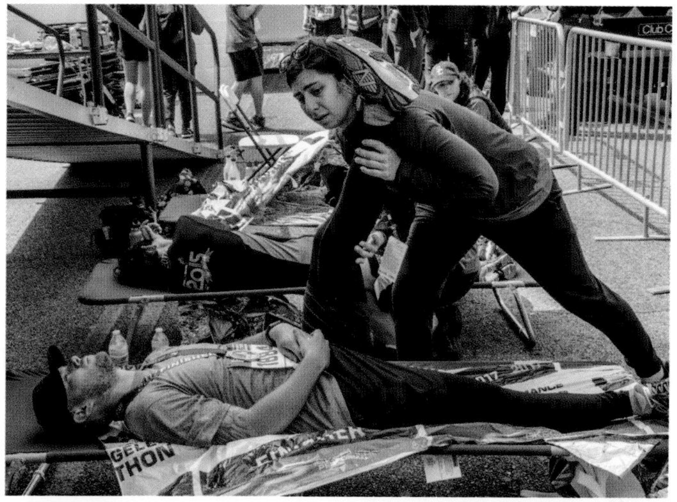

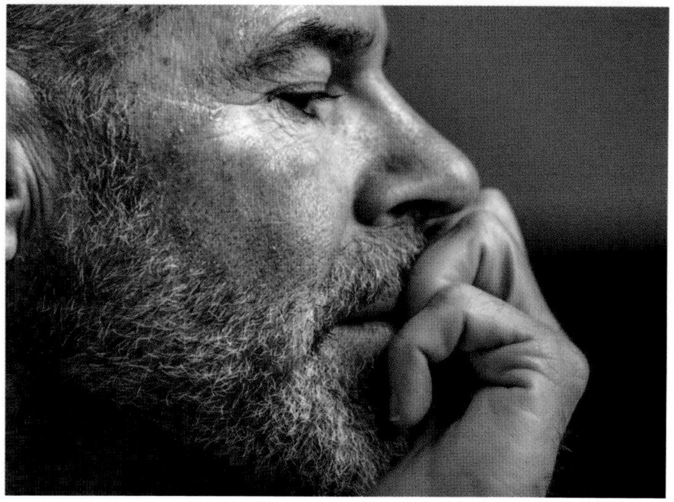

Corita Grudzen, MD

Emergency Physician & Palliative Care Researcher
New York, New York

We all die. One hundred percent of doctors have a 100 percent failure rate, because — as far as I can tell — no one lives forever. It's not about death; it's about how we treat patients at the end of their lives. We assume families should be able to sort through their emotions and make medical decisions based on how a treatment will impact the patient's quality of life; it's an unfair burden. One of the most difficult things a doctor has to say is, "Your loved one is suffering and, based on what you've told me about them, I don't think this is how they would want to spend the end of their life. We should focus on comfort."

More and more, we're seeing an aging population in crisis. These patients have been sick for a long time; it's not a quick fix. We think by doing all these invasive, life-sustaining procedures we're helping people feel better . . . but the mind and the body are mysterious things. More interventions aren't always better. Putting a breathing tube down someone's throat doesn't guarantee they'll live longer. We may, in fact, be shortening patients' lives with some of the care we provide.

Growing up, all I knew was my job in life was to serve others — it was just assumed. At extremes, that's not always the healthiest way to live. In some ways, my parents were so serving of others they didn't take care of themselves — or my sister and me — as well as they could have.

My father was a Catholic priest, and my mother was a nun. They met and fell in love in the late 1960s and felt a lot of the work they wanted to do could be done outside the walls of the Church. They had $300 when they got married, and my dad struggled to find work. He finally got a job at the Episcopal church, but it ended when the monsignor from Maryknoll called to tell them my father had been excommunicated. It was difficult.

When I was a kid, we lived in a big house with a whole bunch of other people . . . there were people in the basement, people in the attic. It was very hippie-esque. I had twelve cavities the first time I went to the dentist. When I was seven, I had to get all my hair chopped off because of all the rats' nests. My classmates thought I was a boy. We had ill-fitting clothes. There was no focus on material goods.

We moved to Central America when I was about thirteen. My parents had friends there who were working with the resistance. We stayed with a family in Nicaragua and basically slept on dirt floors. We lived in a liberation theology-type community. . . . I understood enough about the environment to know it was dangerous. I was lucky to have school, though; it was kind of like my happy place. It was something I could control, something I could be good at. I get bored very easily if I'm not constantly learning.

I started thinking about a career in palliative care when I came to Bellevue. We would get a lot of transfers from the public nursing home on Roosevelt Island. They are the most frail, vulnerable human beings in New York City . . . the sickest of the sick and the poorest of the poor. We were doing a lot of procedures we didn't feel were beneficial, so we started imagining better ways to care for these people.

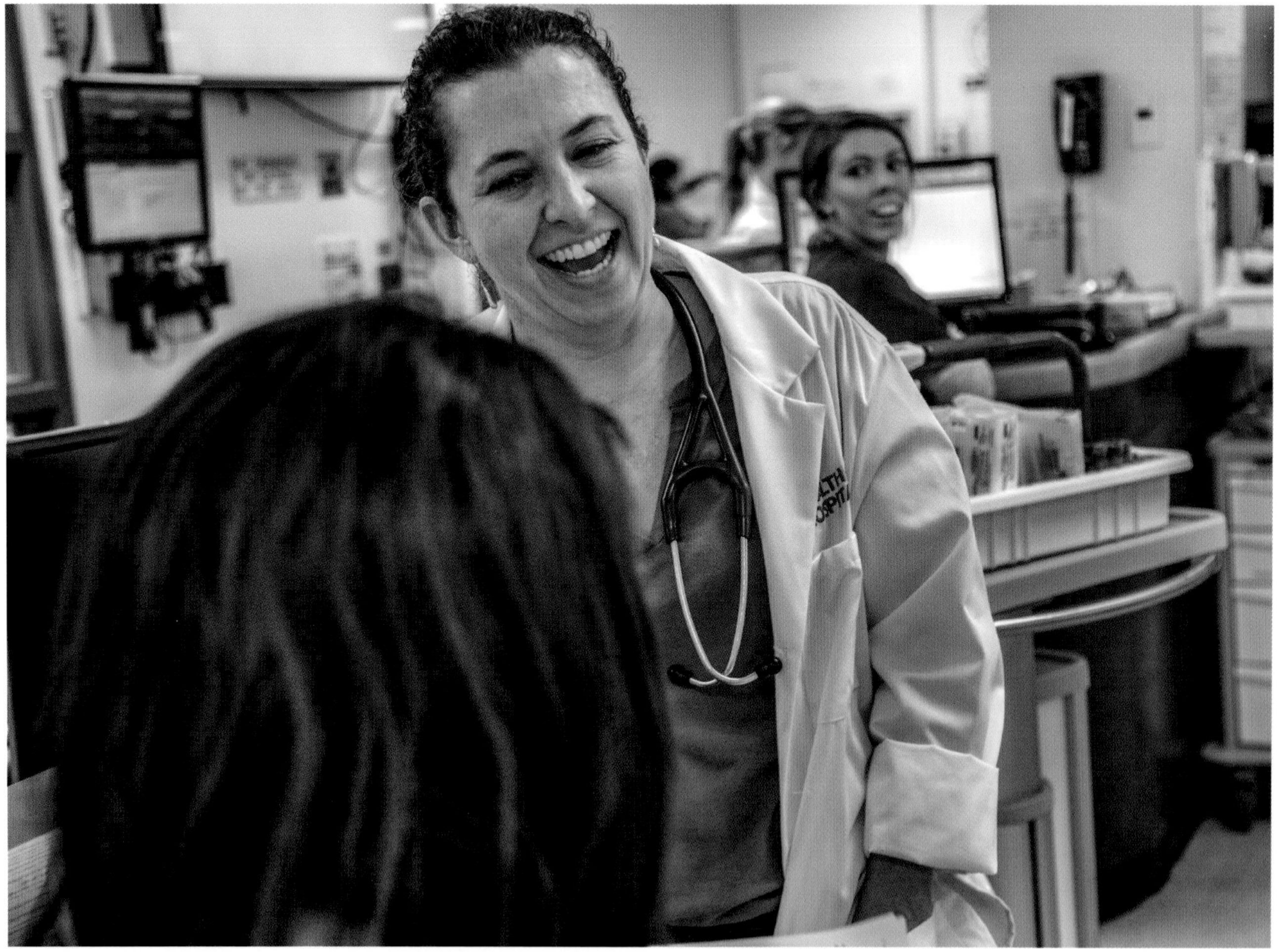

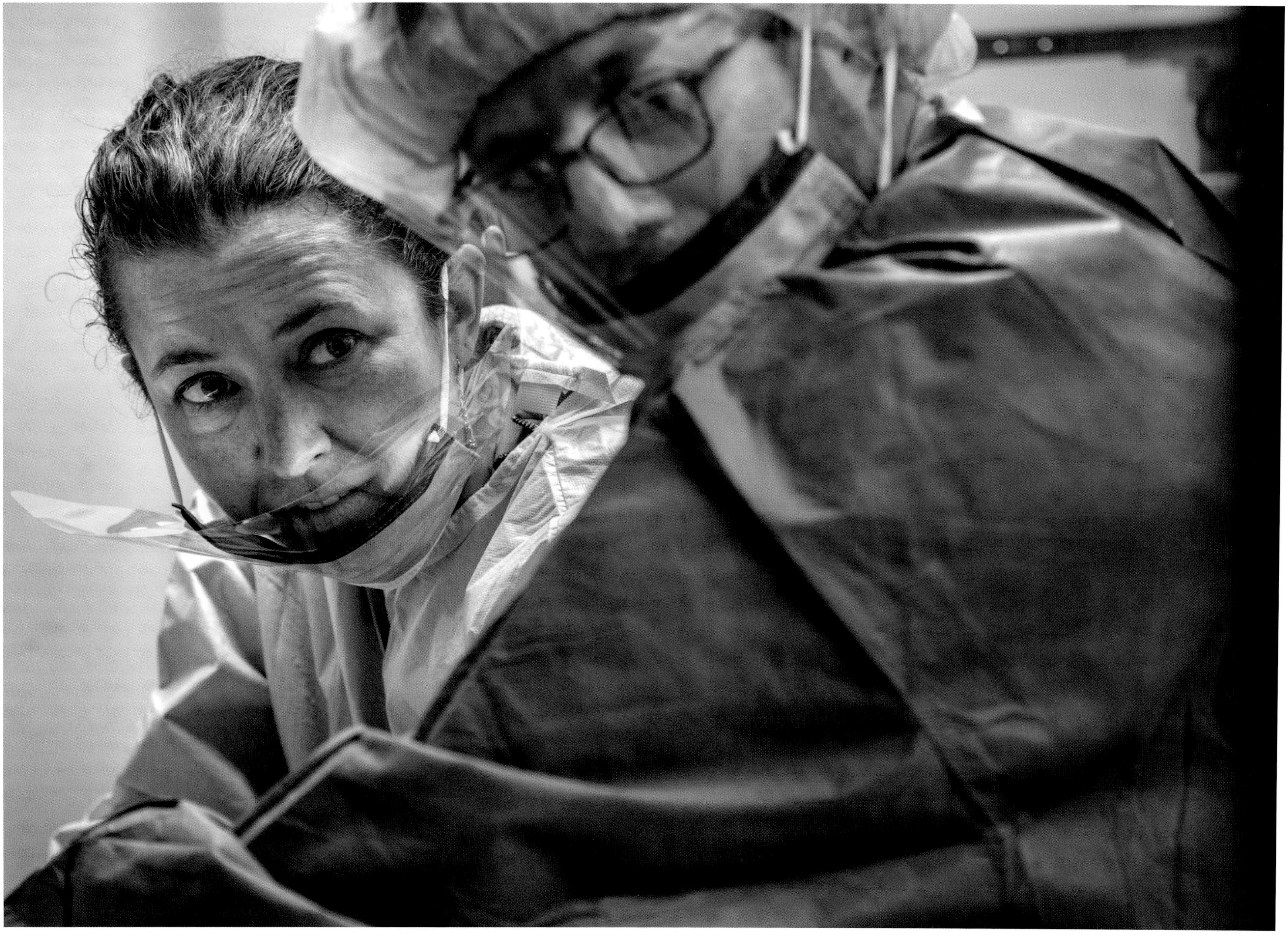

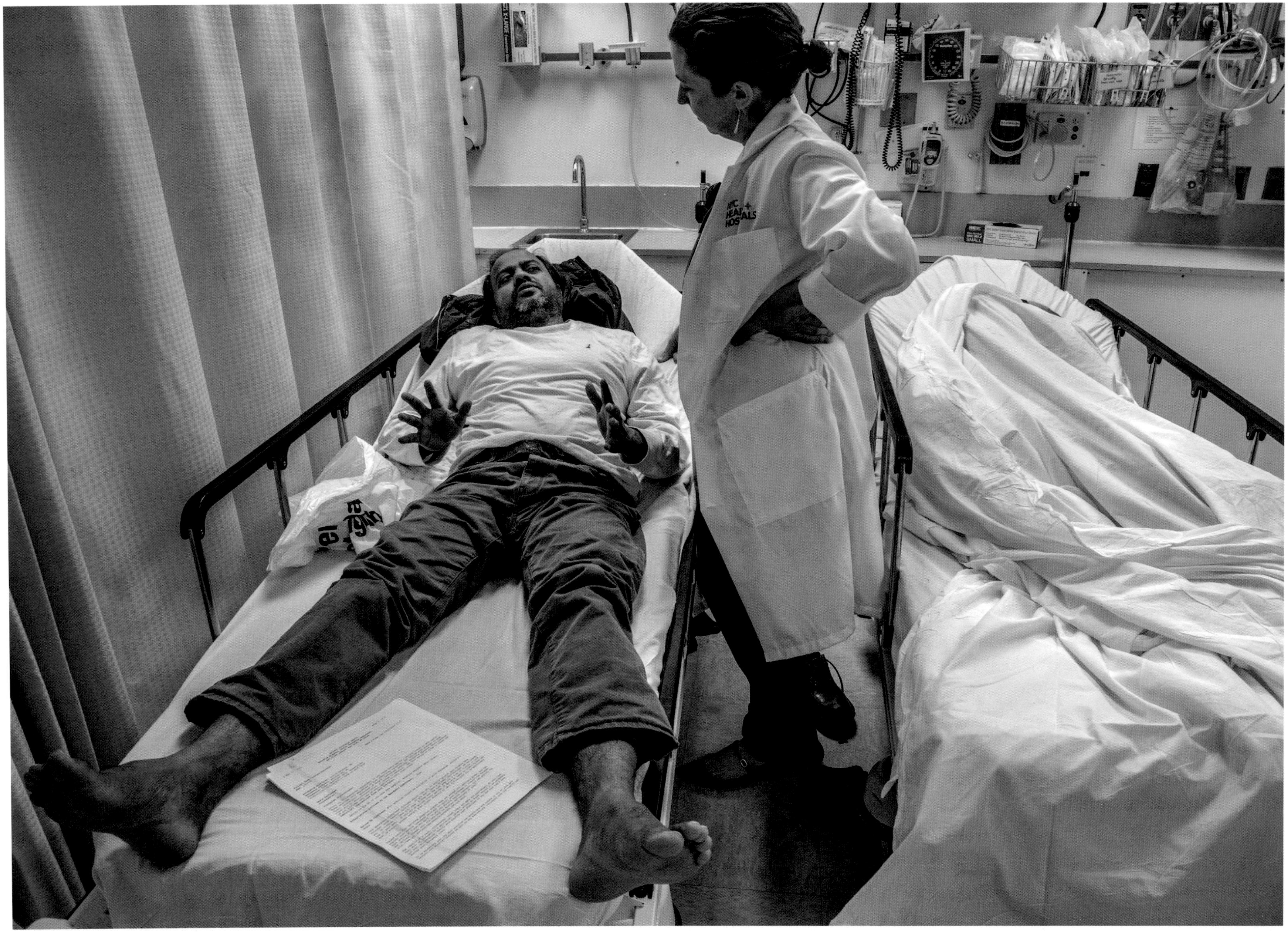

I'd finally found a field that made total sense. I saw palliative care as a *way*. Patients were happier, families were happier, *I* was happier. It renewed my practice, and it made me feel so good about coming to work in the clinical space.

What do I do with my day? I go to meetings. I take care of patients. But mostly what I do is *think*. I love thinking about societal problems — the hardest ones. I love working on issues no one cares about, that people don't want to talk about. That's why I went into medicine . . . to be forever thinking. ✚

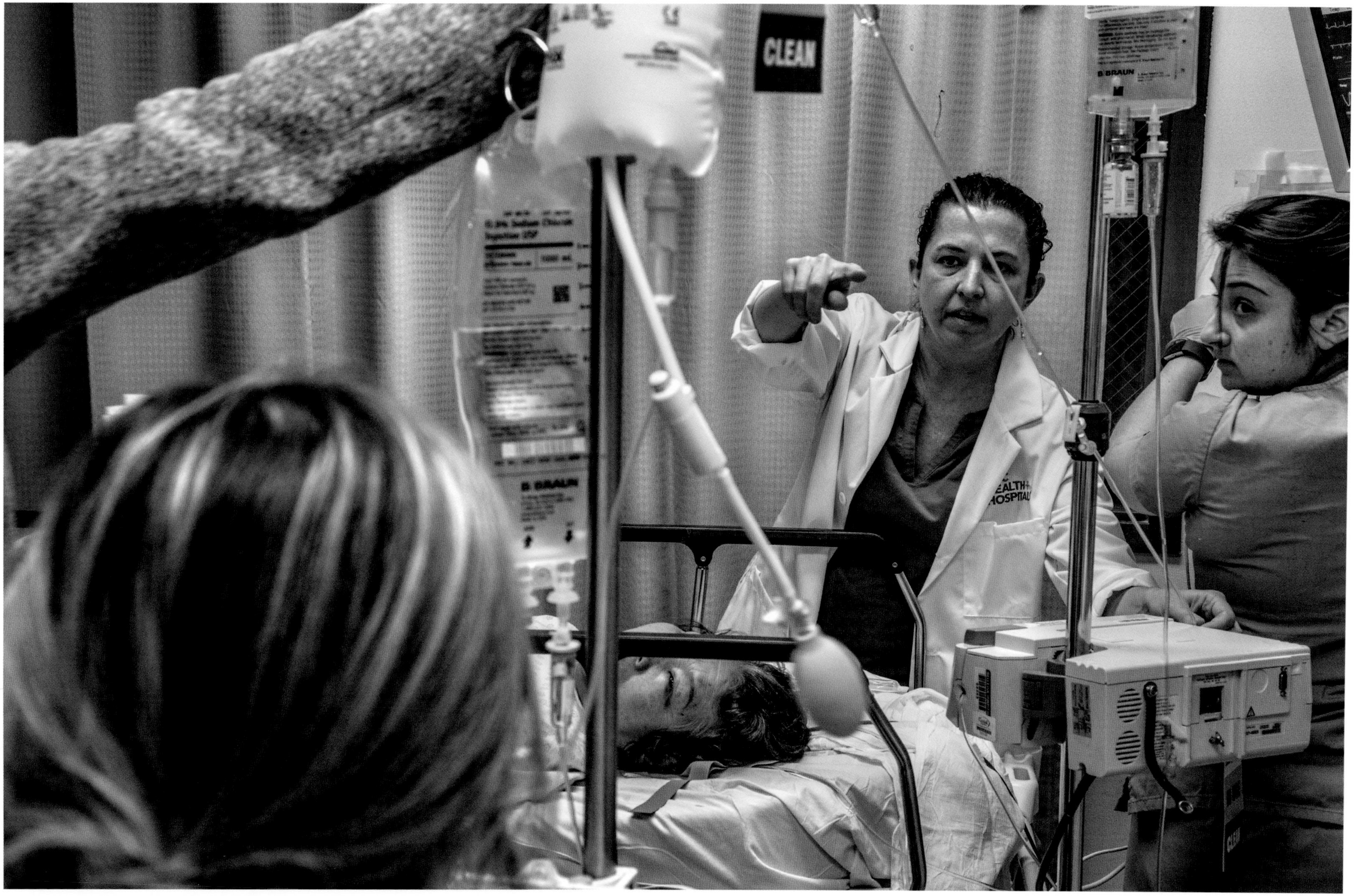

William Lewander, MD

Pediatric Emergency Physician
Providence, Rhode Island

In medical school, they sent us out to Spanish Harlem to track down patients who'd tested positive for tuberculosis. We'd go to an address but find ourselves standing in the middle of an abandoned lot. Those experiences taught me a lot about the pressures faced by inner-city patients . . . stresses I'd never really considered. Just because you know medicine and have some "wisdom" to share doesn't mean everyone is ready to receive it.

In those days, pediatric emergency medicine was just emerging. Children were often cared for by internists or emergency doctors who had some pediatric training — but not nearly enough. Although the training has improved significantly, upward of 80 percent of kids still are treated by doctors who specialize in adult or non-pediatric emergency medicine. This can be problematic because the body of clinical knowledge doesn't always translate.

Developmentally, physically, anatomically, physiologically, and in virtually every other way, kids are unique . . . they're not just little grown-ups. Their bodies and minds continue to evolve dramatically over time . . . it's like the patient becomes an entirely new person at each age. Heart rate and blood pressure in a one-year-old are very different than they are in a teenager. The patterns of traumatic injuries also vary widely, depending on the age of the patient and their physiological response to stress. All of these factors must be considered.

It's one thing to be good with children, but it's equally important to understand how to interact with the families. You spend a lot of time reassuring them that everything is going to be okay or trying to convince them to let you stick a needle in their child. And every situation is different . . . you have to learn how to read between the lines. There are social and economic dynamics that extend well beyond the kid's ear infection. A family might say, "Yes, yes, yes. Thank you, doctor. . . ." But what they really want to say — but are too embarrassed — is, "We don't have any money for the medicine and will never pick it up from the pharmacy." Or you may have a family that questions everything you do . . . wants endless explanations about every move you make. You need to be firm, but you must have patience and be a good listener.

As a last resort — or sometimes even as a first one — more and more troubled kids are referred to the emergency department. We'll get a six-year-old who's been hitting his sibling or running out in the street or the teenager who's feeling the stress of bullying, gangs, substance abuse, sexuality, or whatever. These are issues that, in the past, would have been dealt with by the family.

Emergency providers have always had to be on the alert for signs of child maltreatment and ready to intervene, but we need to be doing a better job with these growing mental health issues. Suicidal gestures and feelings have probably tripled in the last three years, and there's simply not a good network for these patients outside of the hospital. Sure, there are pediatricians, behavioral health services, and psychiatrists, but a strong infrastructure is missing.

You can do a lot of good in a nine- or ten-hour shift. For me, that's the best part. Of course, you never forget the terrible cases . . . the boy hit by a car . . . the teenager with cancer . . . children who, despite your very best efforts, are lost. But you take solace in the balance . . . in the resilience of the kids . . . and in the fact that good things are happening. ✚

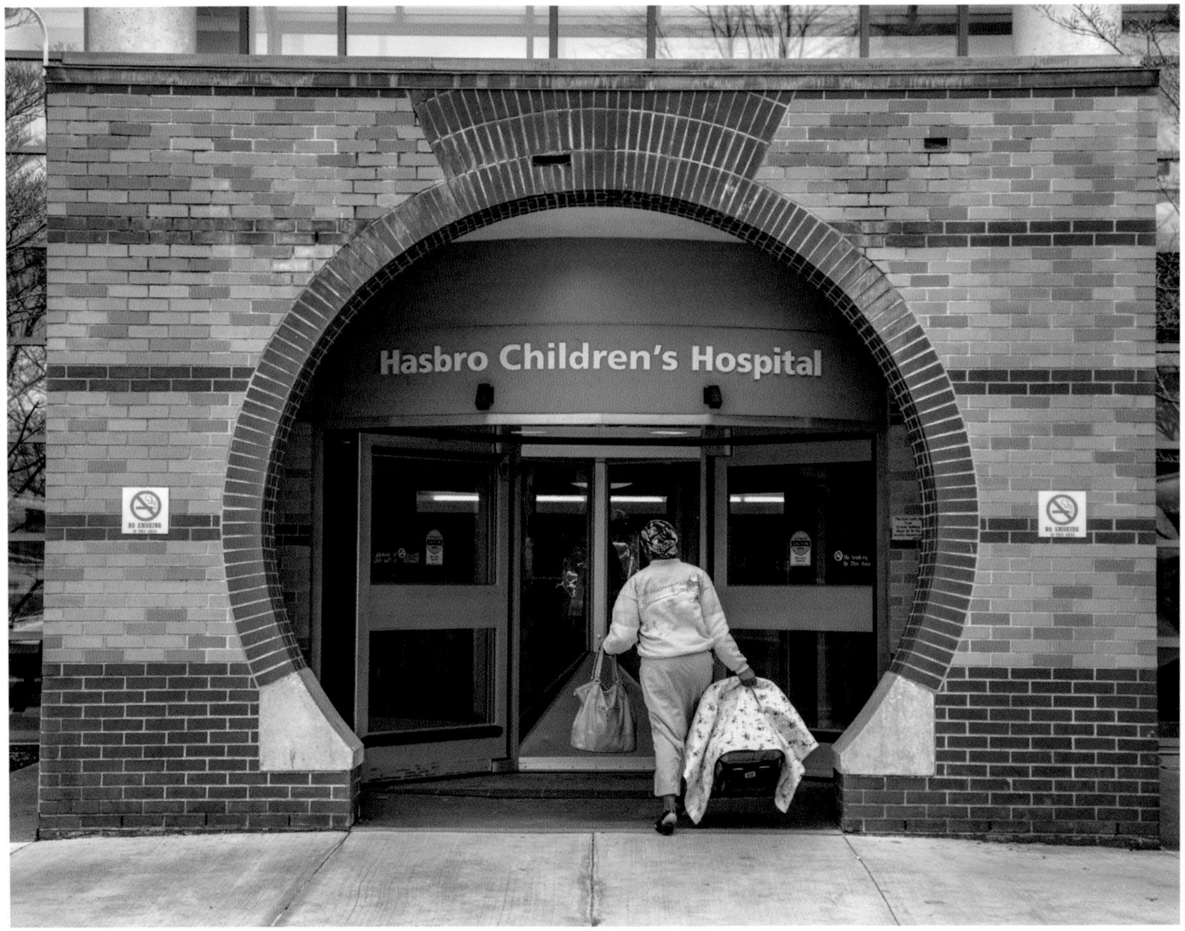

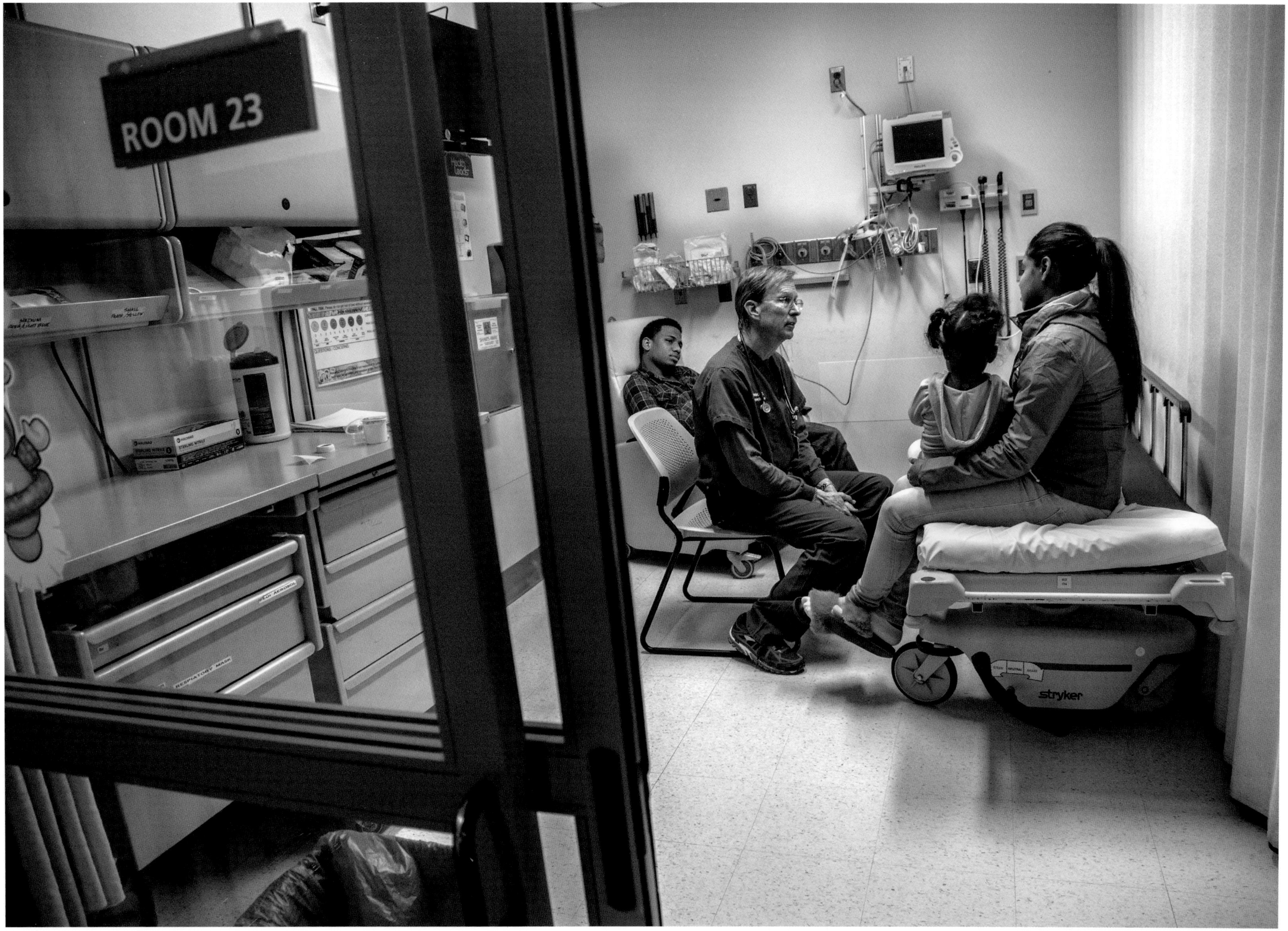

William Lewander, MD

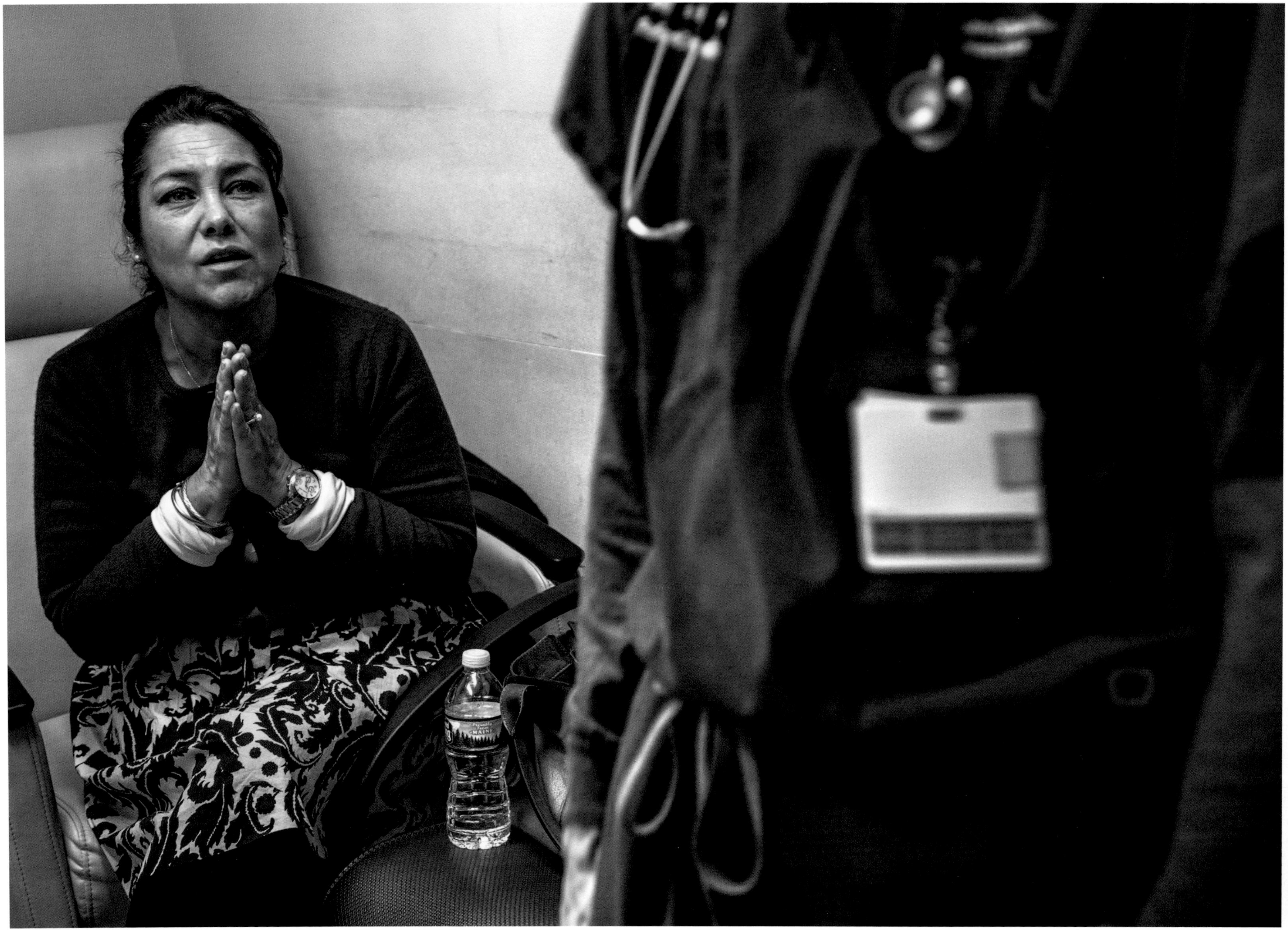

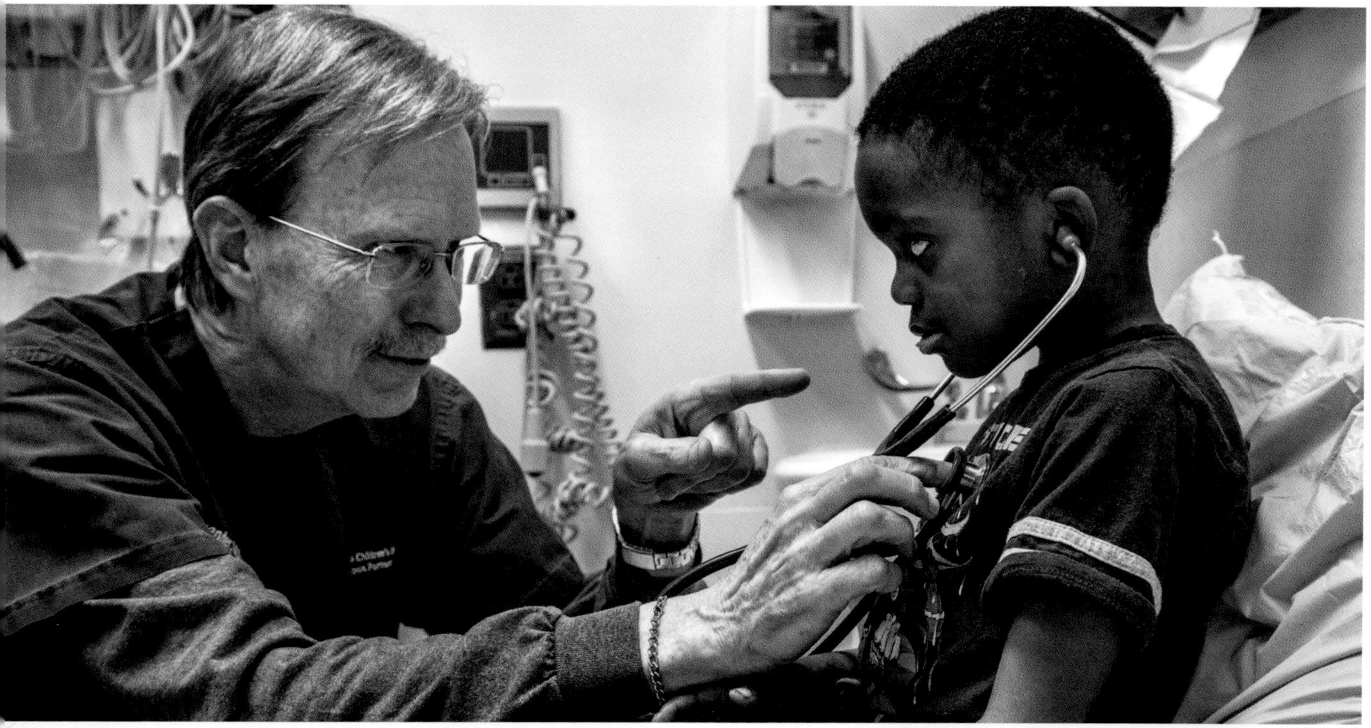

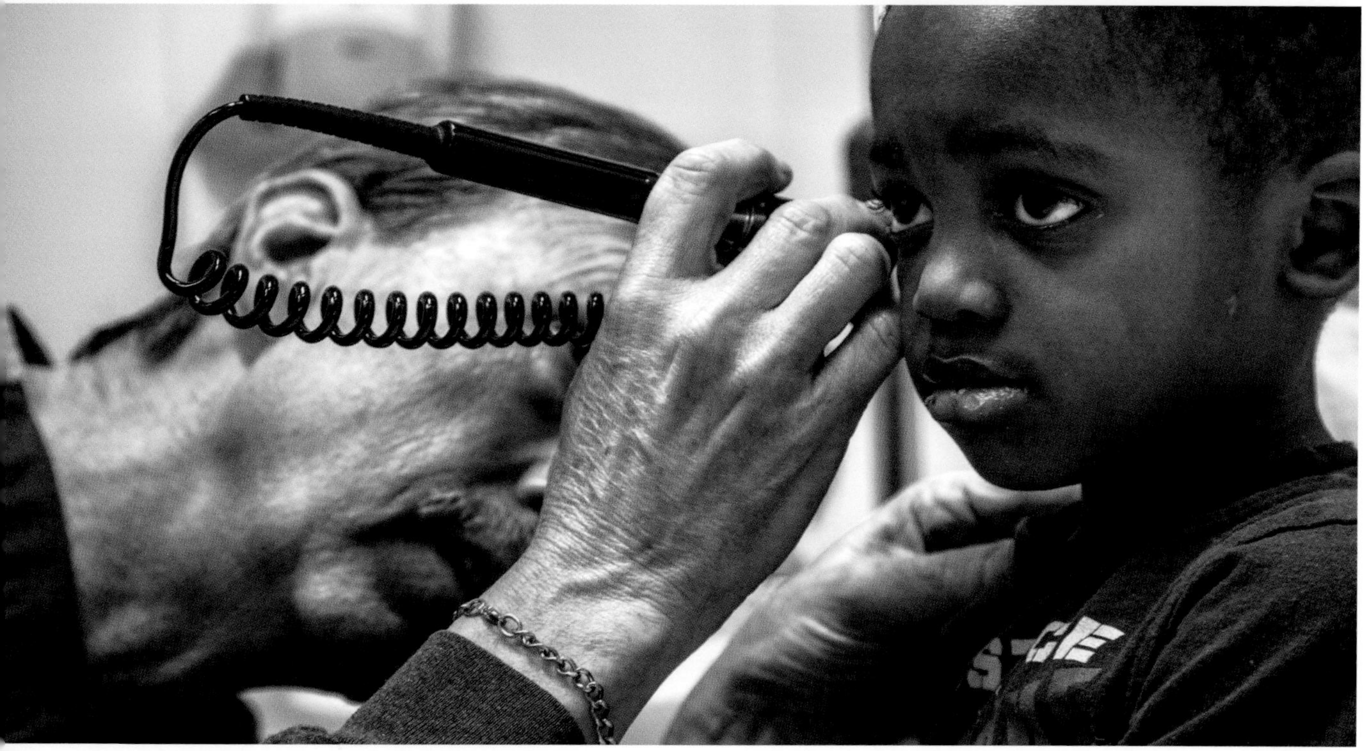

Bret Ackermann, DO

Military Emergency Physician
San Antonio, Texas

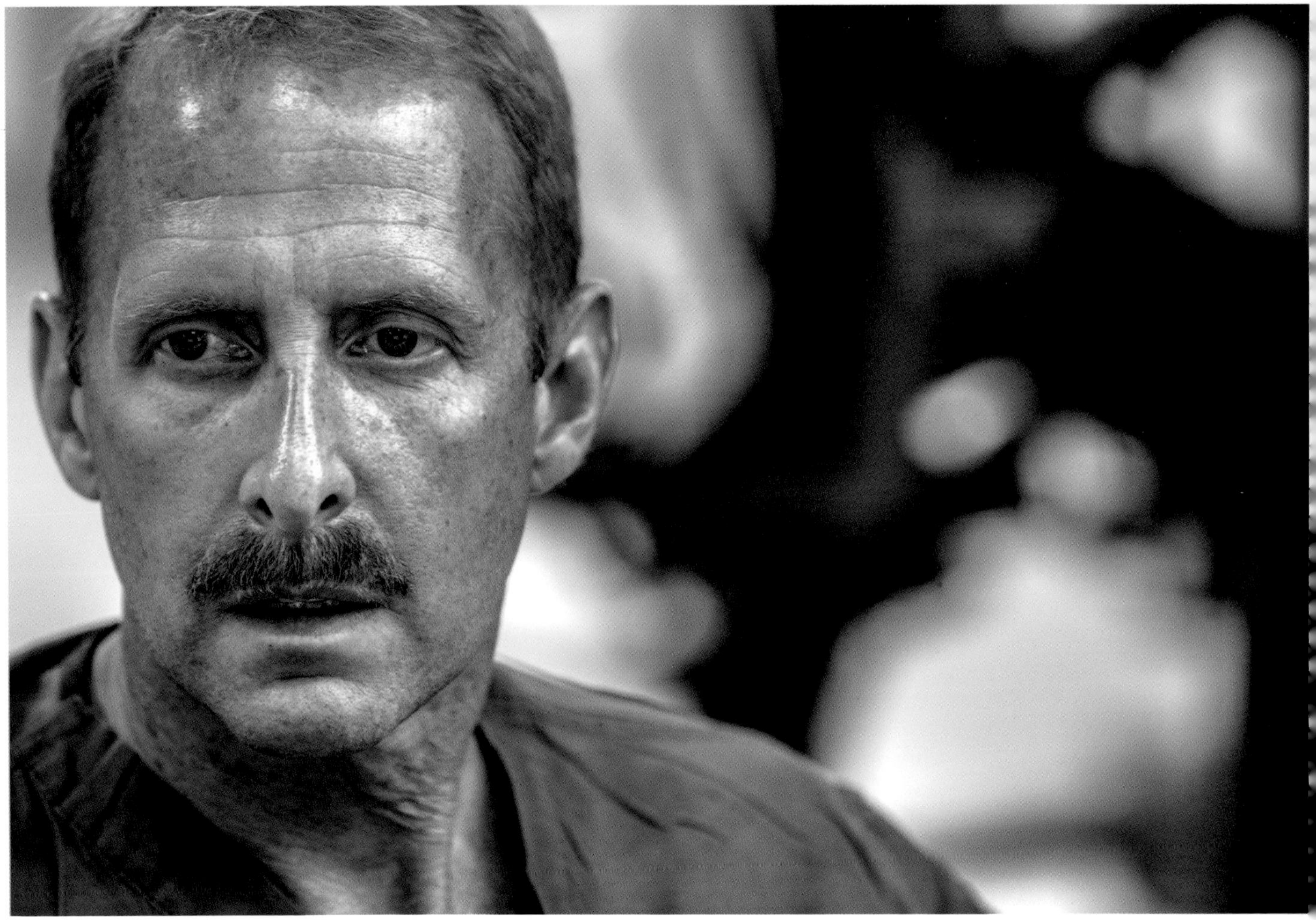

I was a nerd who learned how to do pushups and run. When I was in college, my goal was to work on the Human Genome Project, but the idea of living grant to grant scared me. Around that time, my mother got into a car accident. I was driving home and saw the wreckage in the middle of the road . . . a shattered, bloody windshield. Her injuries turned out to be minor, but when I got to the hospital, one of the ER guys offered to show me around. He told me about an arrest they'd just had, and I saw a little kid getting his arm cast. I thought it looked like a pretty cool place to work.

I was born in 1964 and grew up watching the Vietnam War on TV. Every day, they announced the new tally of wounded or dead soldiers. I joined the US Army during the Cold War, right before starting medical school, so I probably didn't even realize what I was getting myself into. It's different for the kids coming in today, though . . . the United States has been at war for fifteen years. But you can learn a lot about yourself by preparing for combat. You figure out how to lead — and follow — when you're cold, wet, tired, and hungry. You learn how to focus.

In the 1990s, I knew an orthopedic surgeon who'd been selected for battalion command. I asked him once, "How can I be like you?" He said, "Well, you can't." Before I had the chance to bow up and tell him how arrogant he was, he said, "You need to be *you*." He explained the practices and character traits that had worked for him would not work for me and vice versa. Our genetics, our environment, the lives we'd led up until that point . . . they had molded us in very different ways. He told me to just be the best *me* I could be. I take that advice with me wherever I go.

I was in Iraq with a special operations team in 2006 when we heard a helicopter was en route with two rangers who'd been shot during an infiltration. During the handoff with the medics, we got word a suicide vest had just gone off in the field. We were about to receive an unknown number of casualties. The two young infantrymen who'd been shot, Brehm and Barraza, didn't make it . . . I felt nauseated, but I knew I couldn't let up.

What really gets me is those casualties who came in — as busted up as they were — were only thinking about the guys who'd been shot. We just had to tell them the bad news . . . and watch as they tried to process it. No training can prepare you for that loss, for the day a fellow soldier isn't there. Just that morning, we'd been joking around in the gym. One of them had said, "Hey, sir, when are you gonna work out with *real* weights?"

We had a small service and paid our respects, but we all knew the best way to honor those guys was to get right back to work. I'll never know if their sacrifice was worth it. I'm not sure how you measure that. I just know we did everything we could to save them.

One time, a family friend asked me very innocently, "Did you ever see anything that bothered you while you were over there?" I just shot right back, "Of course I've seen . . . where the hell do you think I've been?" I later apologized because I knew she didn't mean anything by it. But, my god, I don't think people understand what these kids go through . . . the hardships they're willing to endure to serve their country. ✚

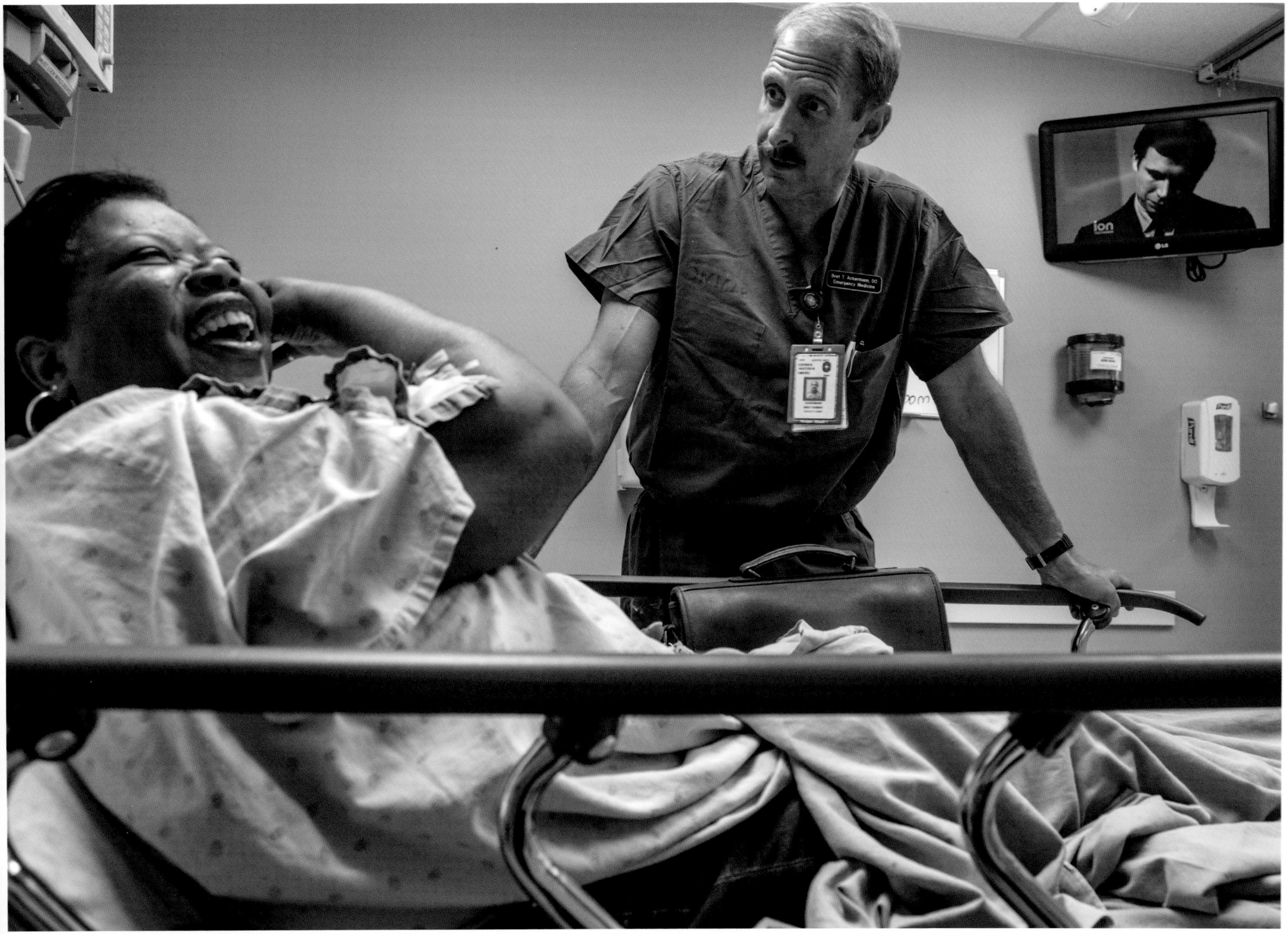
Bret T. Ackermann, DO
Emergency Medicine
ion
LG

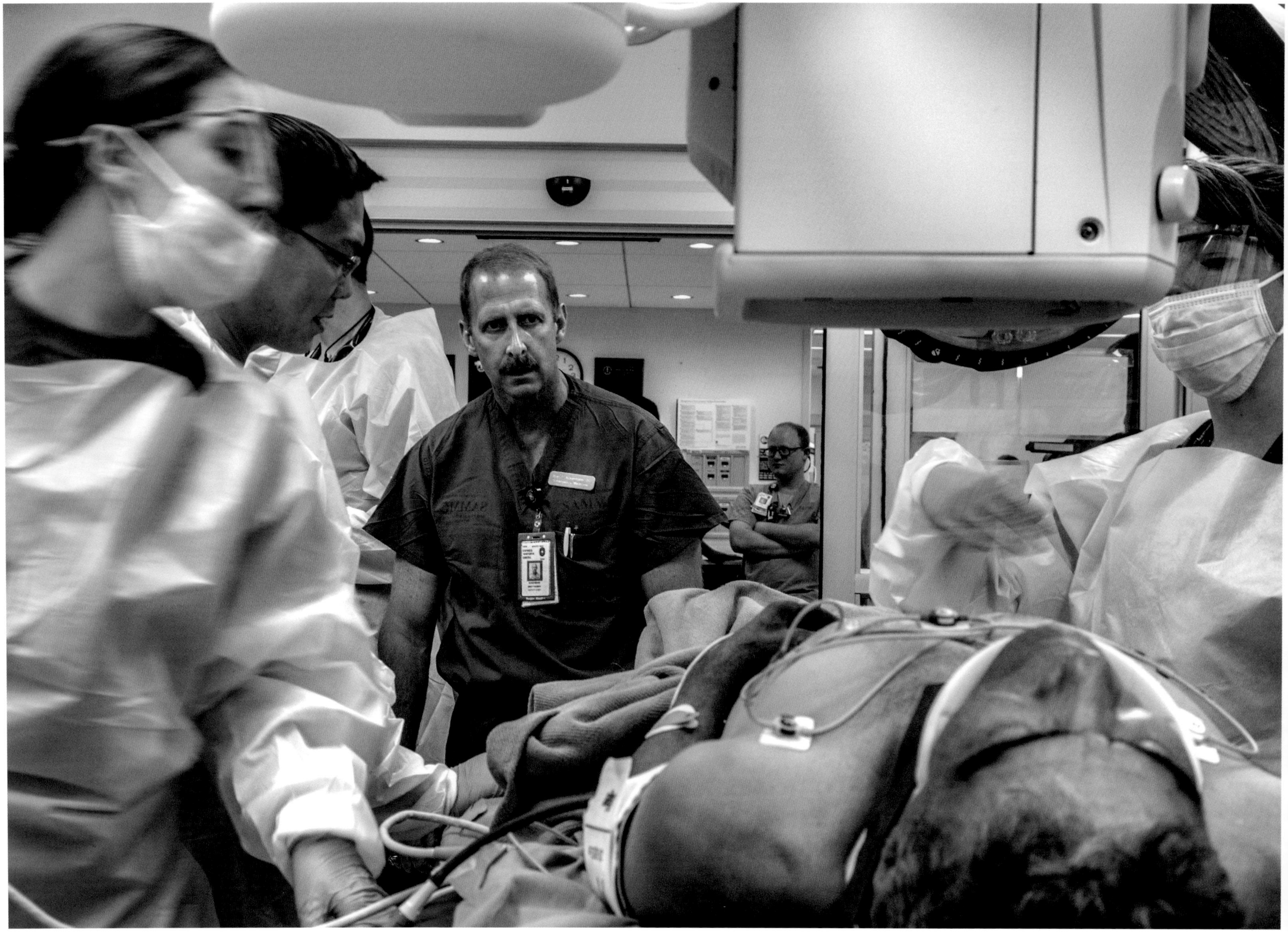

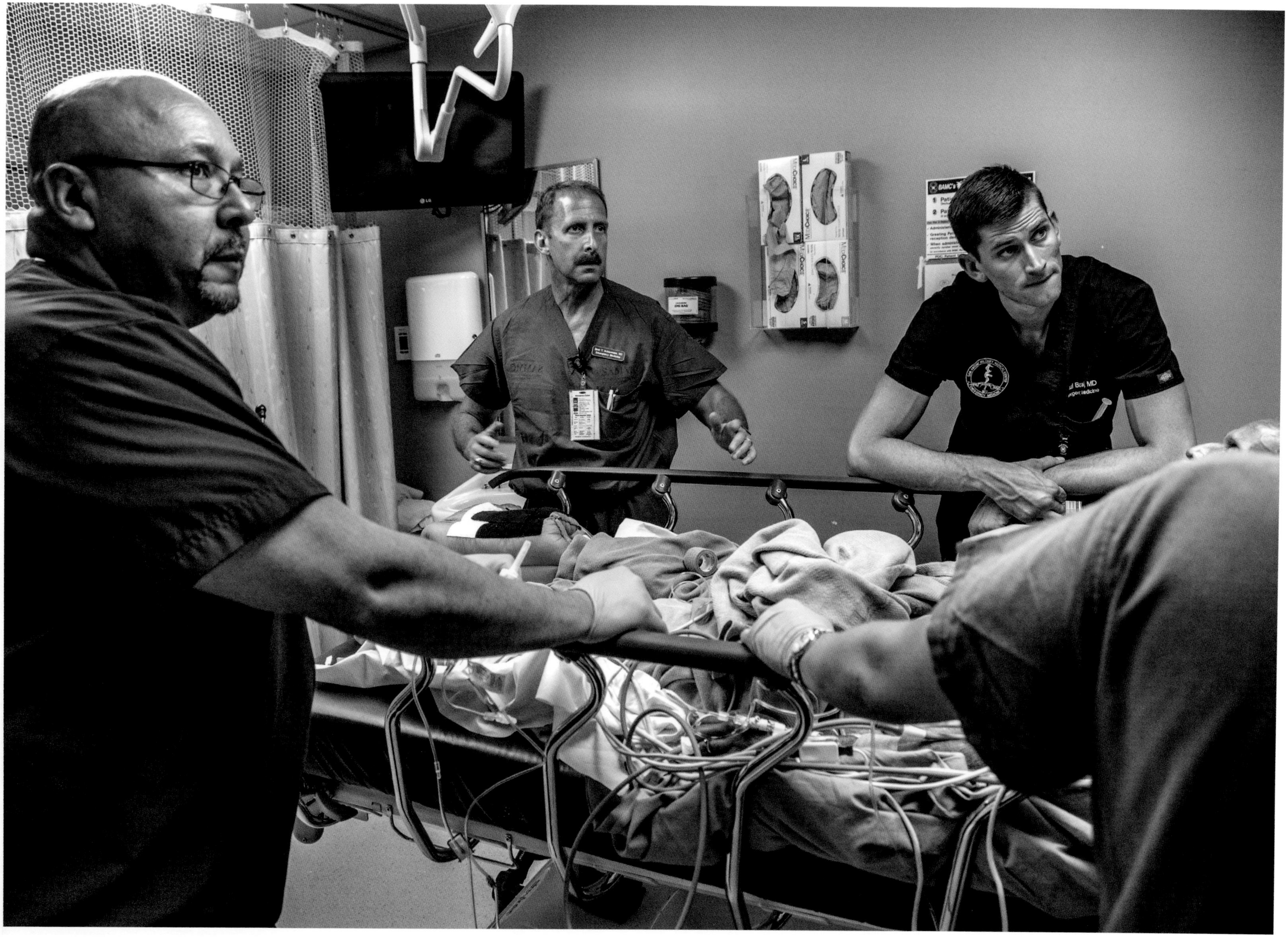

Gina Hurst, MD

Emergency & Critical Care Physician
Detroit, Michigan

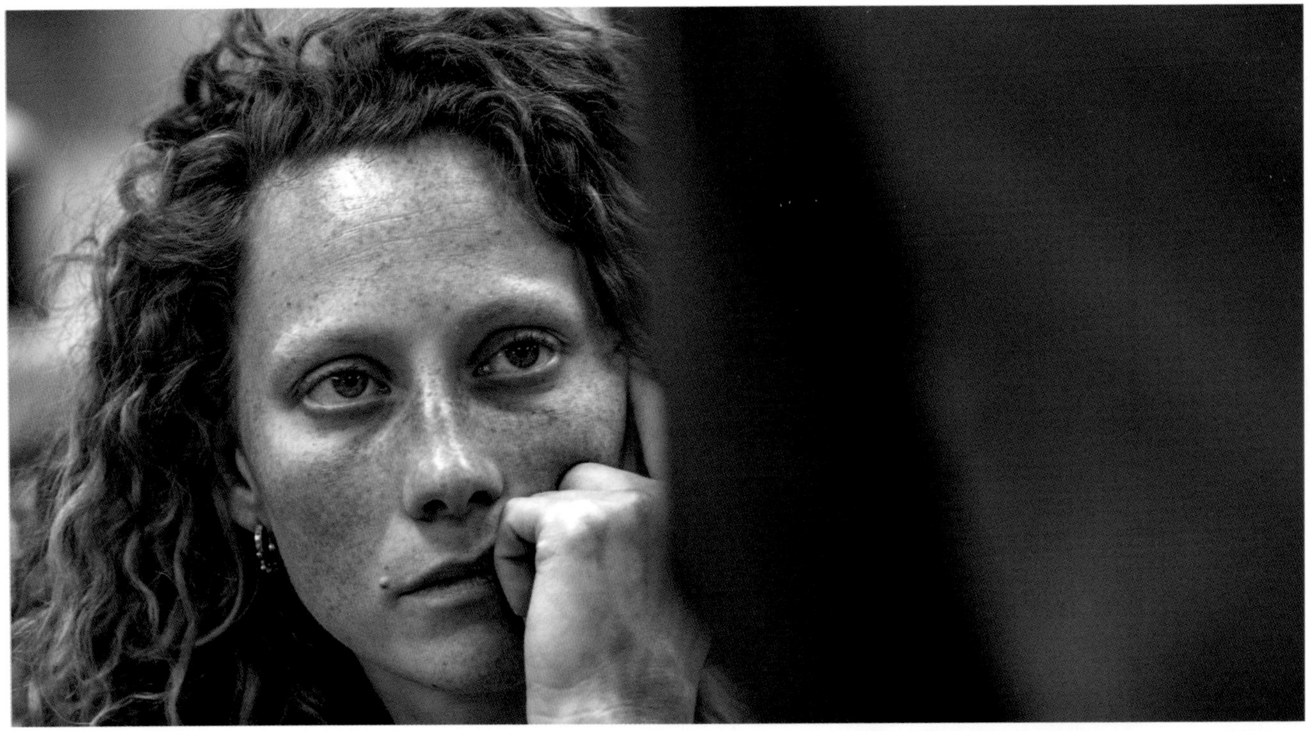

"Rise to the occasion, Gina. There's nobody else here to do it." That's what my mom used to tell me when I was growing up. I'm one of thirteen children — six of them adopted from China, Russia, and Kazakhstan. We were homeschooled, so each time a new child was brought into our household, our history and social studies lessons would revolve around their culture. No two siblings had the same learning style . . . one was dyslexic, one had an auditory processing disorder . . . everybody had their own struggles. I think that shaped the way I teach residents today.

I graduated high school when I was sixteen. I thought I was going to be a professional singer, but my parents were very practical people. They warned me it would be hard to make a living that way. Who knows? Maybe I just wasn't as good as I thought I was. Fortunately, I also really liked science. I started medical school at eighteen, which meant I was in a different stage of life than most of my classmates. Every time they went to a bar, I got left behind . . . so I just buried my nose in the books.

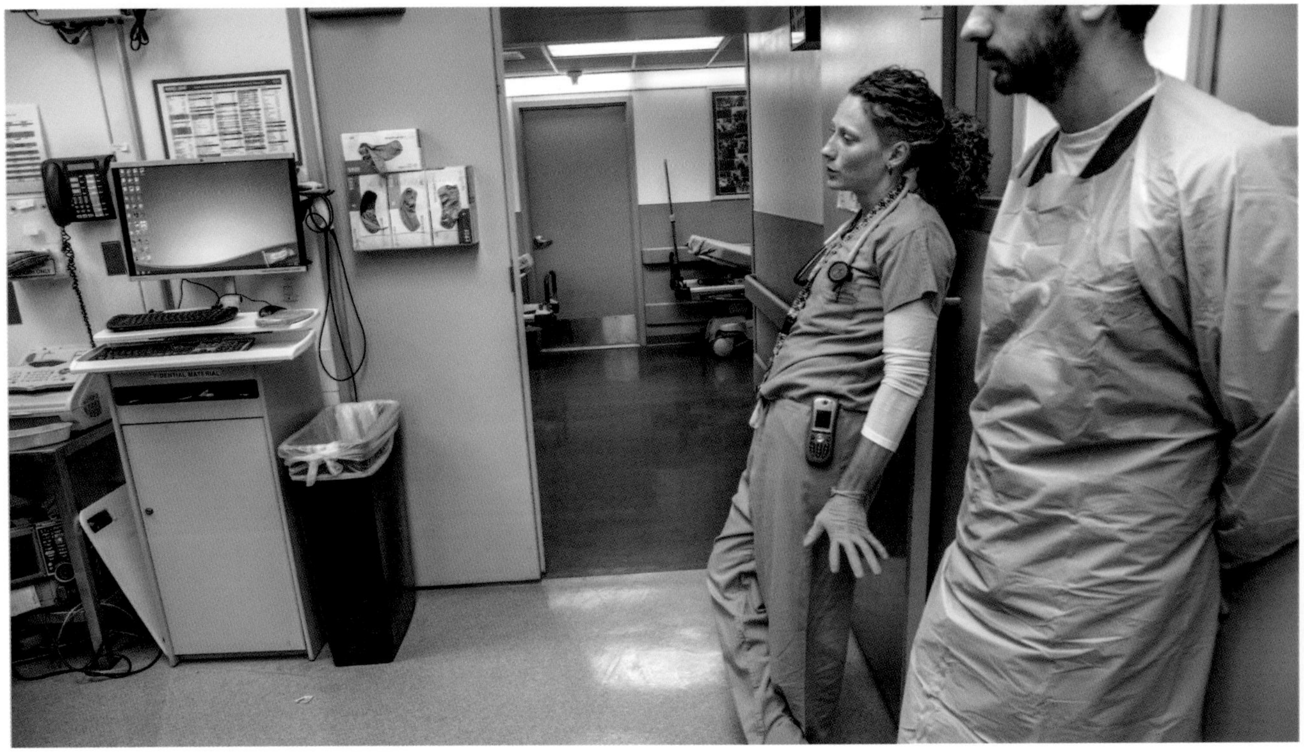

You can strap any yoke around my neck, and I'll keep moving along. I have no problem with high patient volumes or lack of sleep. The only thing I can't handle is mind-numbing boredom. That's why I love emergency medicine. I'm happiest when I'm bouncing around. I've never been the type of person to shy away from a challenge. When something is hard, I view it as an opportunity to grow.

During residency, I was always asking myself, "Who are you going to be when this is all over?" The people charged with your training have enormous influence . . . you look to them for guidance just as you would a parent. You observe their behavior . . . take in their feedback . . . decide if their words are strong enough to defeat you.

I try to be mindful of that responsibility. I remember an instance when I was particularly harsh to one of my junior residents . . . I really upset her. I just thought, "I cannot be this kind of person." I do not have to repeat others' bad habits. If you're going to choose someone to emulate, you can pick someone who is discerning and wise with their words — or you can pick somebody who's not.

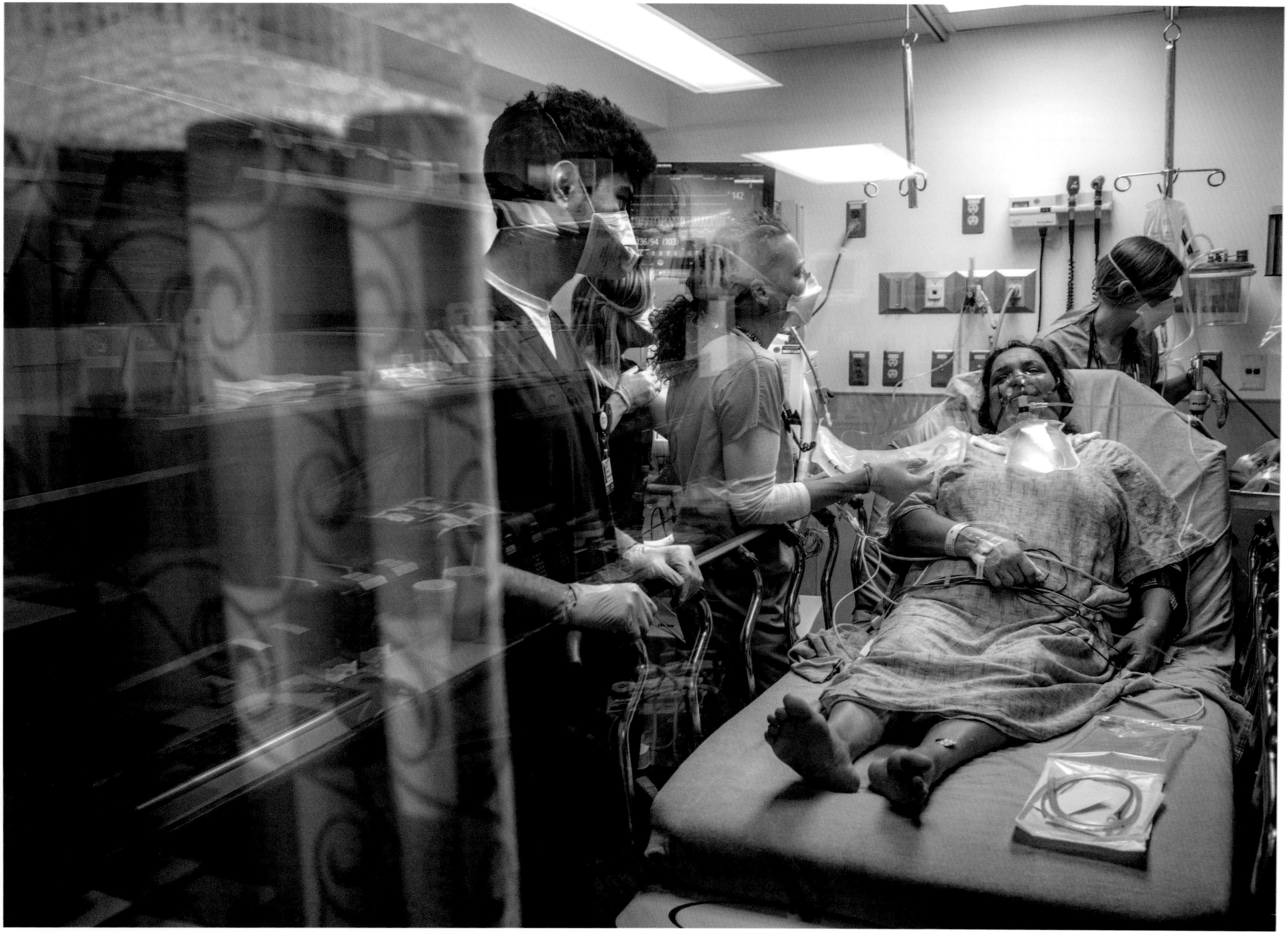

Gina Hurst, MD

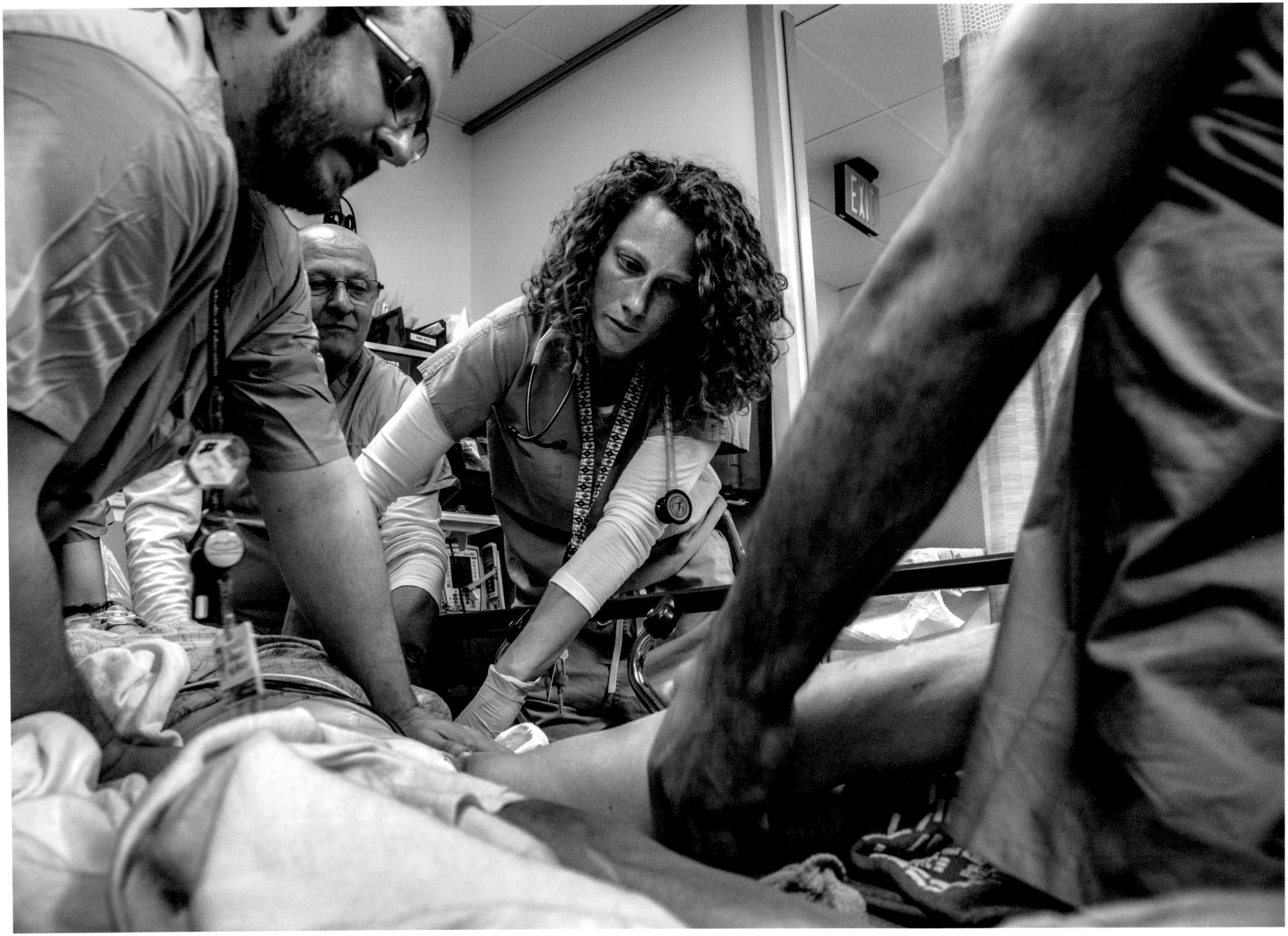
EXIT

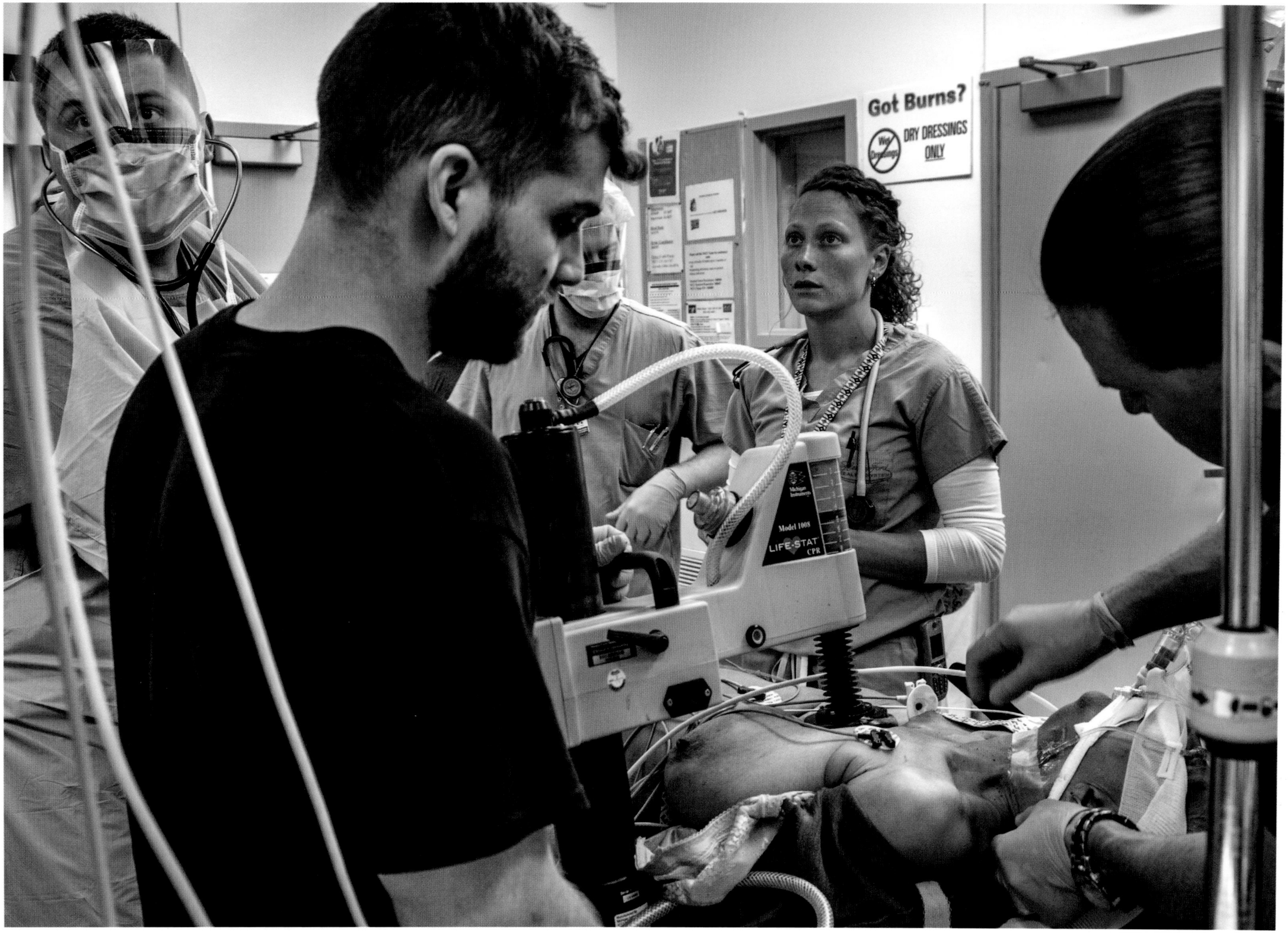
Got Burns?
DRY DRESSINGS
ONLY
Michigan Instruments
Model 1008
LIFE-STAT
CPR

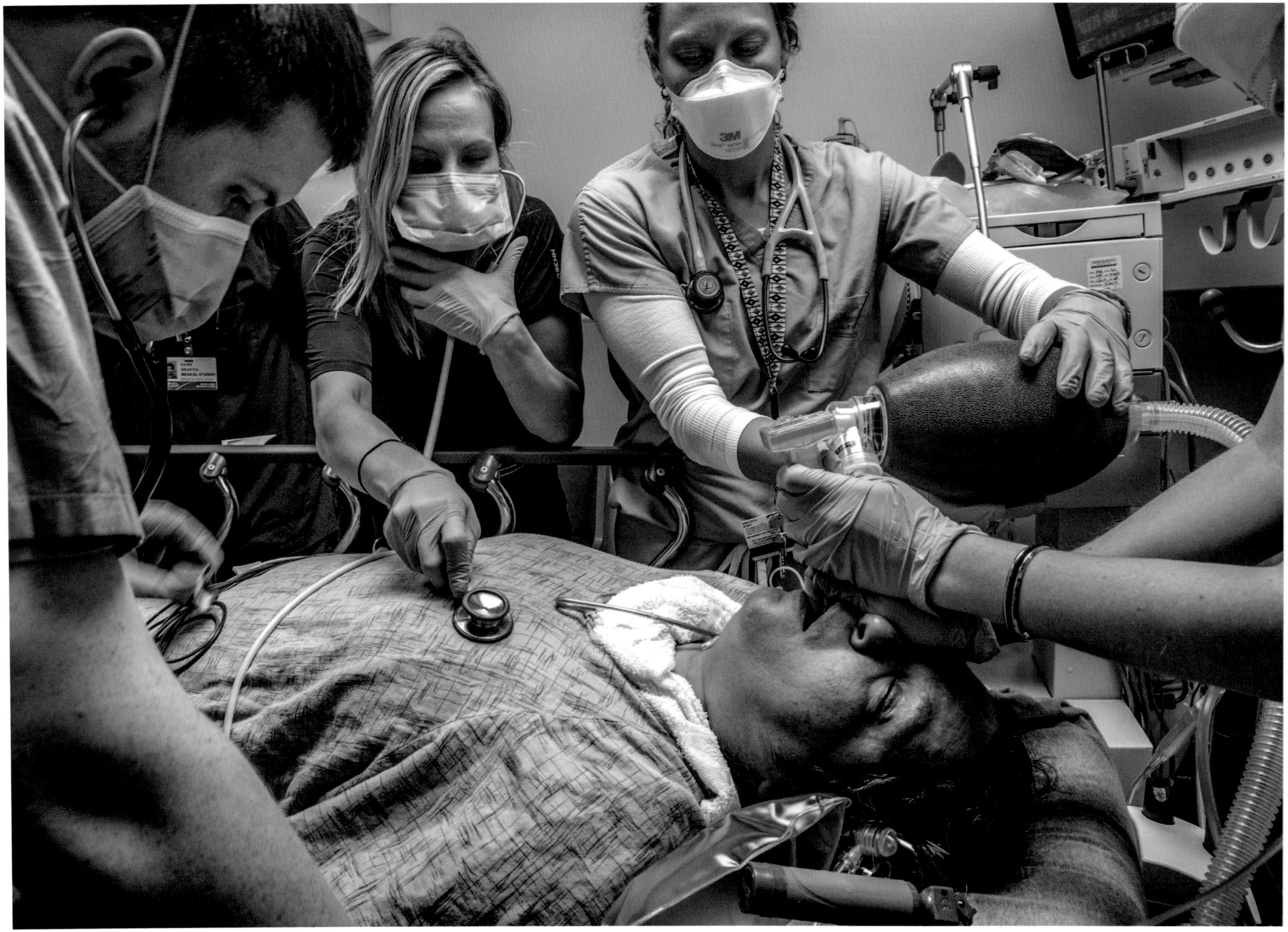

We have a lot of difficulty accepting death in our culture. Patients come through these doors, hoping — expecting — we'll give them life. But *life* may not always be the right answer. Being hooked up to machines . . . hauled around in a wheelchair . . . that's not "life" for everybody. As an ER doc, I'm blown away by the privilege of being able to fix people, but some of the most meaningful conversations I've ever had have been with patients who couldn't be fixed.

I recently treated a man who had end-stage cancer that had metastasized from his colon to his skin. He told me, "I have a new grandson, and I just want to know how long I can be his grandfather." We talked about how he probably didn't have more than a couple of weeks, maybe a month. It was a very emotional experience, but he came to terms with his illness and we formulated a plan that included modifying some of his pain medications and providing close follow up with palliative care.

I didn't save his life. In fact, I told him it had come to an end. He was in tears, but he said, "Thank you for having this conversation with me. Thank you for being able to tell me the things that I couldn't tell myself." ✚

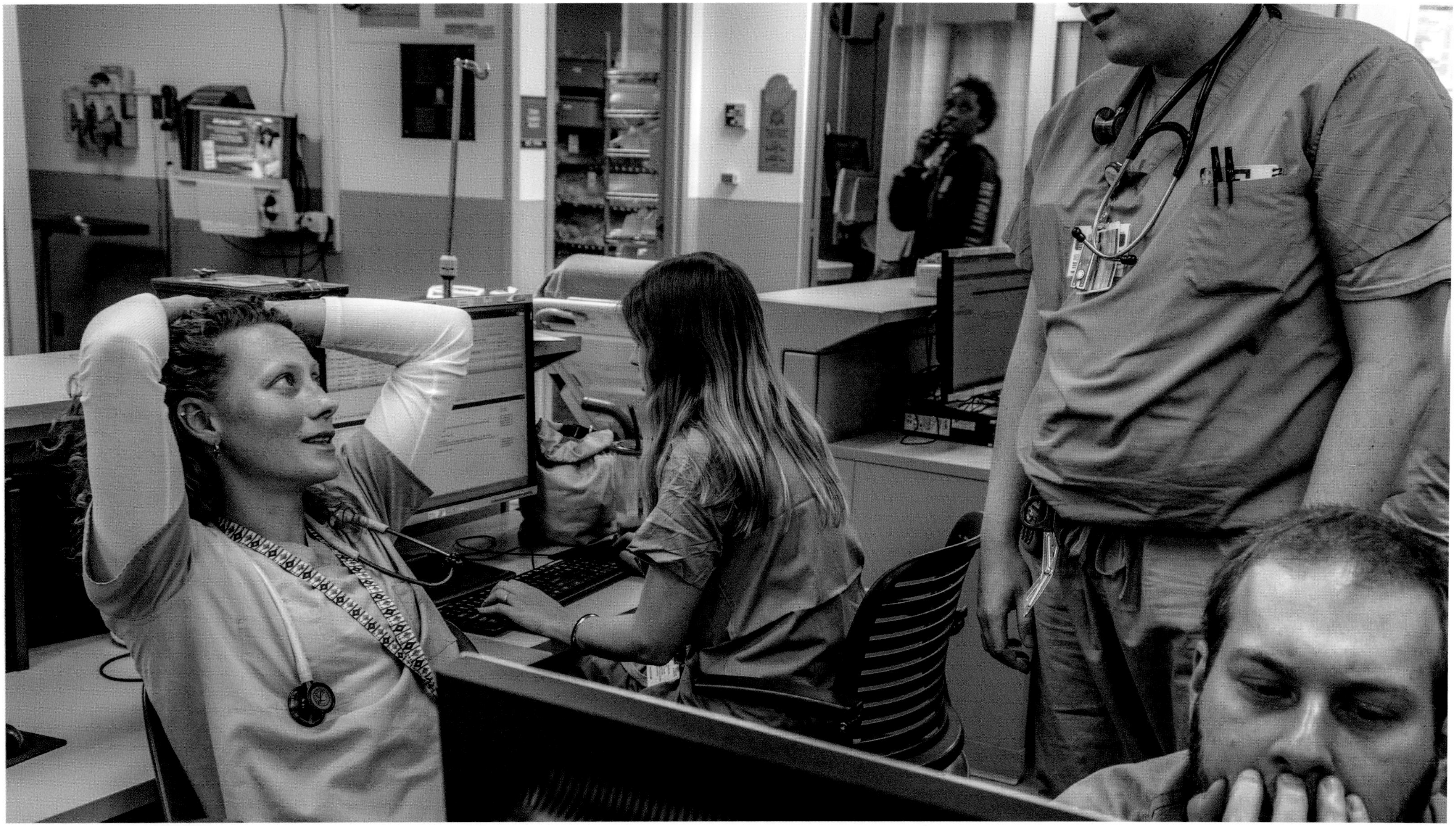

Michael Alter, MD

Emergency Physician
Palmer, Alaska

When you come out of school, you're pure of heart but before long, you're jaded and jilted by satisfaction scores, hospital administrators, and patient complaints. You just get drilled down. It's unfortunate, but doctors get to the point where they're like, "Okay, whatever — here's the Z-Pak you don't need. Just don't complain because I don't want to get in trouble when the Press Ganey survey comes back."

Sadly, I became complicit, too. If you came with an injury, you were probably gonna leave with a prescription for painkillers. That's just what was expected. Gradually, I started suffering from this thing called "compassion fatigue;" basically, I was sick and tired of drug addicts trying to scam me. I stopped hiding my intolerance — I'd go toe to toe with every patient.

I had this one guy who came in with strep throat; he was the world's biggest wimp. He says, "I'm in pain! So. Much. Pain." I give him some ibuprofen, but he says it's garbage — says he needs something stronger. I'm like, "Yeah, *right* . . . I don't think so." I'm a pretty vocal guy, so whatever comes out of my pie hole comes right from the heart. I finally tell him, "Dude, you need to grow a set. You're not getting narcotics for a sore throat." Anyway, he complained to the administration, of course. He got his movie tickets or whatever, but he still didn't get any opiates.

People want immediate gratification, but good medicine is not Walt Disney World. When you come see me, you shouldn't expect the royal treatment . . . you're here for my education, my expertise, and my advice. I'm being paid to do what's in the patient's best interest. You're not doing your job if you don't piss off 10 percent of the people you see. Sometimes you need to say no; sometimes you need to say things people don't want to hear. Sometimes you need to tell a guy with back pain to lose fifty pounds and hit the treadmill.

I mean, life has a certain amount of pain associated with it. We have to learn how to tolerate some measure of discomfort. I learned that lesson on my own when I was in Hawaii a few years ago. A fat boy shouldn't bodysurf in big waves. I got destroyed and ended up with ten broken ribs, a flail chest, a collapsed lung, and a broken shoulder. I was thankful for the opiates when I was in the throes of pain, but when things settled down three or four days later, I took myself off them.

The problem with opiates is we're losing people. I've pronounced five patients dead on a seven-night stretch. About a week ago, I took care of a young guy with back pain. He's been seeing a clinic doctor, who has him on morphine. Now the guy can't get enough of the stuff. He's crushing his pills and shooting up . . . it's just a natural progression. If the doctor ever cuts him off, he'll be on heroin in a flash.

The only solution is prevention. We need to re-educate doctors, and we need to take our profession back. Screw the government telling us what to do . . . pharmaceutical companies pumping money into congressmen's pockets . . . giving bad information about the non-addictive nature of opiates. We followed them like a friggin' flock of sheep; we knew better.

I got involved with the Alaska Opioid Policy Task Force two years ago and, boy, it changed my world — my whole calculus. I've had a lot of role models in my life, but I never imagined some of them would be ex-addicts. It's just amazing to see the transformation these people have made. Back in the day, a lot of them were my patients; they were the kind of people you'd want to poke in the eye with an icepick. But here they are now . . . they've turned their lives around and have dedicated themselves to helping others. They're the most selfless bunch I've ever met in my life.

Working with these folks inspired me to start a pilot program for ambulatory detox through our urgent care system. We've been successful at getting people off heroin and pills, so we're expanding the project — taking it into the hospital. That's what I'm going to do with the next few years of my life. I'm retiring from emergency medicine to pursue my passion. I'm turning my healthy six-figure income into a minimum wage job, but I'm hoping to make a difference in our community. I think it will be a great challenge — and it needs to be done.

I'm a heathen, but I need to get to heaven somehow. Maybe this'll be my way in. ✚

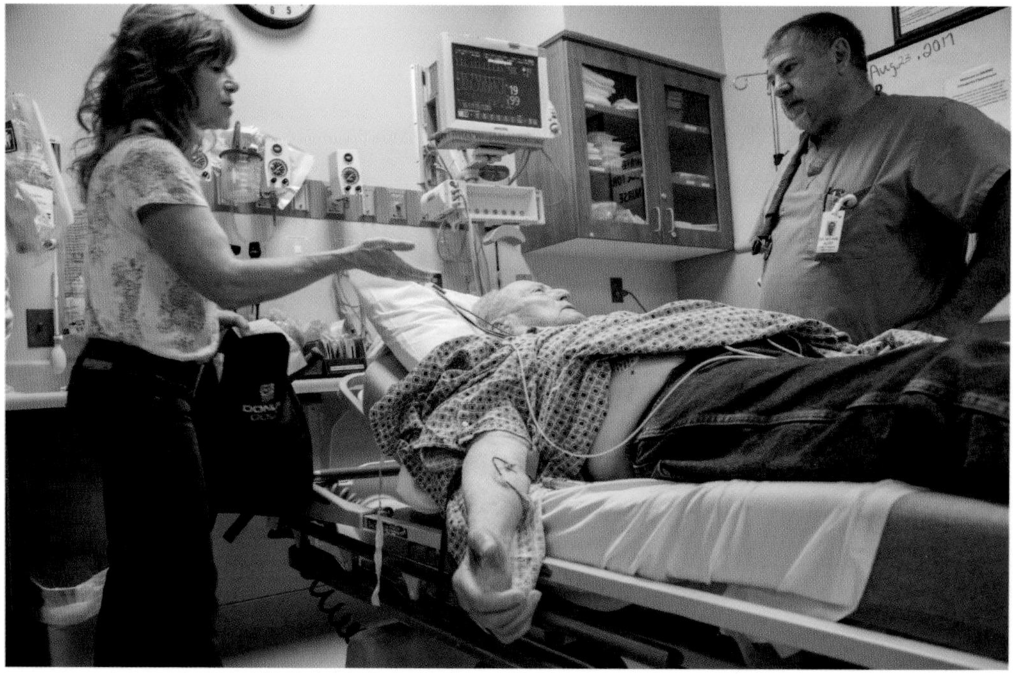

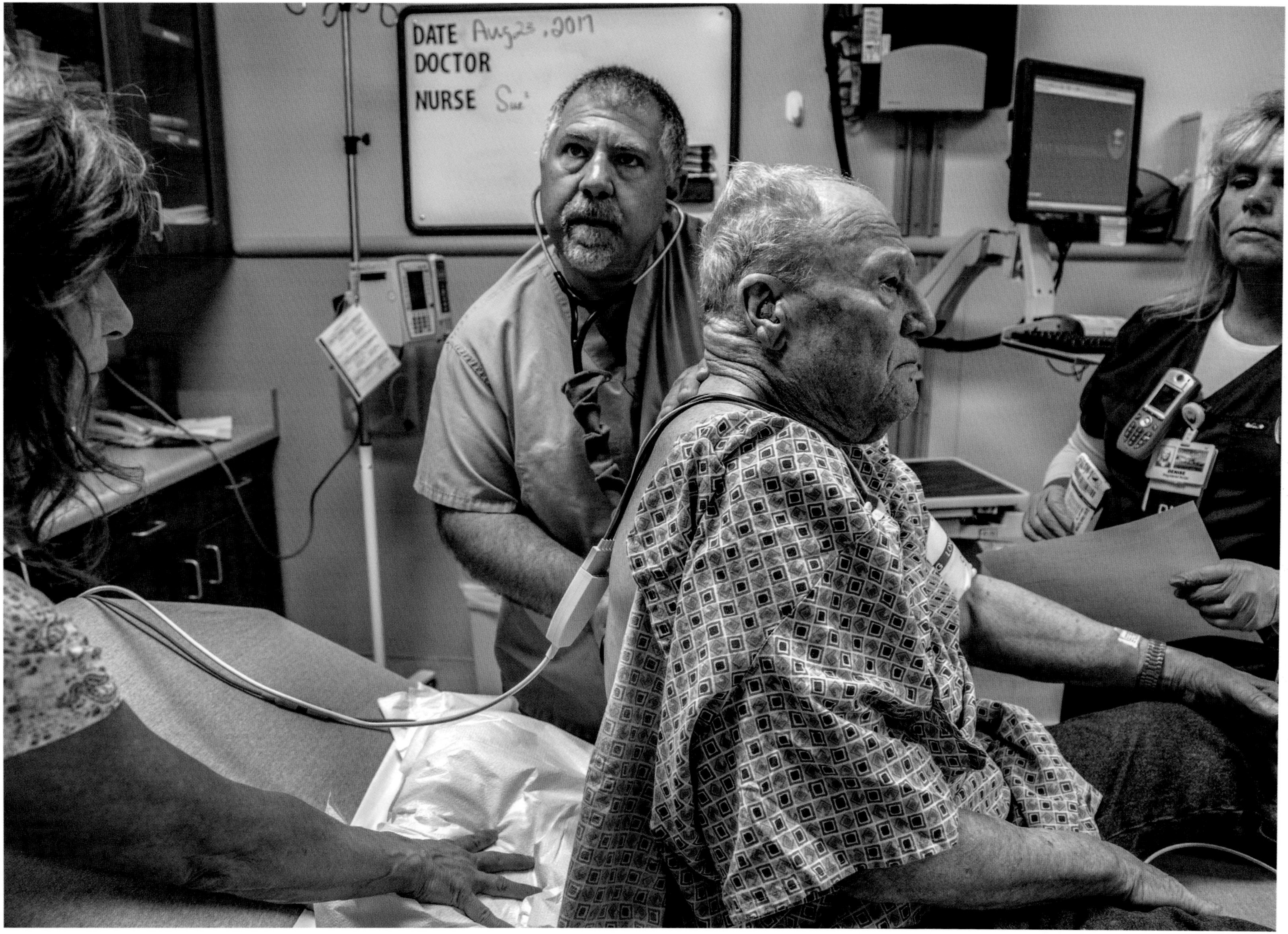
DATE Aug 23, 2017
DOCTOR
NURSE Sue

Marc Eckstein, MD

Emergency Physician & EMS Bureau Commander
Los Angeles, California

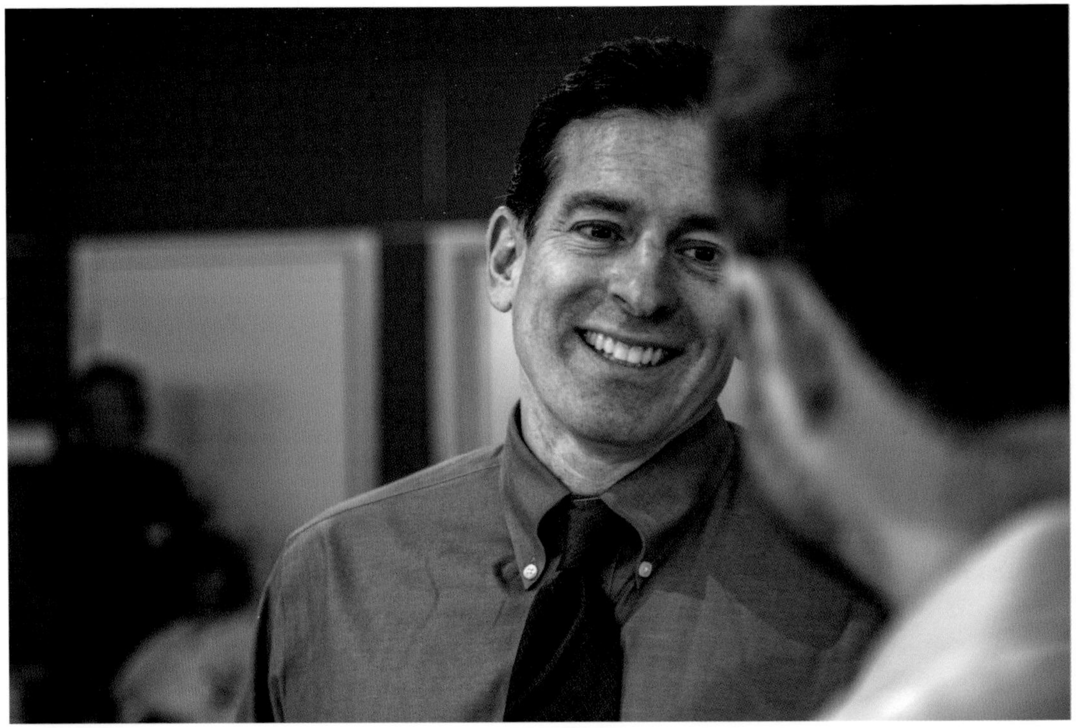

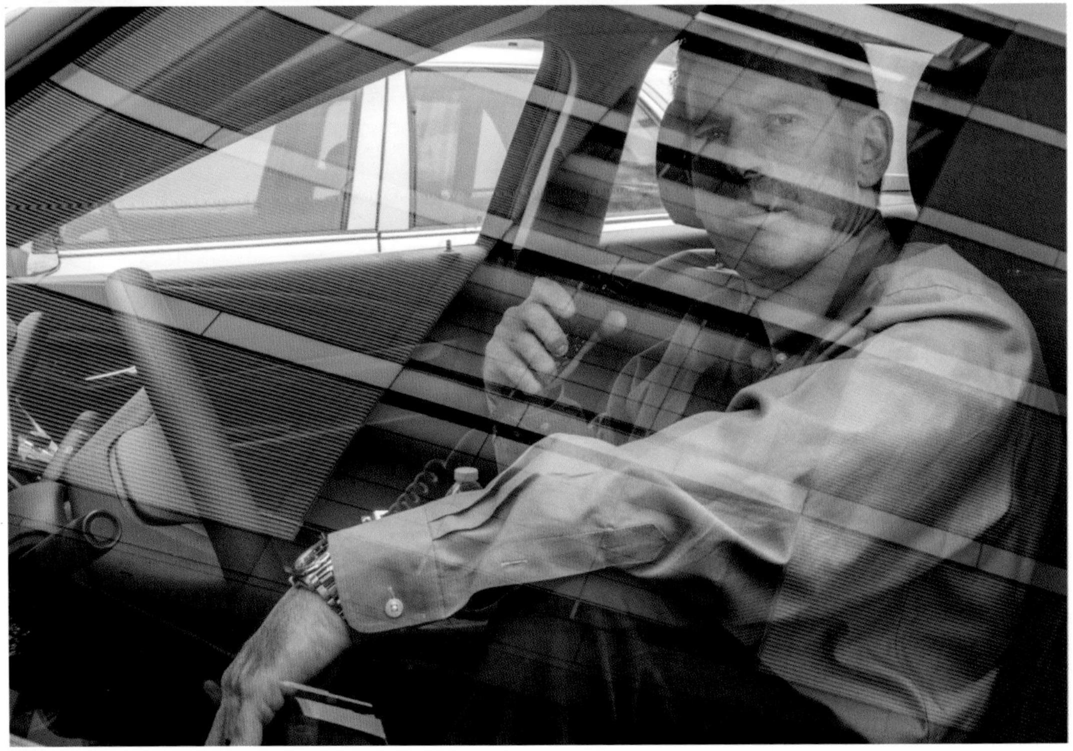

I was a medic in New York when crack cocaine hit the streets. The violence was incredible; the city was just a bloody mess. You never knew what was going to roll through the door. You could have moments of boredom followed by absolute chaos. To me, the appeal was getting order from that chaos — to play medical detective, come up with a presumptive diagnosis, and treat without having all your data points. Even after thirty years, I find that aspect very appealing. I've always liked the concept of helping people, tying science and biology and all those types of things to the human body. I've always been a bit of an adrenaline junkie, too.

I was a senior chief resident in Los Angeles in '92 when the city set a record for homicides. We had about 1,200 that year — it was insane. We also had riots and gang wars, and the emergency department would get what we called the "homeboy drop-offs." Typically, there'd be a car-to-car shooting. Gang members would drive their buddies right up to the ambulance ramp. They'd hit the emergency buzzer and bail. We would run outside and see a car riddled with bullet holes, blood and brain matter in the front seat, and some poor gang member lying there dead or agonal. We'd get those pretty routinely.

Other times, we'd get a bus crash, but there'd also be patients with heart attacks, strokes, and everything else. Meeting those kinds of challenges requires multitasking to the nth degree. "So, what do you do for a living?" "I'm a professional juggler."

Then, of course, you have the emotional component if there's a kid involved. You must be disciplined to keep that separate and take care of business; you have to deal with the emotions afterward. Obviously, kids are the toughest. You just can't let it distract you.

OxyContin is the scourge here, and meth is virtually ubiquitous. We're seeing obvious deaths and 911 calls from opioid overdoses. I'm about to launch a pilot program thanks to a donation of thousands of doses of nasal Narcan spray. We've started training LAPD officers, typically in high-impact areas like Skid Row and Hollywood and Venice, how to recognize an opioid overdose, give a squirt of Narcan, and save these people's lives before we even get there. The [opioid crisis] gets into moral, ethical, and political issues, but we have a lot of support. This work with the LAPD is evolving into a public health model.

In the last twenty years, I've also helped the push for more specialty EMS centers. In the past, people would call 911 and you'd take them to the closest ER. Now we have STEMI centers, primary and comprehensive stroke centers, and centers that specialize in neonatal care, sexual assault, and trauma. What literature has shown, and it's not unintuitive, is when you do something frequently, you get good at it.

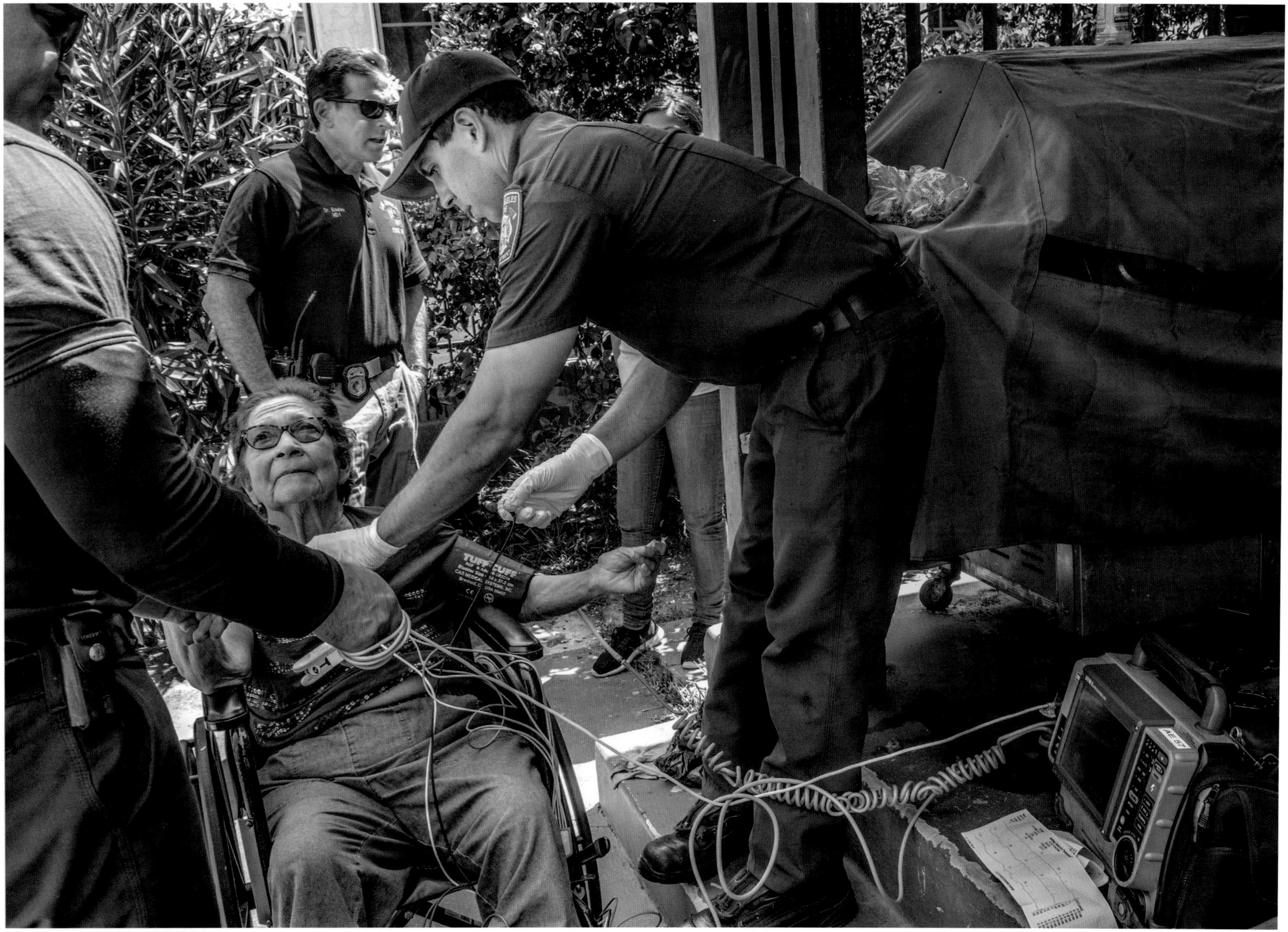

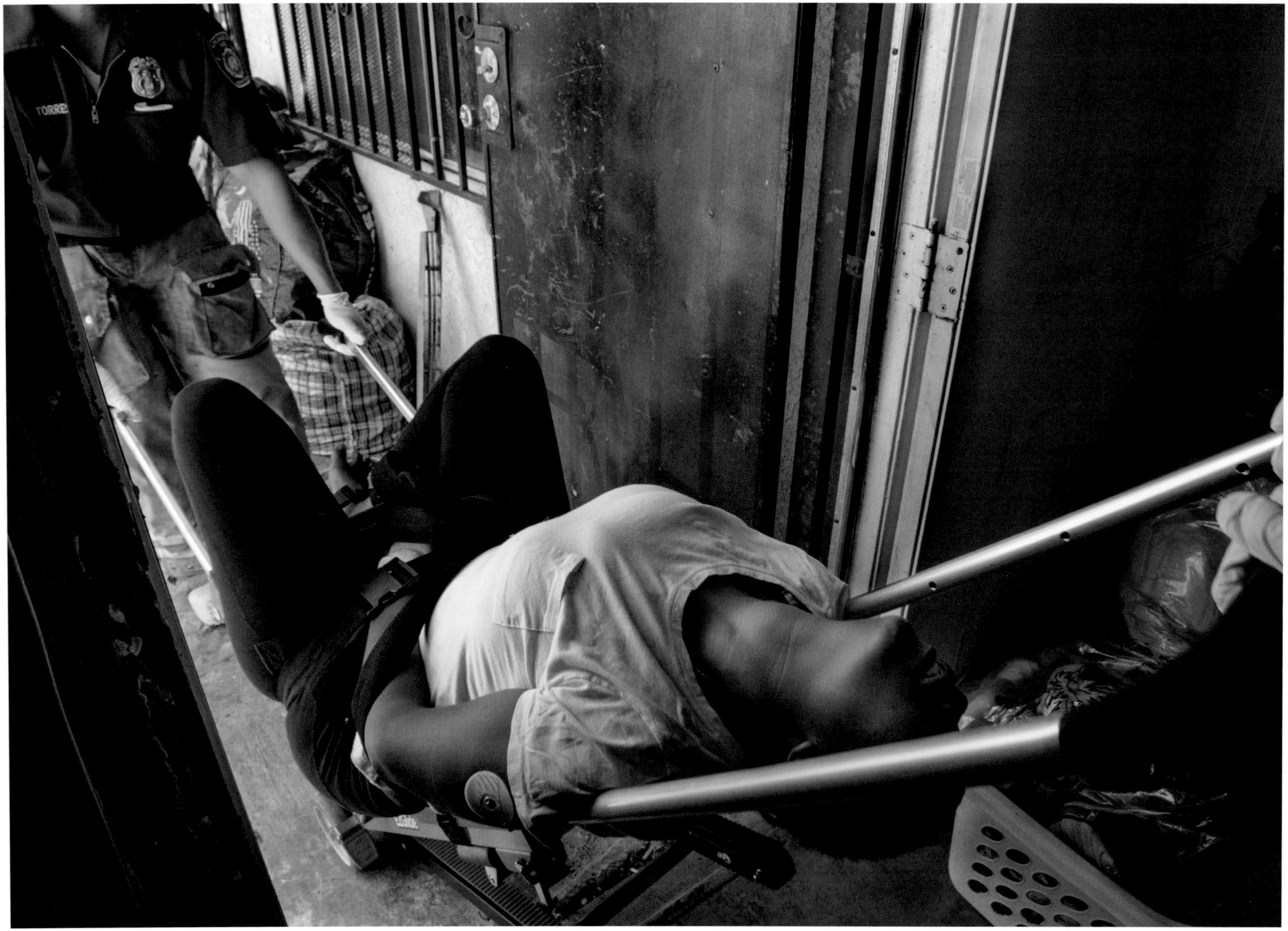

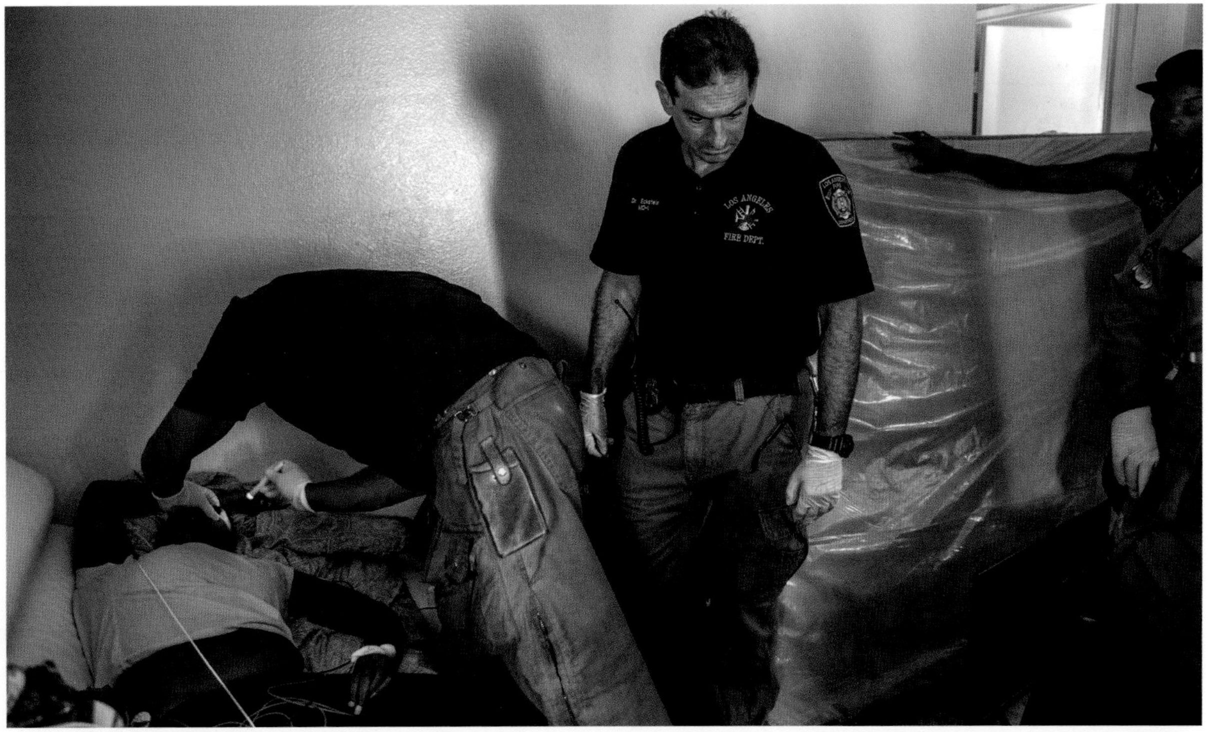

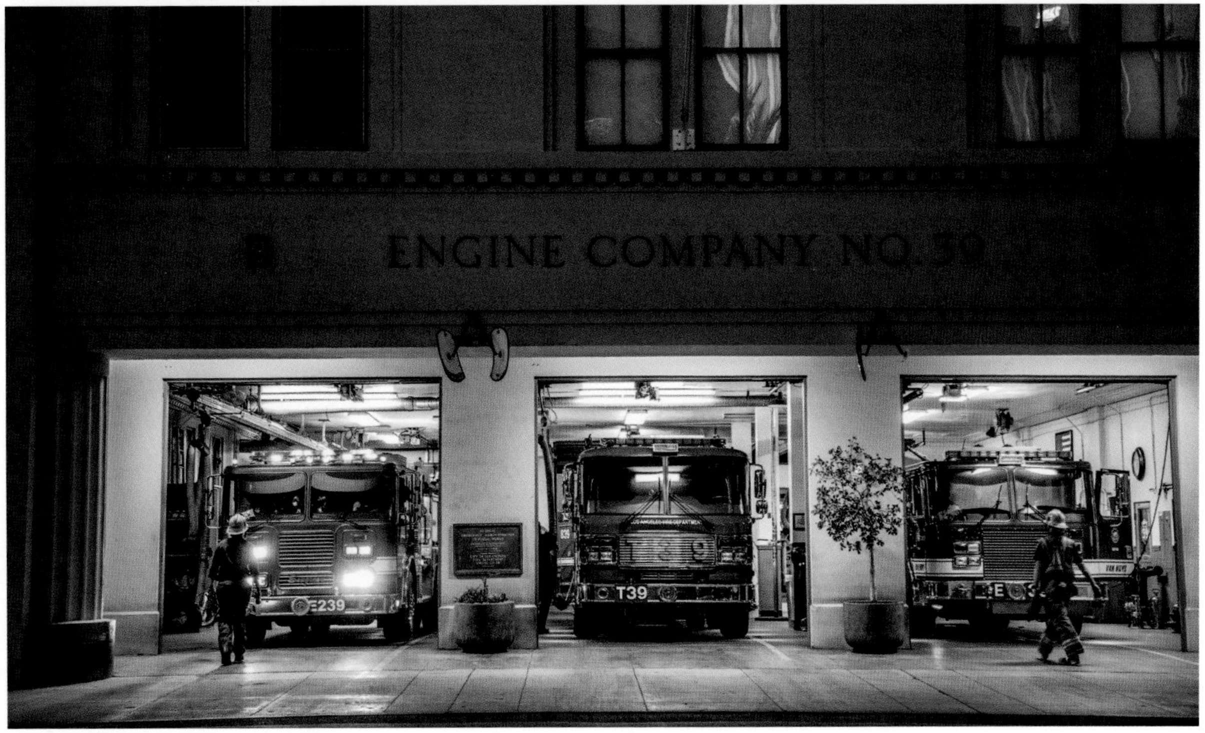

Certainly by the twenty-year mark — no matter what specialty you're in — things get pretty routine. But in emergency medicine or EMS, field saves come along once in a while. They just stick with you and make it all worthwhile. Very few professions allow you that, very few.

I went back to New York to work at the World Trade Center site after 9/11. As a New Yorker, it was very poignant for me. I remembered my parents taking me to the Windows on the World restaurant when I graduated from medical school; it was a big event. On our first full day there, it was pouring, just pouring. It almost was as if God was crying. It was absolutely surreal. Glass continued to fall from the surrounding skyscrapers. The closest we came to finding somebody — and we had very experienced cadaver dogs who were used to earthquake drills — was a torso buried a couple of feet down in debris. We found a wallet, so we were able to give closure to one family, but most of the bodies just basically vaporized. That was very demoralizing.

Being on scene for so many big incidents, including the Metrolink train crash in LA, has just . . . well, I'm grateful to be able to help and render care under the very worst circumstances. ✚

Susan Rowell, MD

Trauma Surgeon & Critical Care Specialist
Portland, Oregon

I worked my first shift as trauma chief on the same night I got back from maternity leave. My mother was watching the baby, but she refused to take a bottle . . . would only nurse. My mom calls and says, "Claire won't eat. She's been screaming all day!" I tell her to bring the baby to the hospital, but as soon as they arrive, I get a level-one trauma — a stab wound to the heart. The guy is under, and he's in arrest. We head straight to the OR.

I get on top of the gurney, so I can plug the hole in his heart with my finger; his chest is wide open, and there's blood everywhere. I'm rolling down the hall with my hand in this guy's chest, and, of course, the elevator opens up and there's my mom. She just looks at me.

I call her later and she says, "Susie, what was *that*?" I tell her the guy had been stabbed but lived. I'm so excited! I tell her I sewed up his heart. "You sewed up his heart?!" I was like, "Yeah, that's what you have to do." And she says, "But, Susie, you don't know how to sew."

I've thought many times maybe I should do elective laparoscopic surgeries instead . . . you know . . . something more "regular." But the truth is, I like not knowing exactly what's coming in next. I get bored if I'm doing the same thing all day. In trauma, you have a chance to save the lives of people who are dying. When you don't succeed, though, it really sucks. I always question myself. "Could I have done something different? What if I would've done this? What if I would've done that?" It's just the nature of the job.

I later found out the first guy I ever saved was a pimp. My first response was, "Oh, that's unfortunate." But you know, I'm not the one to judge. You just have to do the best you can and leave the personal circumstances out of it.

One of my worst cases was this eleven-year-old girl who was brought in after a car accident. She was in cardiac arrest. Her mom had died on the scene. I did everything I possibly could . . . opened her chest, her belly, all of it . . . but I just couldn't save her. The car they were in had been hit by an eighteen-year-old kid who had run a light. When they brought the girl to the ED, they also brought the guy who'd killed her; the only thing dividing them was a curtain. He didn't even have a license, had already gotten it taken away. That was a hard one. It made me think maybe I should do something else, find another job.

But that same day, out of the blue, I got an email from a patient I'd taken care of in my first year — a fifty-year-old guy who had been crushed by tractor equipment. He had ten kids. I probably operated on him twenty times; he received more than three hundred units of blood — our largest transfusion ever. Our chief of anesthesia warned me I'd exhausted the blood bank and told me to stop. But I said, "I'm not stopping until he dies." I didn't know it then, but the patient's wife heard the whole conversation. She thanked me for not giving up.

After a couple months in the hospital, he was able to go home. He doesn't have a brain injury; he's totally fine. His email read, "I just wanted to let you know that we wouldn't be here if it weren't for you. We just wanted to thank you again, and tell you how wonderful you are."

That's why I do this job. He's the reason. ✚

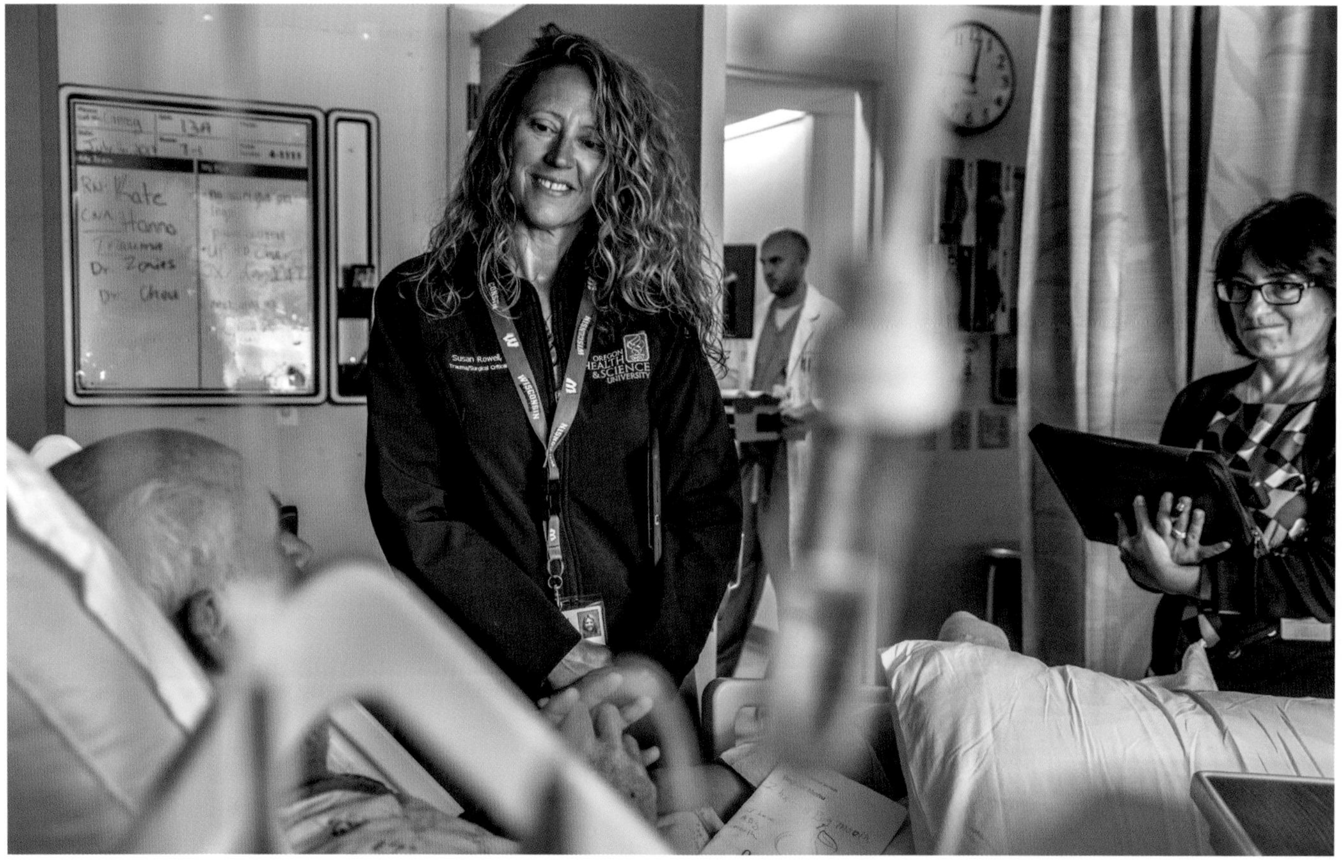

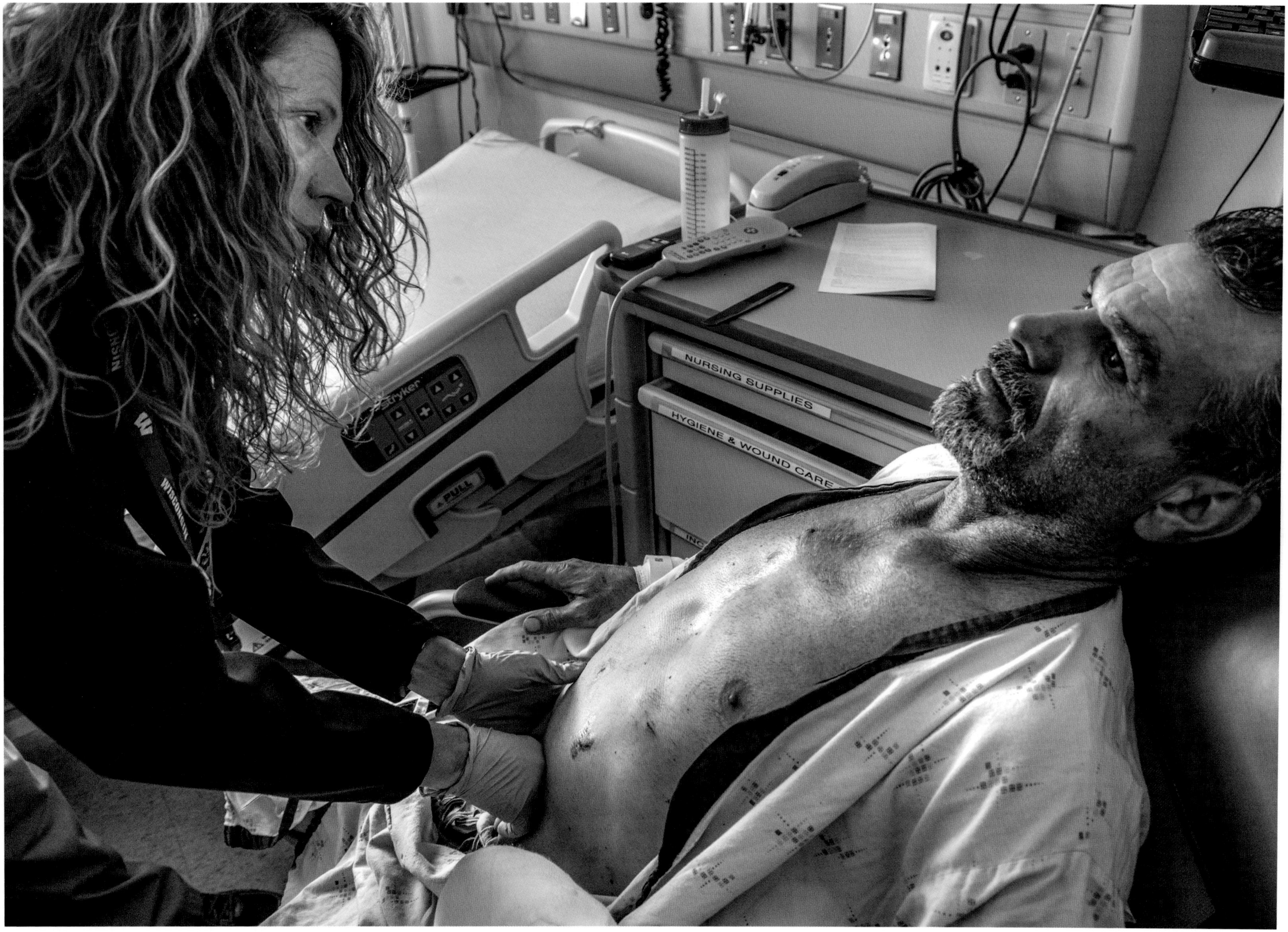
NURSING SUPPLIES
HYGIENE & WOUND CARE
PULL

Lewis Goldfrank, MD

Emergency Medicine & Toxicology Pioneer
New York, New York

Everything goes on here. Everybody comes here. We see everybody who gets in trouble, get to speak every language imaginable, get to see every culture imaginable. You come to an emergency department when you can't wait, when no one else is going to do what has to be done. The poorest guy comes in with the same kind of problem as the richest guy. Here, they get the same care.

We've made progress but sometimes not as much as we'd like to believe. Change is not constant. Like Obama said in his farewell speech, "You take two steps forward, one step back." I think we neglected the extent of the divisiveness and anger that is now so prevalent in our country — hatred that was just waiting for some next event. I mean, Americans have a lot of primitive values.

Patients come in because they're high on drugs . . . some are sociopaths . . . and we've got to care for them. But we've also got to find ways to support our staff, who are being humiliated and hated because of their names, because of what they look like. We've got Muslim residents, and suddenly you have someone who doesn't want to be cared for by them. These same patients like to think of our people as porters, as opposed to doctors. We have had staff say their white coat isn't enough to hide their black skin.

It's a discrimination of the old days, and passivity makes it worse. Martin Luther King said the problem lies less with those leading the racist efforts and more with the vast majority of people who sit by, let things happen, and don't say a thing. So, we're working on it — preparing for the psychological consequences of the new climate of hatred. We held a staff meeting around the concept of Camus's *L'Étranger*, which is better translated as "the outsider" rather than "the stranger." I mean, everybody feels he or she is an outsider. The question is how to bring people together.

My mother was a writer and an activist. She spent a lot of time in the mines of West Virginia and Pennsylvania. My father, like his parents, was involved in the development of the Ethical Culture Society, which was responsible for a lot of progressive activities. Together, they wrote a lot of children's books. We lived way out in the country during the '40s, so all I really had were the dog and nature — and I did a whole lot of reading. Plus, there were lots of intellects who spent time at our house, talking about mathematics, science, everything imaginable. I remember when I was maybe ten years of age, I read "The Annals of Medicine" by Berton Roueché and lots of books on Darwin and Marie Curie. I came away understanding the purpose of life was to find a problem in the world and solve it.

It was the McCarthy Era. In time, my mother would be investigated and both my parents would lose their jobs. Still, they were optimists. Issues like race and the health of the coal miners were consequential, and you worked on them. You didn't worry about what might happen to you, as long as you were doing the right thing.

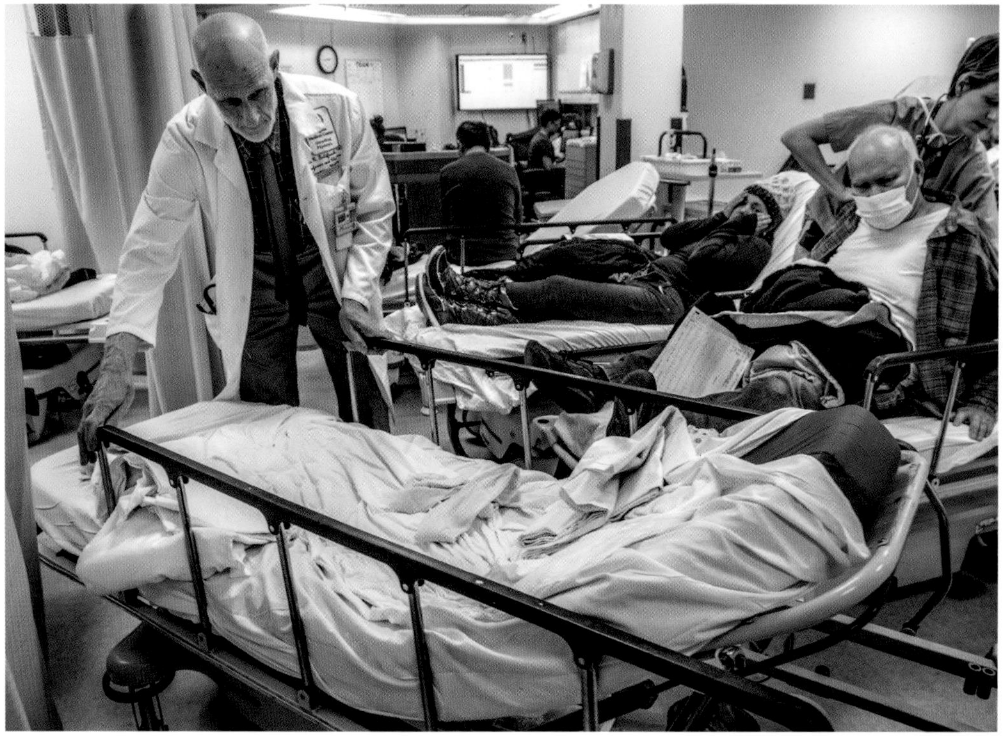

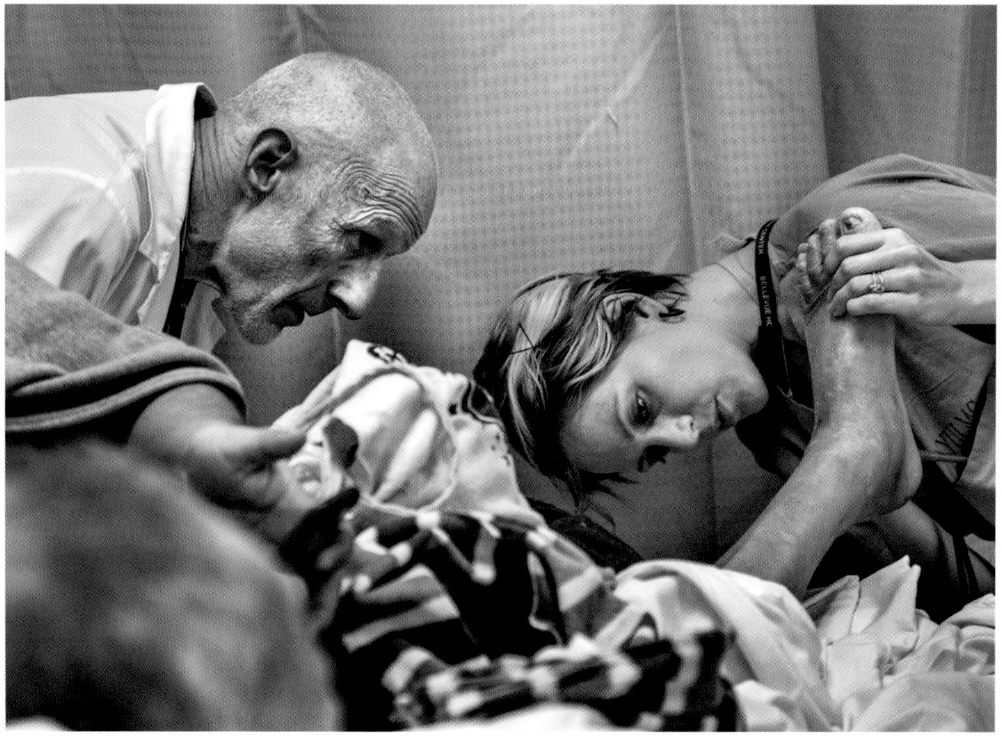

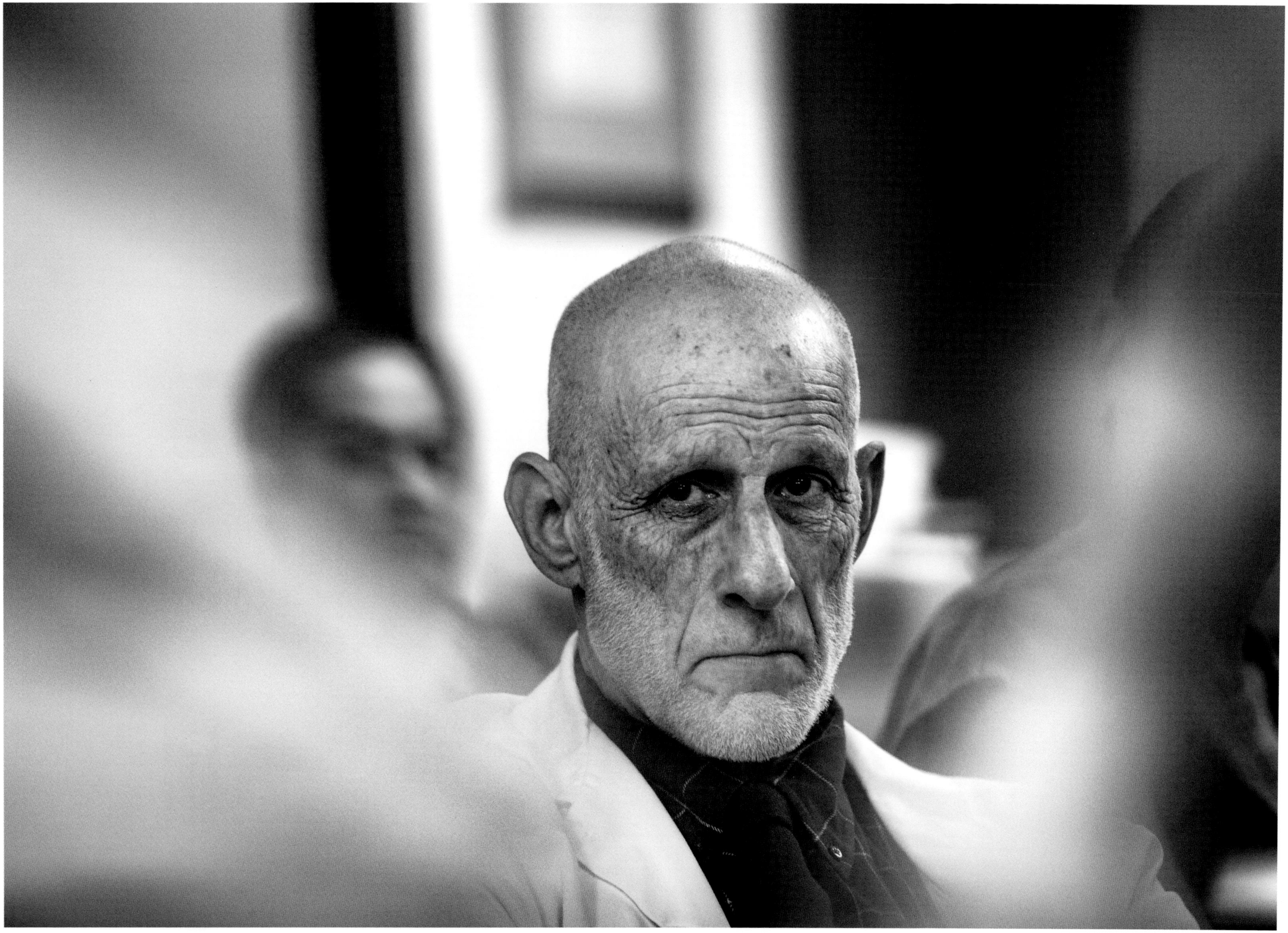

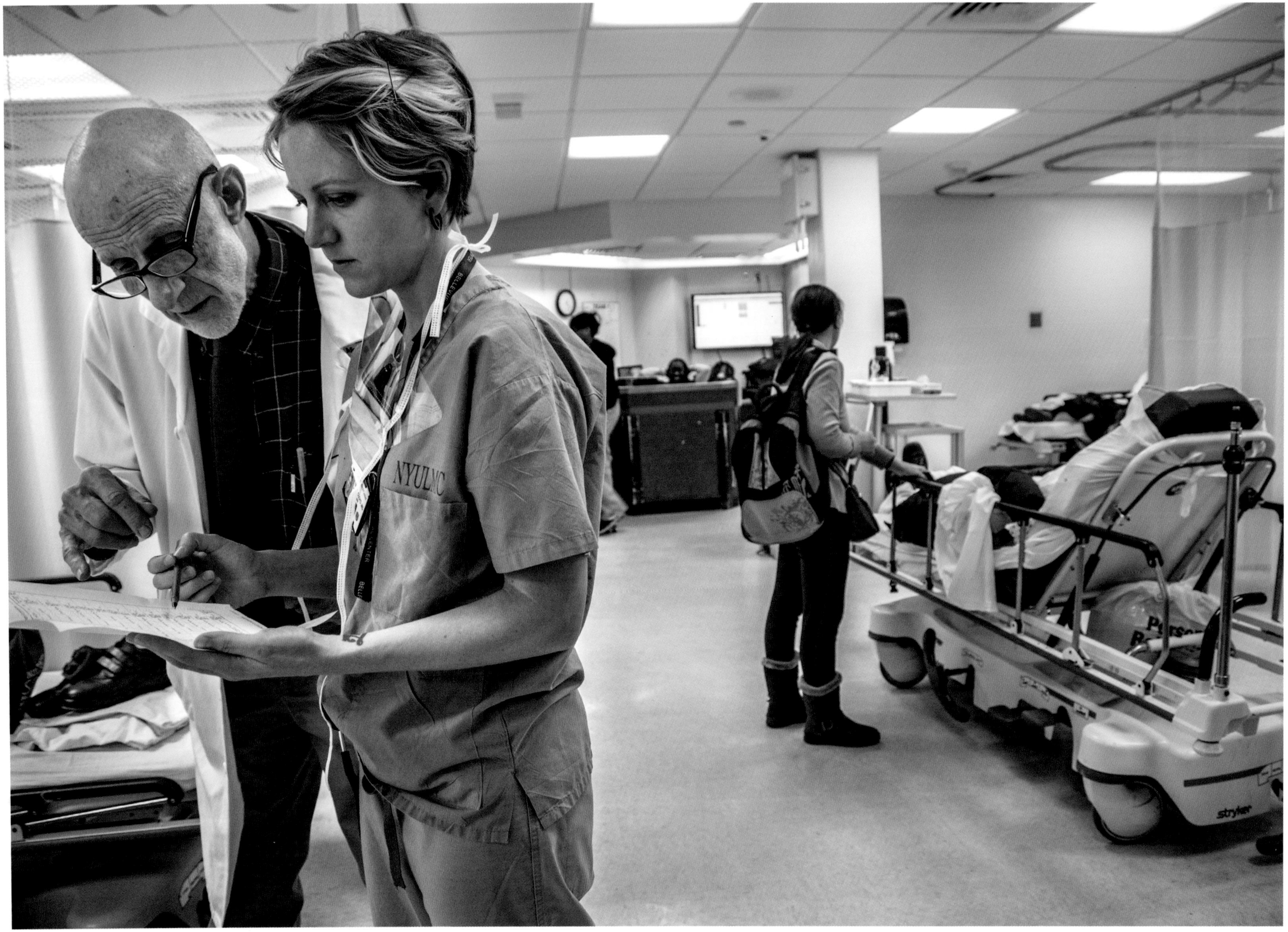
NYULMC
stryker

Those threads of a societal problem and people working to solve it, that's where I was heading. After graduating from medical school in Belgium, I interned in Connecticut. One of my first rotations as a resident was in the South Bronx. It was 1972. It was a very small space, and we had 100,000 people going in and out of there. By the end of my second year of residency — it was in internal medicine — I recognized what I wanted to do. I wrote a grant proposal to become the leader of the emergency department. I said we would develop a department that fused public health, primary care, and emergent care.

There were no ambulances at the time . . . only hearses the city used to transport the dead. Patients walked in or were dropped off. These were people no one was interested in supporting — they were the totally disenfranchised. The way I saw it, the poverty in the South Bronx was a public health crisis, a human rights issue. There were tremendous knife and gun injuries. We saw heroin overdoses and lead poisoning every day . . . septic abortions. And there were no textbooks, nothing much in the literature at that time to say what emergency medicine would be. We were starting from the ground up. ✚

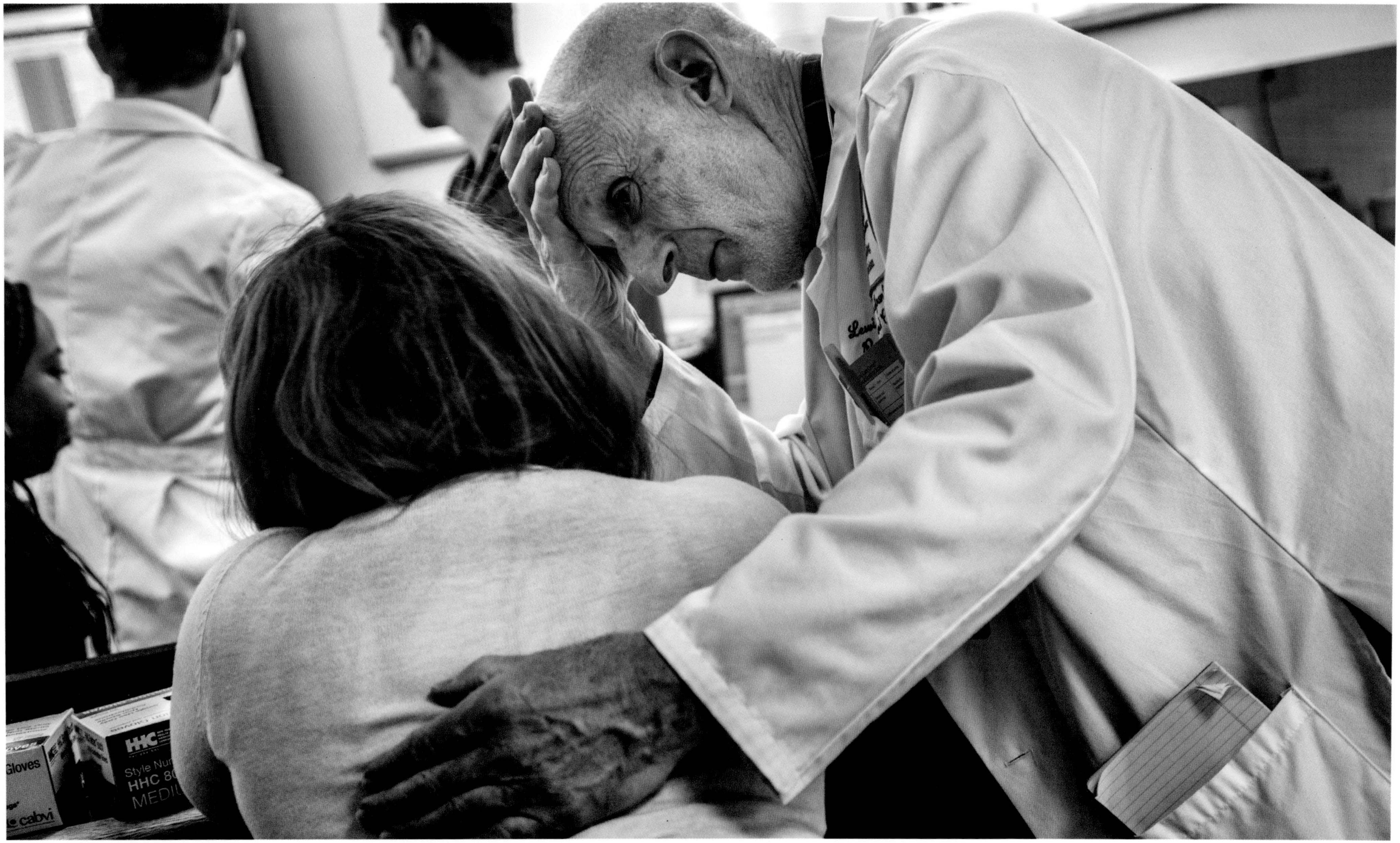

Glen Lee, RN

Emergency Nurse
Los Angeles, California

I love bedside patient care. If a family goes to hospital, they are nervous all the time. It's a new environment . . . you know, needle and knife. They think about the hospital as really formal, not fun. My thing is different. If my patients are freaking out or have a lot of pain, I make jokes. And then I dance and sing for them. They love it. They open mind. We have a really famous song in Korea, "Gangnam Style." I still use that one. When I care for patient, they are laughing, crying, laughing, like that. I think laughing together is good medication, smiling together. The residency school pin me up as nurse of the year. I ask, "Why you choose me?" They said, "You're a good dancer!"

I'm from Kunshan, South Korea, a small town. I immigrated here in 1998 after I graduated from law school and finished a mandatory three-year military service. I was a Taekwondo instructor in the Korean Army. I have a fourth-degree black belt. When I was a new nurse, they called me "Crazy Kung Fu Panda." They know I love martial arts. I'm good at kicking and dancing. I really enjoy all my work, every single day . . . sometimes too much. Mentally, I'm not that exhausted. But after twelve hours, I don't have much physical energy. After work I go to gym; I have to reset button. In the morning, I take quiet time. All the time I think about balance, physically and mentally.

We have a bunch of very good nurses here. I'm just average, but I do my best all the time. Some patients need water, but you cannot give it, right? Other nurses, they tell patients they are not allowed water. I don't say it like that. I explain why you cannot drink water. You may be going to surgery. If you take water and then get anesthesiology, it can make you choke. I not nurse for money. I focus on person first.

We get big accidents with kids. They are drowning, they are hit by car — some by their parents' car. I'm really sad for pediatric patients, but I'm really happy saving lives. I remember one of my former patients. He got multiple gunshot wounds — shoulder and chest and optimal area. He almost died. One month later, he complain of chest pain and came back to ER. I tell him, "I remember you." He told me, "You guys saved my life. I really appreciate that." That's why I love my job.

I've been to Korea. People ask me, "You want to be a senator? You want to be a lawyer? You want to be some businessman? Which one you like?" I would choose nursing again. I'm proud of my job that much. ✚

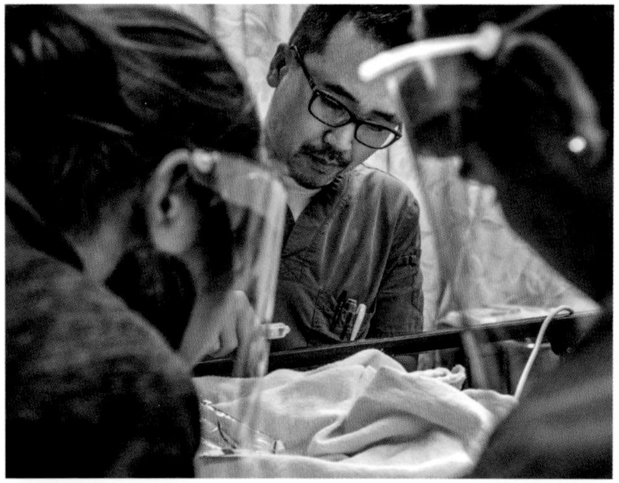

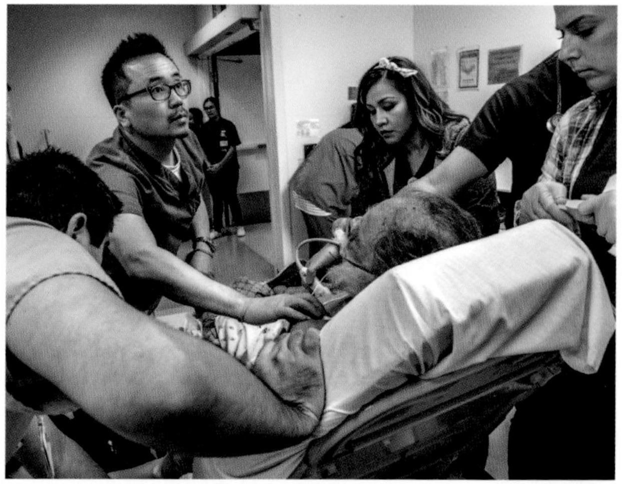

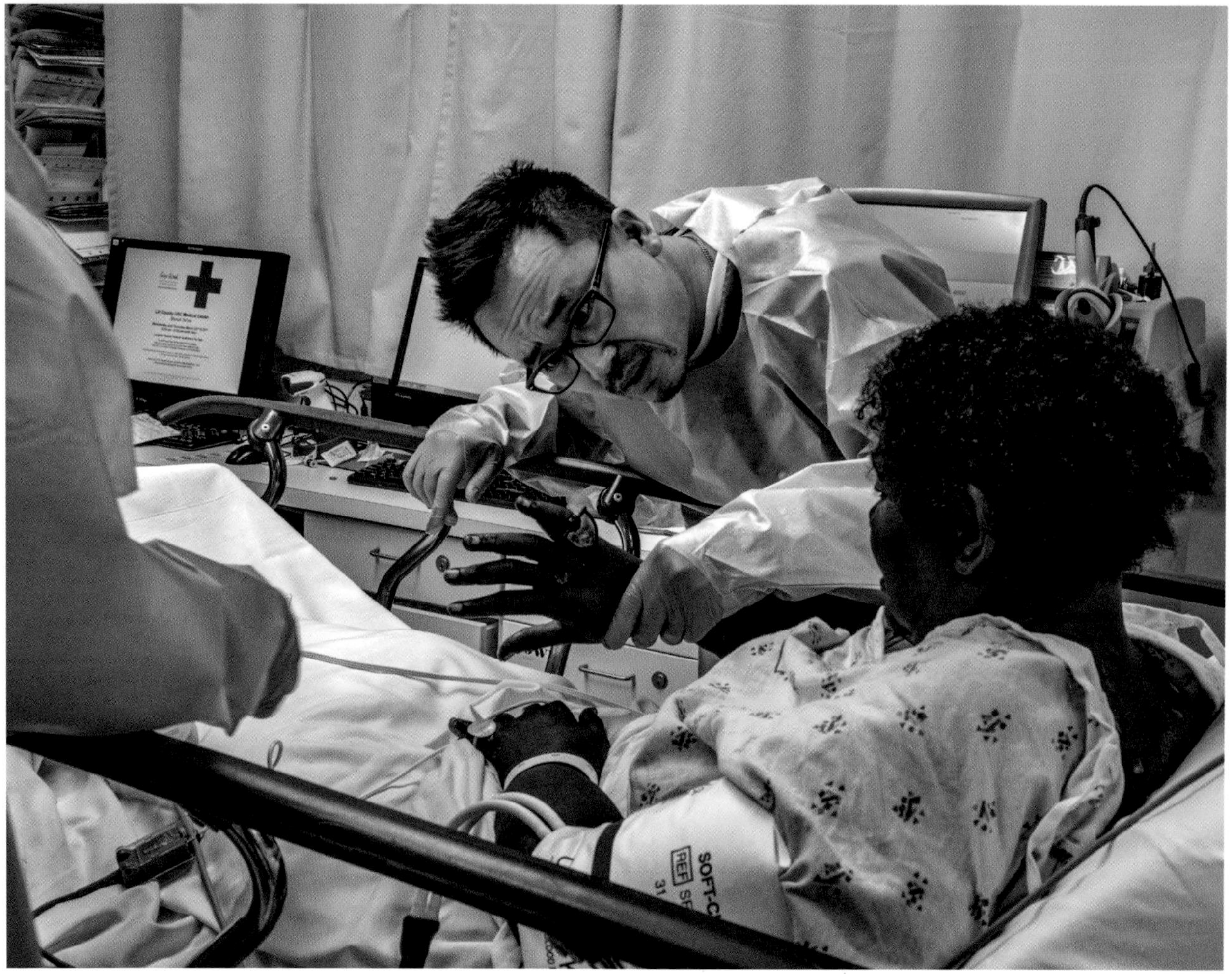

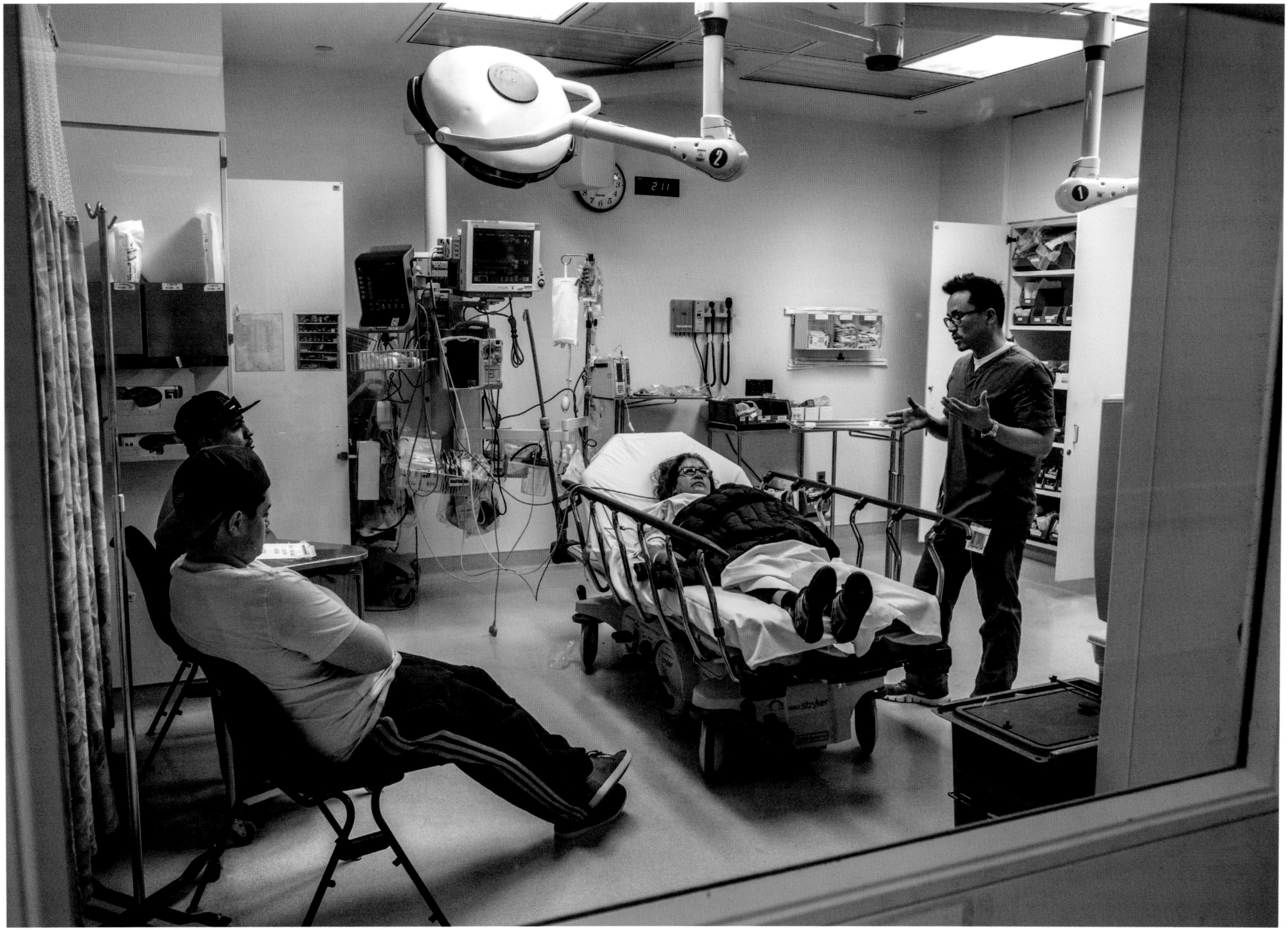

Glen Lee, RN

Jeffrey Keller, MD

Emergency & Correctional Medicine Physician
Idaho Falls, Idaho

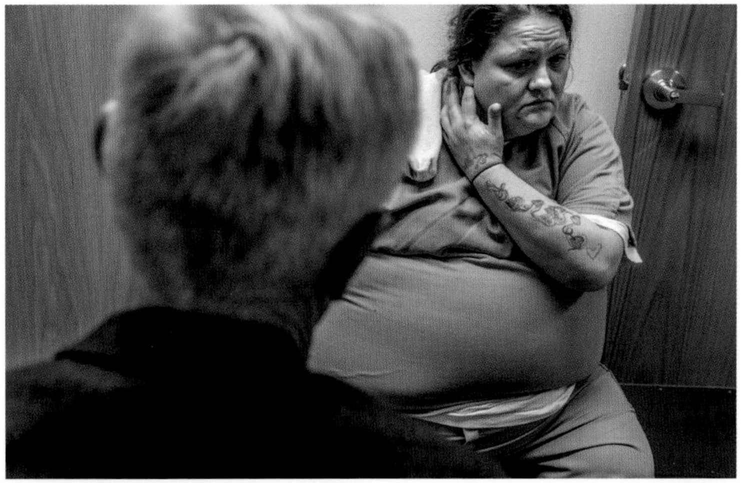

Part of the issue with correctional medicine is people aren't lining up to go into it. Back in medical school and residency, nobody said, "You know, you really ought to think about prisons and jails. *That's* where your talent would be best utilized."

I got a call from the county commissioners in the mid-1990s. They needed a doctor for the jail, and my name came up because I worked with paramedics and the paramedics were good friends with the deputies. They asked if I would be willing to take the job. Being the civic-minded good ol' boy that I was, I said, "Hell, no! What, are you nuts? Who'd work in a *jail*?"

After I'd already turned them down twice, the commissioners came back a third time about a year later. They said, "We're desperate." The jail was under an ACLU consent decree; they had lost a legal battle related to conditions there. A good chunk of the court order concerned the way medical care should be delivered, but the doctors were refusing to abide by the decree. It was a miserable, horrible place.

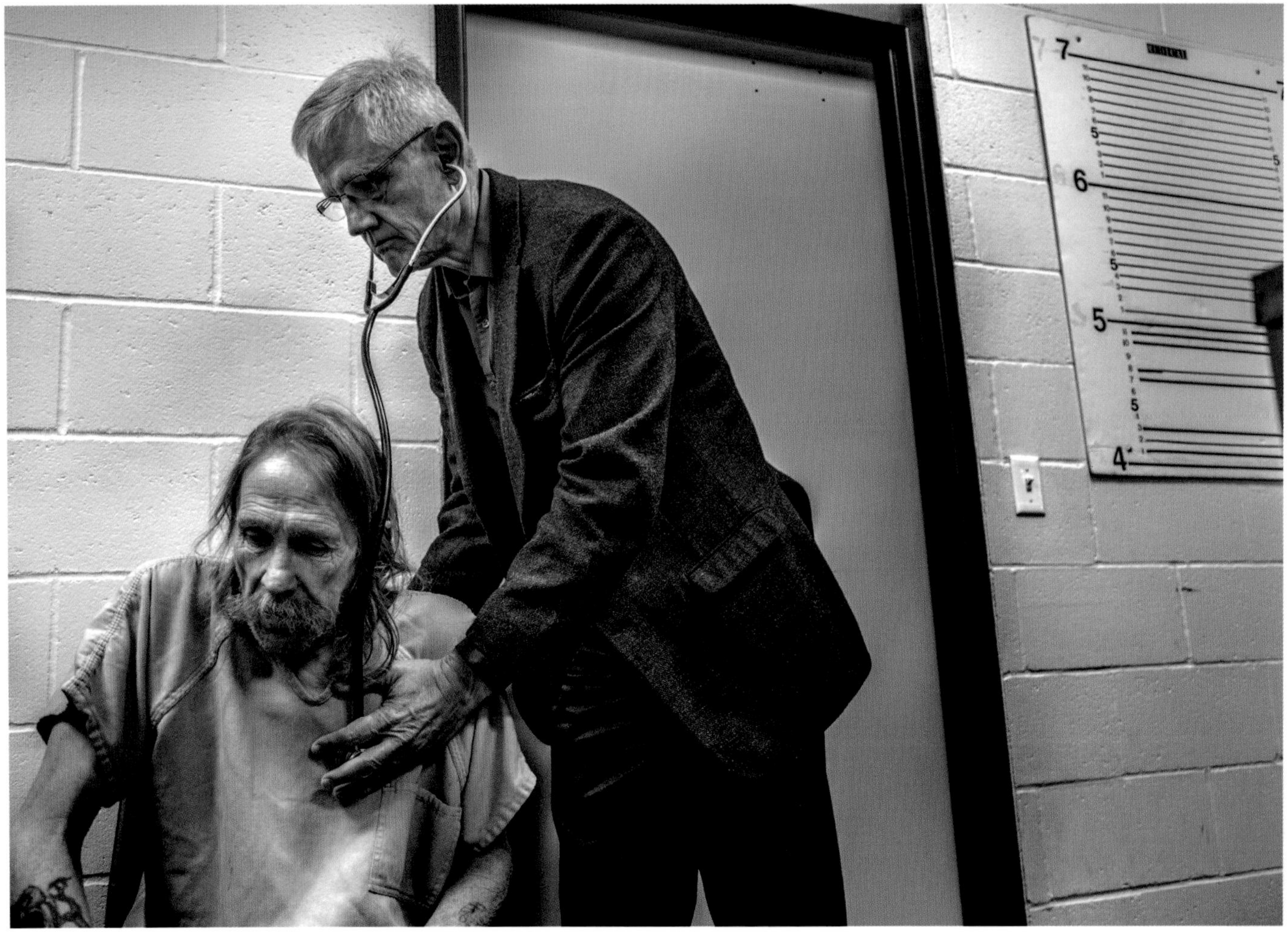

I finally agreed to bail them out but only until they could find somebody else. I found out two things that year. One, I liked it. Two, my phone wouldn't stop ringing. "We're the Bingham County Jail down the road and we need a doctor." "We're the Jefferson County Jail down the road and we need a doctor, too." All of a sudden, I was in charge of five, ten, then fifteen jails.

When I took over the first one, there wasn't a medical room, so we commandeered an office — maybe a classroom. A folding table covered with a sheet became the exam table. There were no cabinets; everything had to be carried in. We had to figure out how to dispense medications properly. The other doctors weren't willing to tackle any of those issues. Even though the jail was decrepit and old, it took four attempts before the city could pass a bond issue to build a new one. But I bet nobody would have thought twice about funding a clinic in Haiti. Things are improving, though. We expect better in the United States — and we should have better.

Jail doctors have the same stigma ER doctors used to have. Back in the 1950s if you said, "I'm going to be an ER doctor full time," people would ask, "What's wrong with you that you can't have a real practice?" The other residents looked down on us. Their opinion was, "I can do your job

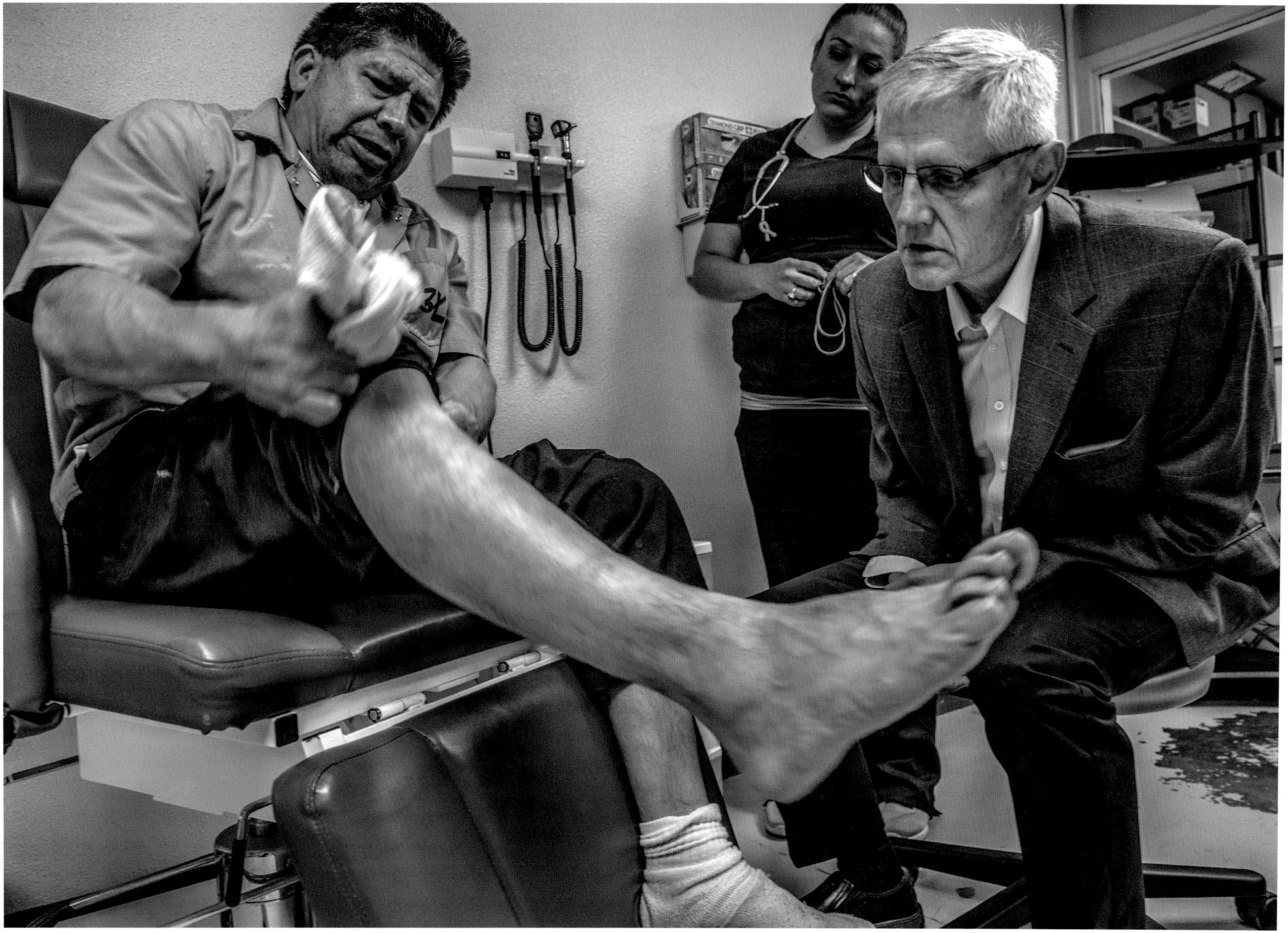

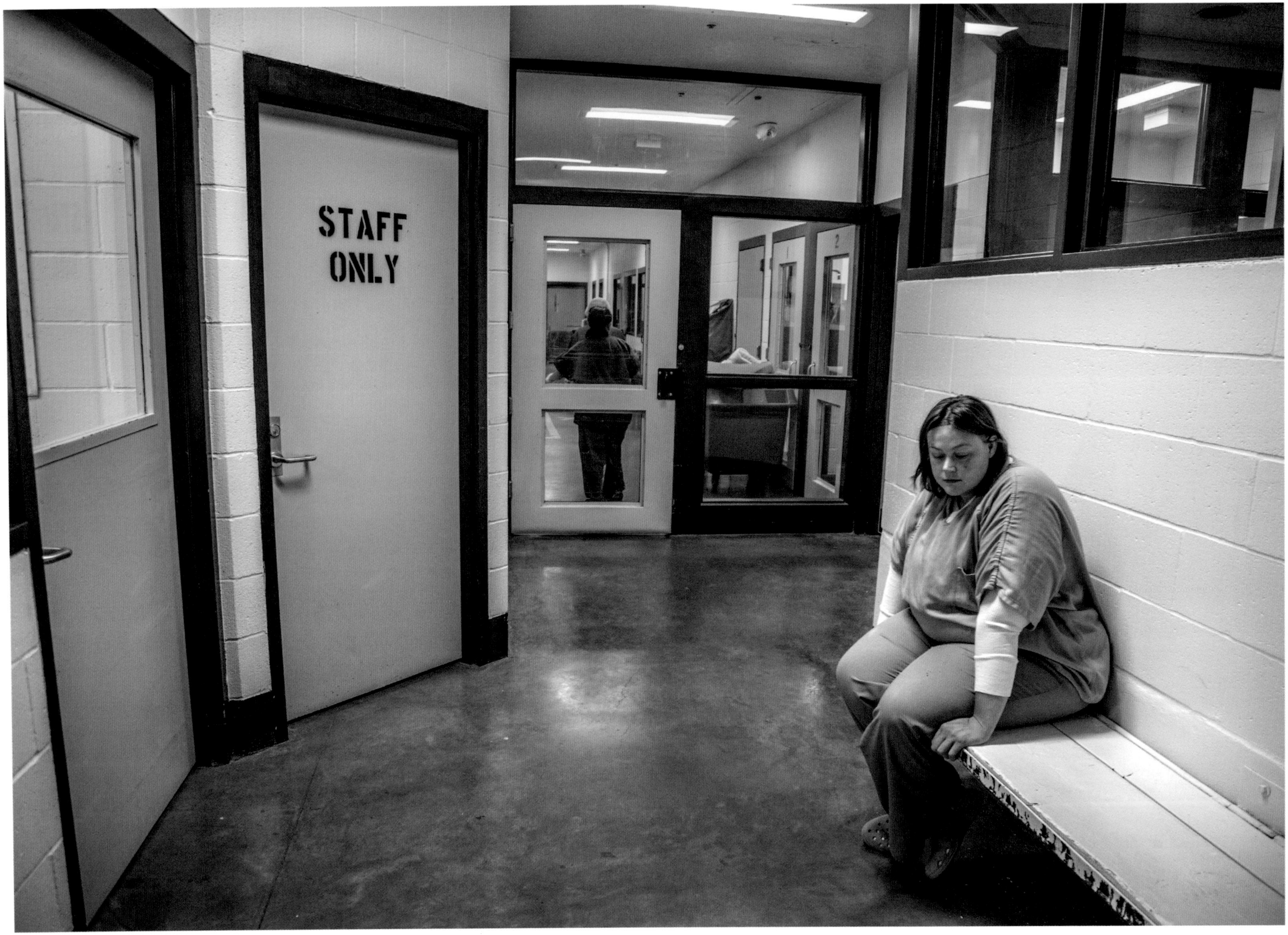
STAFF
ONLY

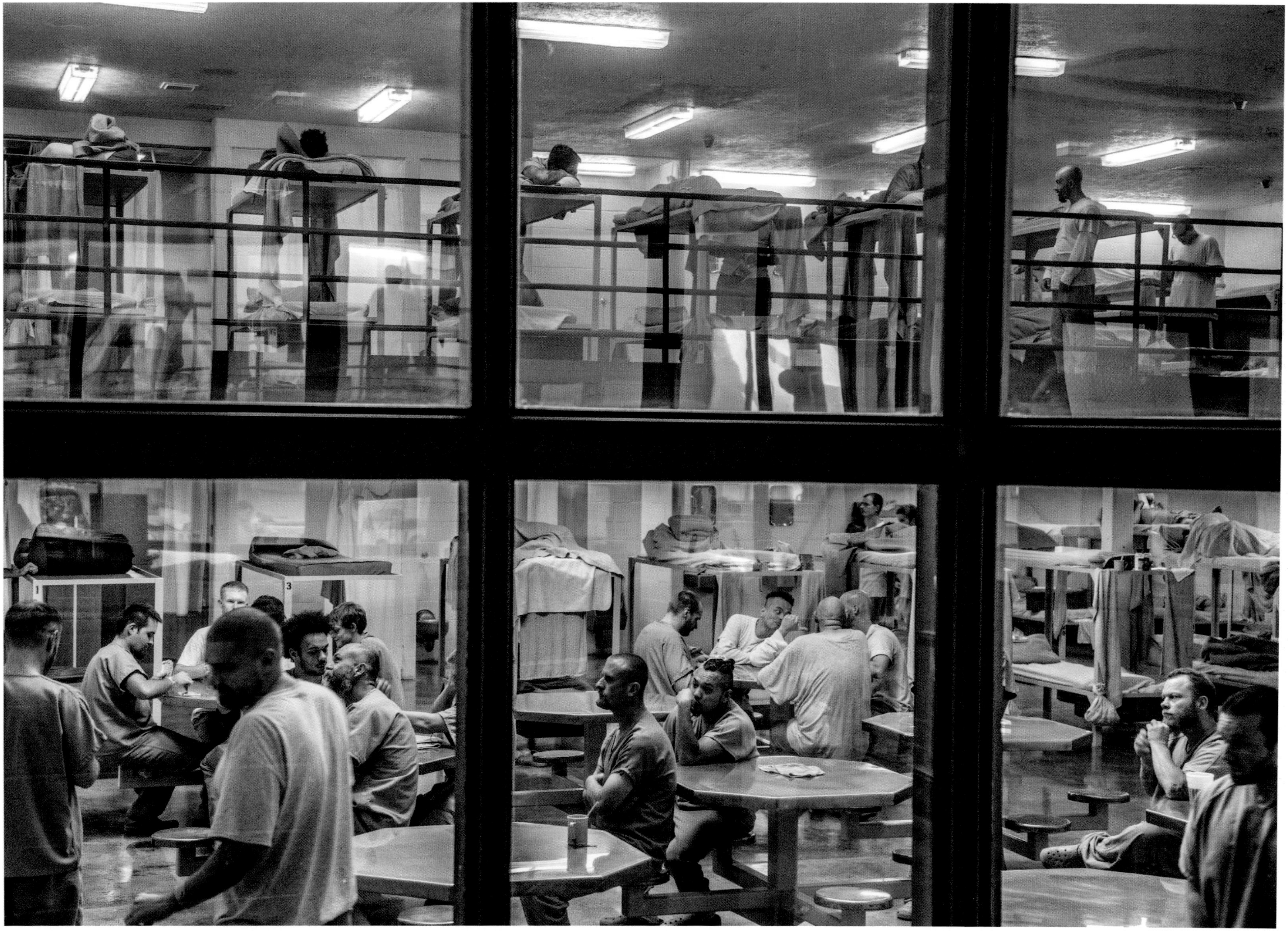

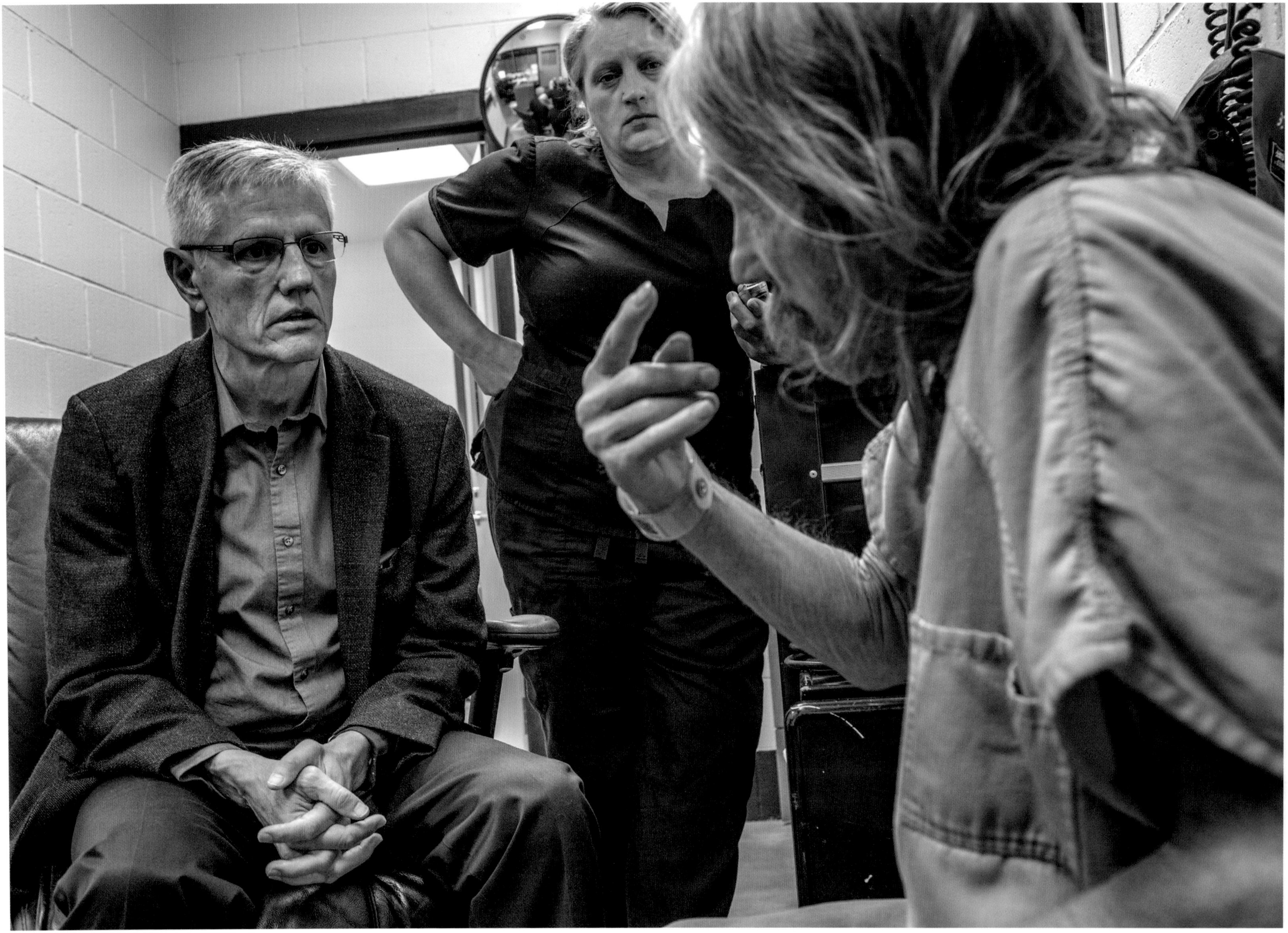

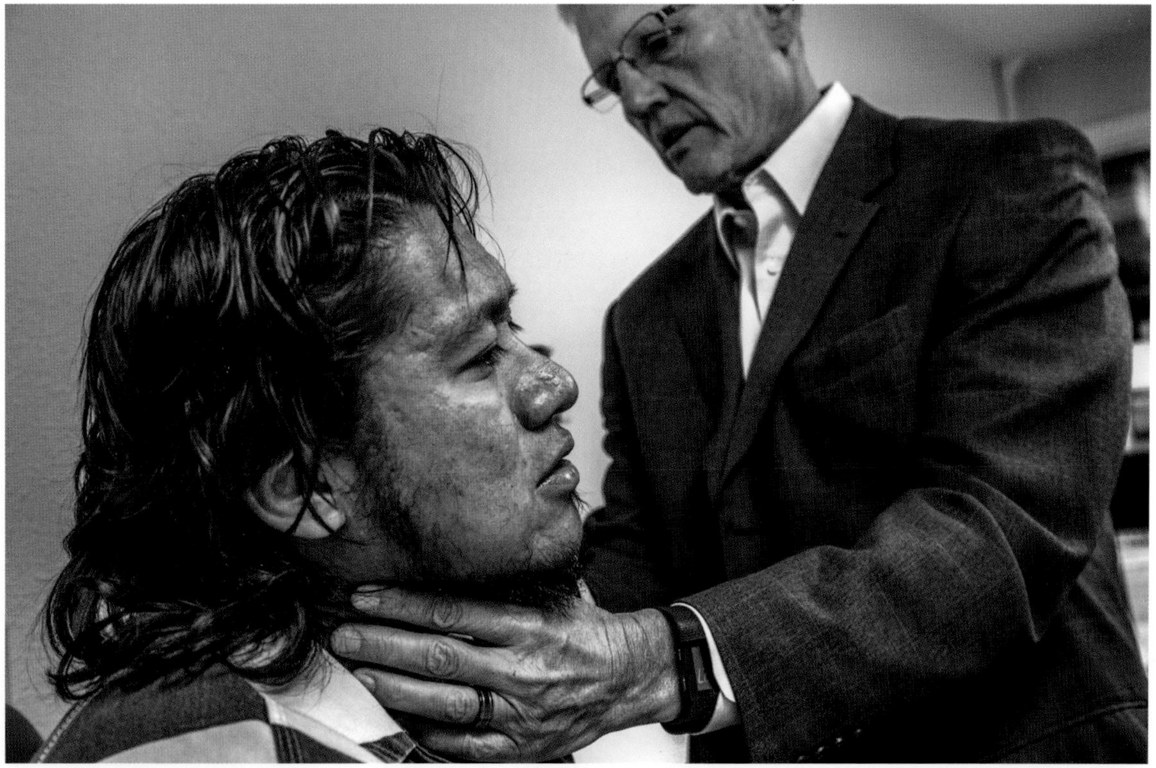

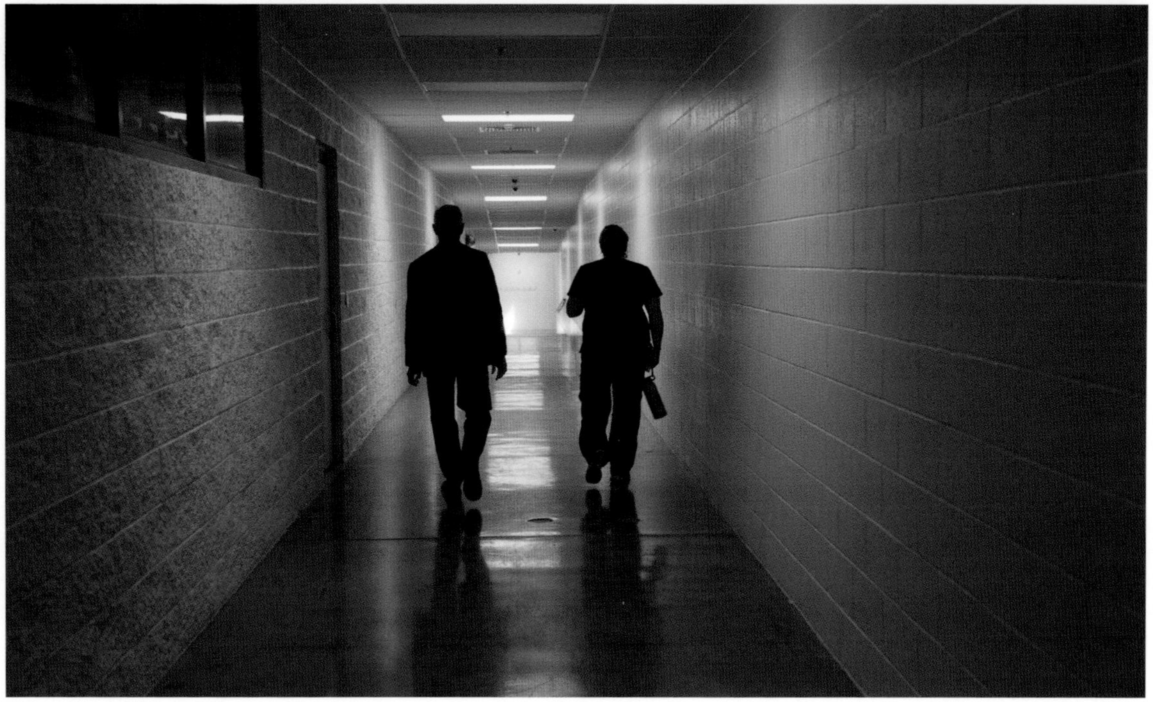

and mine. You're just glorified triage nurses." That attitude has changed toward ER physicians but not toward correctional doctors. They ask, "Do you have a restriction on your license that prevents you from being around children? It's got to be something like that."

I've been thinking about what causes that emotional reaction. Many assume people are in jail to be punished, and therefore have no right to health care. That's not right, of course. It's also not right to say people are there to be punished. Most of them are pre-trial detainees, so they're innocent until proven guilty. Unlike prisons, where the inmates have all been sentenced, people are held in jail pending trial.

Correctional medicine is different in a lot of ways, and it took me about two years to get comfortable with all the nuances. I had to learn how to deal with psychoses. I had to learn the drugs. I had to learn how to diagnose. I had to learn the difference between true mental illness and a personality disorder.

A lot of jail medicine isn't medicine at all. An inmate will say, "I've got this bad back, and the mattresses are really hard. I need you to give me a medical authorization for a double mattress." (I've never seen anything in a medical textbook about treating back pain with a double mattress.) Or, "I have a knee injury and these jail shoes are horrible. I need medical authorization to wear my own Air Jordans." On and on. These are comfort issues, not medical issues.

Safety and security come before medical care in this setting. You cannot be alone with a patient, ever. It has to be that way. A guy was here for about a year and a half on an attempted murder charge. His presence made the hair on the back of your neck stand up. He hated women; he tried to murder his mother with an ax. We brought him into the clinic, and he leaned over and bit the nurse on the breast when she was taking his blood pressure. He even faked a seizure to get the attention of a female nurse. Women stopped responding to his emergencies. There are lots of stories like that. Still, I'm safer here than I was in the ER.

Some doctors can't deal with the inmates who get in their face, the verbal jiu-jitsu. But I like this job; it's very satisfying. I feel like I'm doing good. The down side is the physical plant — clanging doors, having to push a button every time you want to go through one. You can't get patients delivered; everything is locked down. It's cold, even in the middle of summer. And the smell, it stinks sometimes.

The Supreme Court ruled in *Estelle v. Gamble* that inmates have a right to medical care; denying it violates their rights. Inmates can't go out and find good doctors. Good doctors have to come to them. ✚

Meghan Lindstrom, MD

Emergency Physician
Palmer, Alaska

Some of my earliest memories are in Anchorage hospitals, peeking through a doorway, watching my dad at the bedside. I grew up thinking the hospital was a wonderful place, where the nurses were kind and there was an unending supply of graham crackers and chocolate milk. It was where people were healed. My dad was an internist, and his patients just adored him. He had one speed — *slow*. He walked with his hands behind his back, always whistling. He was incredibly patient, which is not one of my virtues, but I always wanted to be just like him.

I put myself through college partly by winning a scholarship pageant my mother signed me up for. And then when I was in my thirties, I got into bodybuilding. I'd been a lifelong athlete, but I could feel myself begin to atrophy after I had kids. I found my time in the gym could be a great defense against burnout. That one hour a day seemed like a vacation — my respite from work and responsibilities at home.

When I entered my first bodybuilding competition, I had to wrap my mind around the idea that it was not a bikini contest — it was a sport. I trained hard, ate clean, and — really by accident — started to win. But I don't feel like I'm competing against the people flanking me; it's more personal. *Have I reached my goals? How far have I come? How can I do better next time?* Sure, it's fun to win trophies and bragging rights, but I feel like I've won just by trying something new.

Emergency physicians fill a unique role in Alaska, servicing a community that is really close knit despite the fact its people are separated by many, many miles. Certainly, every ER receives patients from many walks of life but, in Alaska, I can see a world-famous musher, followed by a climber off the top of Denali from who-knows-where in the world, followed by the local high school principal. I love the variety, the challenge.

Out here, you don't have to wander very far to really realize you're in the middle of nowhere at the mercy of Mother Nature. We see a lot of aircraft wrecks, but there are certain cases that stand out — one involved two pilots who had been missing for three days. Everybody had written them off, but — miraculously — they managed to crawl out of the wilderness, injured and covered in blood. They spent hours shimmying down ravines and across rivers . . . fended off a mother bear and her cubs . . . until they were rescued by a couple of guys who were out four-wheeling.

I finished assessing one of the patients and remember hearing the beep and the opening of the door as the family was buzzed through. I'll never forget the sight of his wife running down that hallway . . . the shriek and the thrill . . . the mixture of joy and terror . . . the release of fear that came with the realization her husband was alive.

Even on the worst days . . . the *Why am I doing this?* days . . . the shifts full of drug seekers and perfectly healthy patients who think they're dying because of something they read on the Internet . . . I think about the cases with happy endings. And I remember how grateful I am to have found myself here . . . on the frontier serving my community. ✚

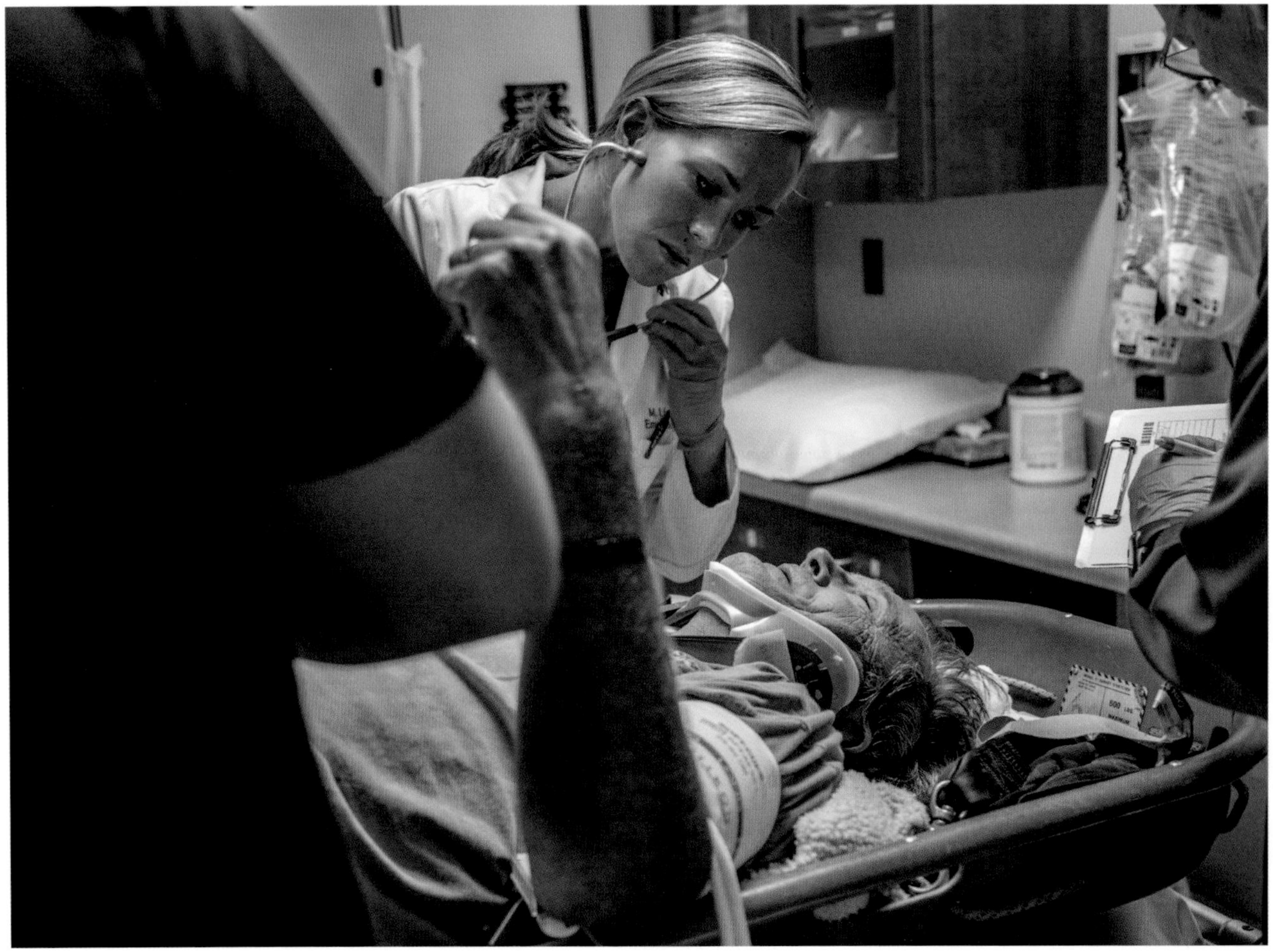

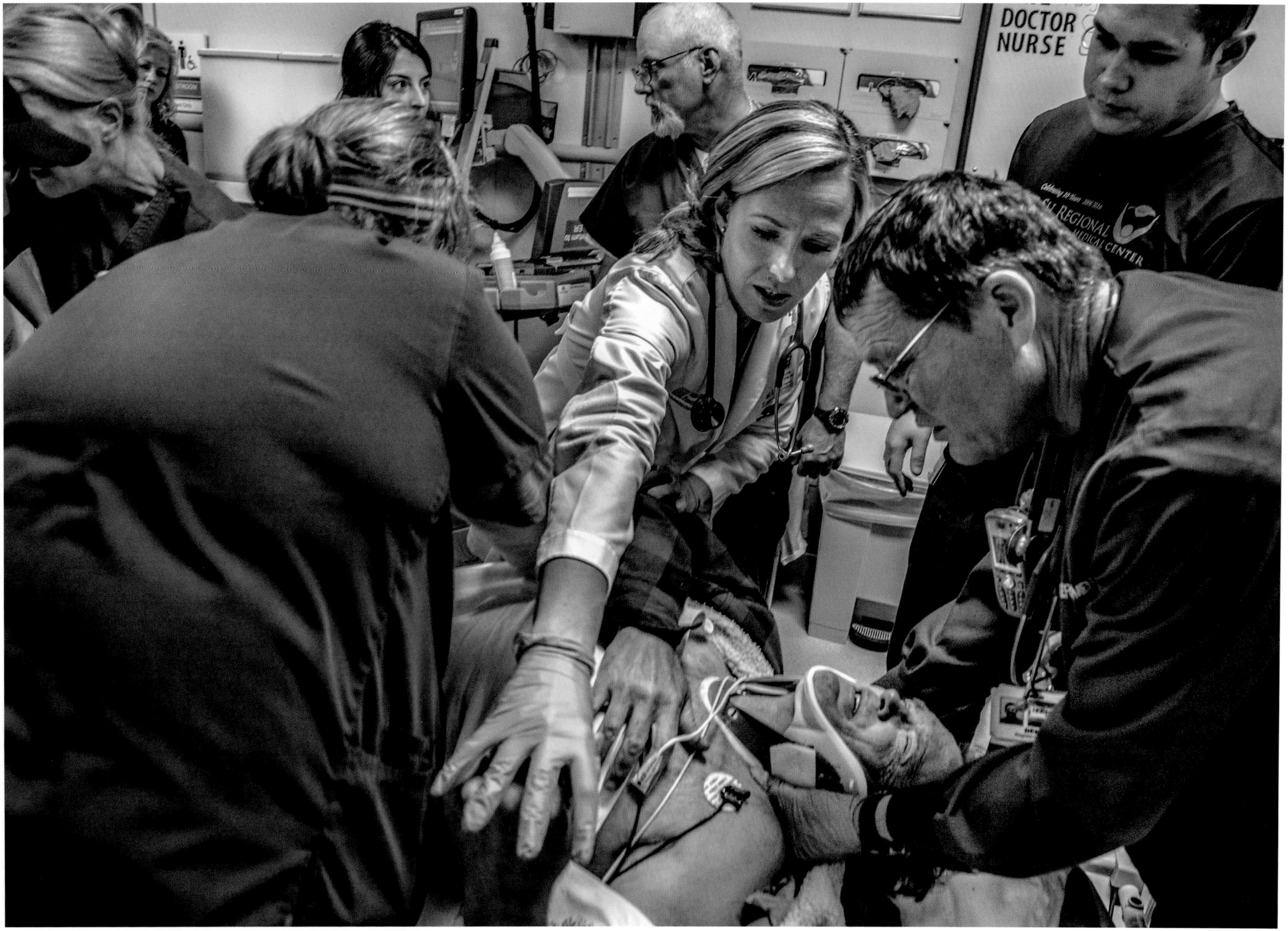

Meghan Lindstrom, MD

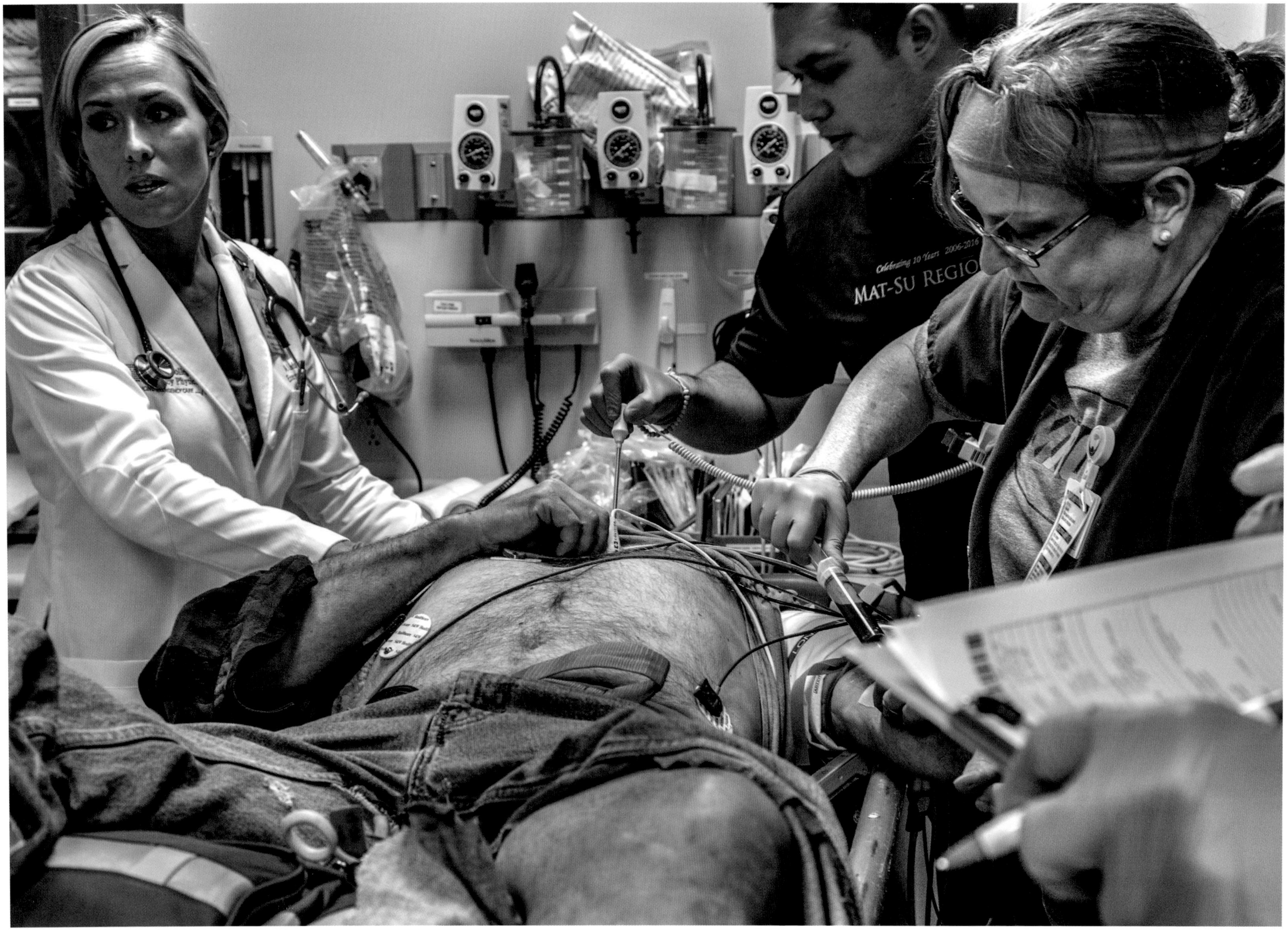
Celebrating 10 Years 2006-2016
MAT-SU REGIO

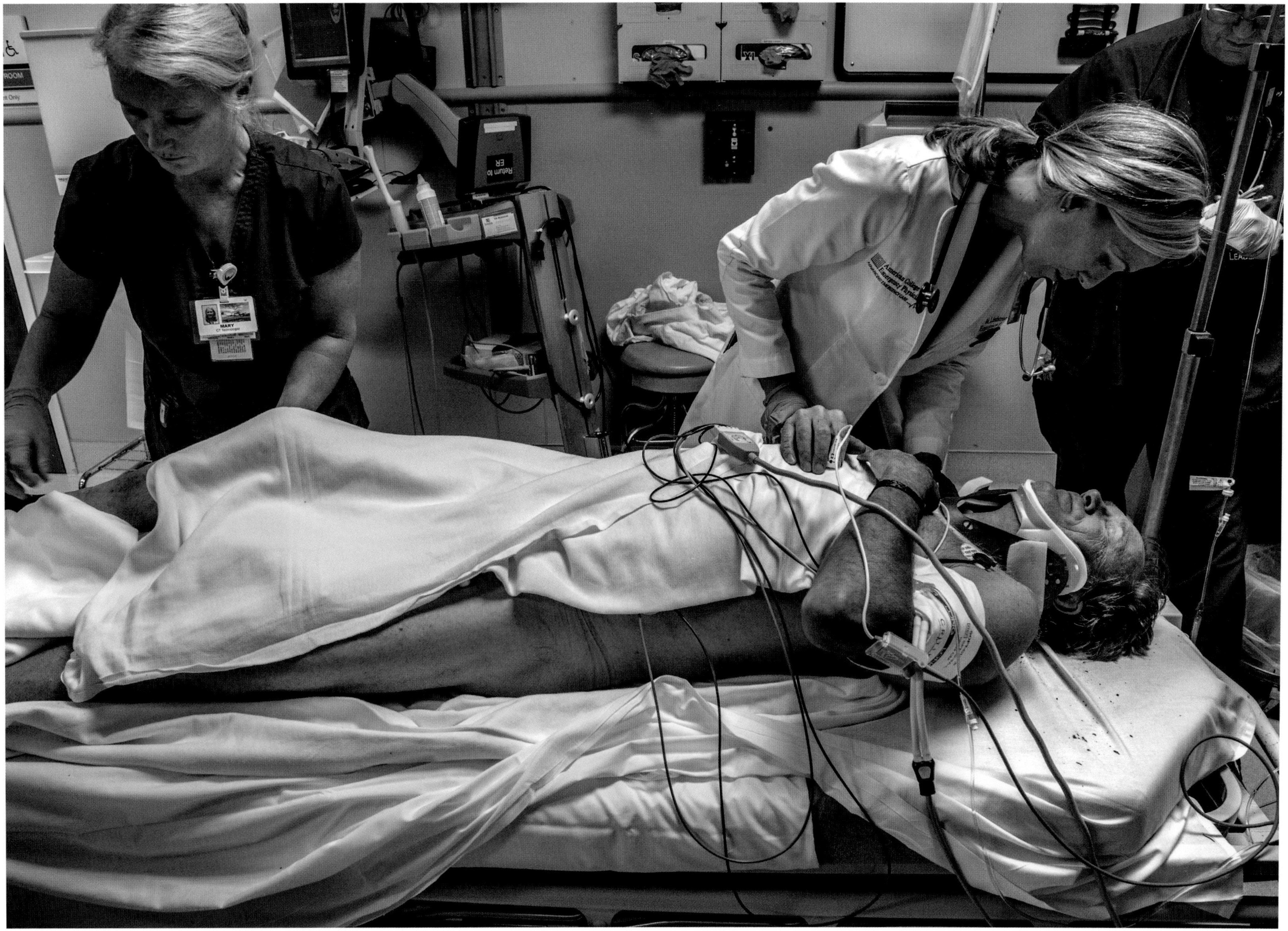
Return to
ER
MARY

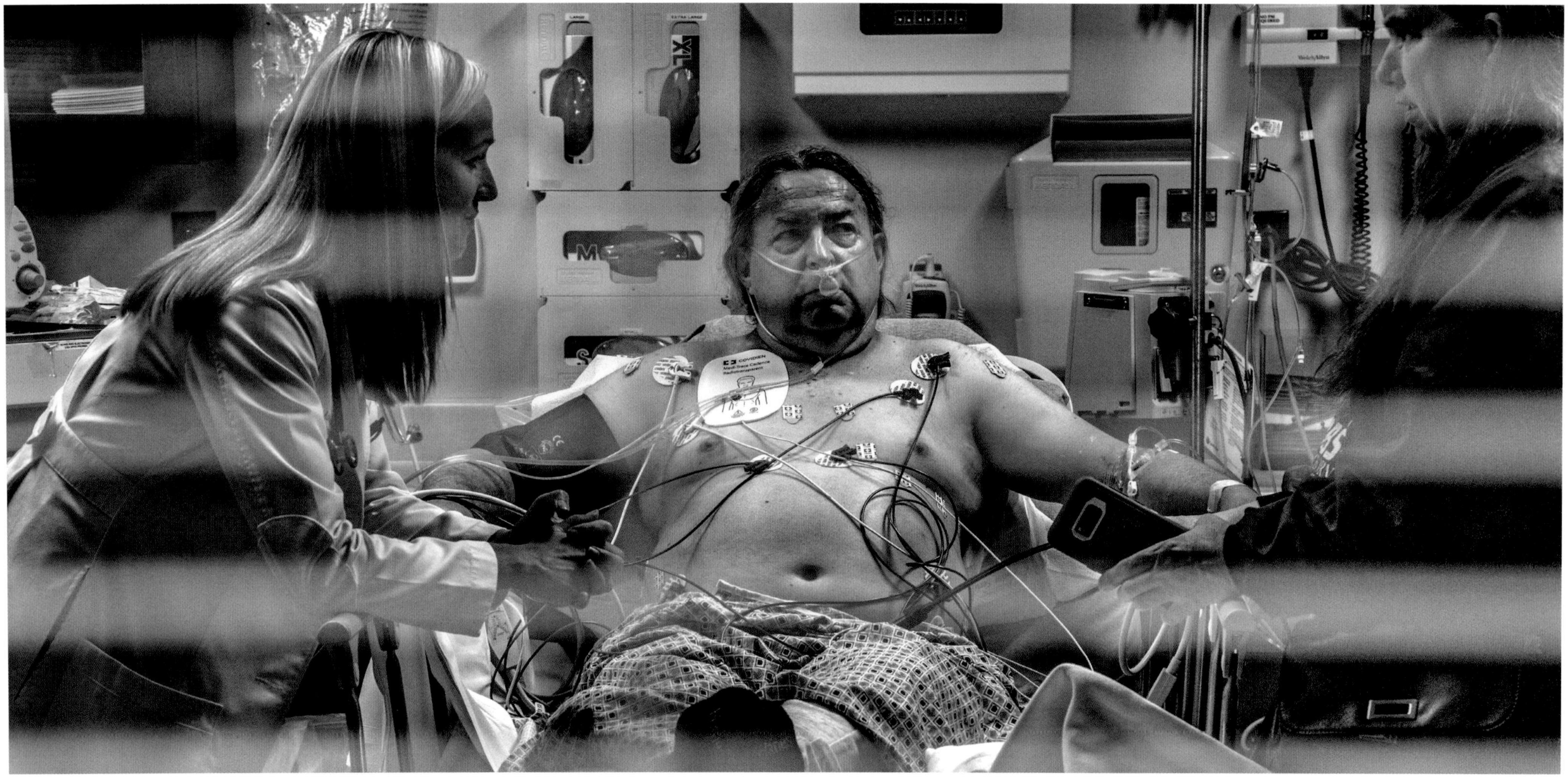

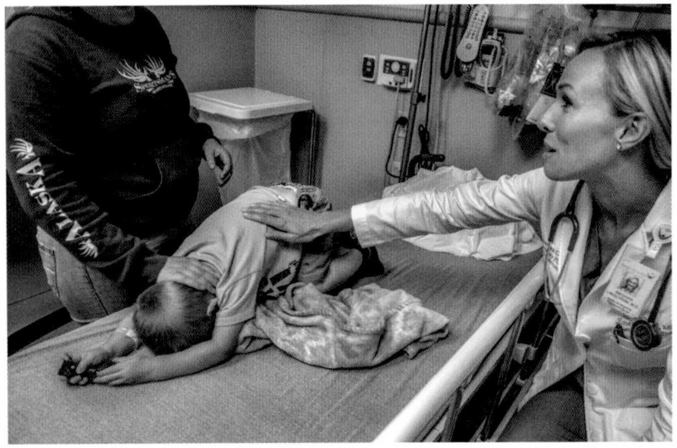

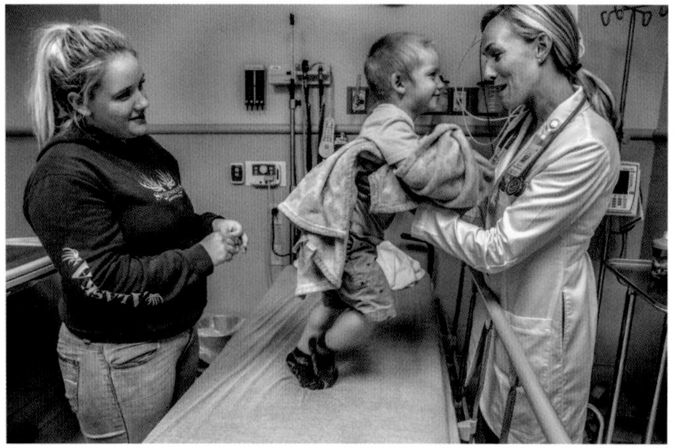

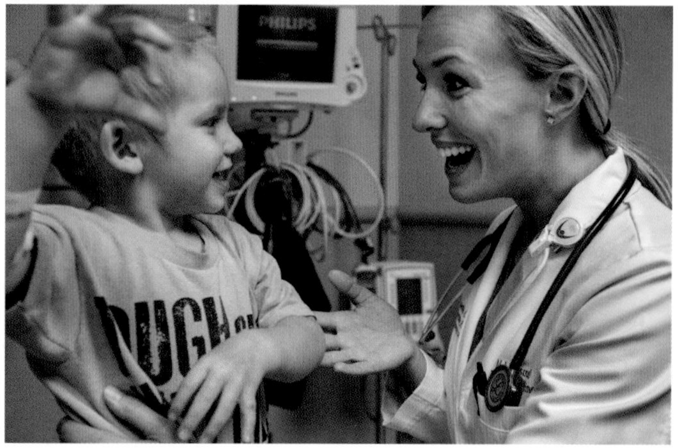
PHILIPS

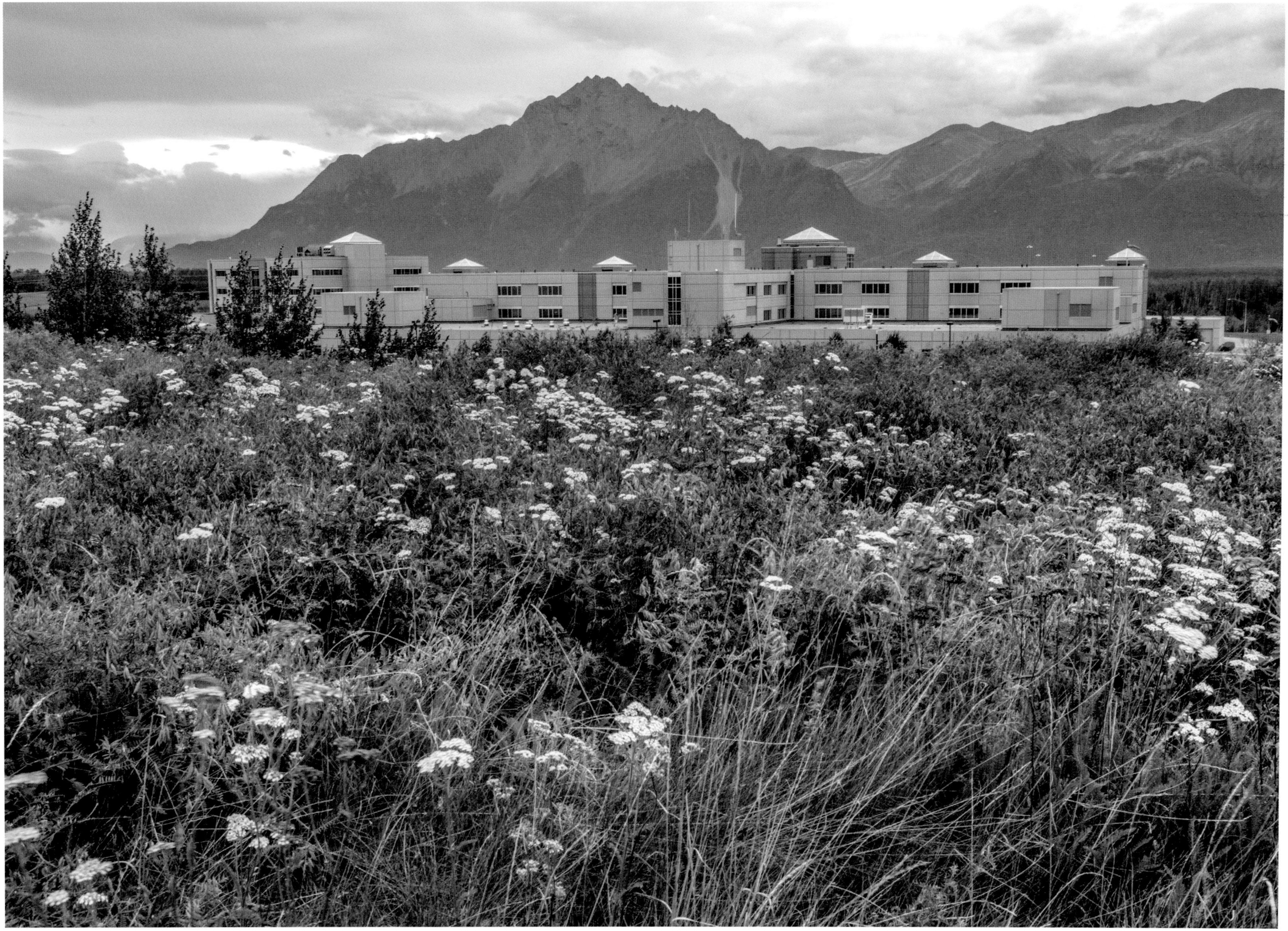

Ronald Stewart, MD

Emergency Medicine & EMS Pioneer
Nova Scotia, Canada

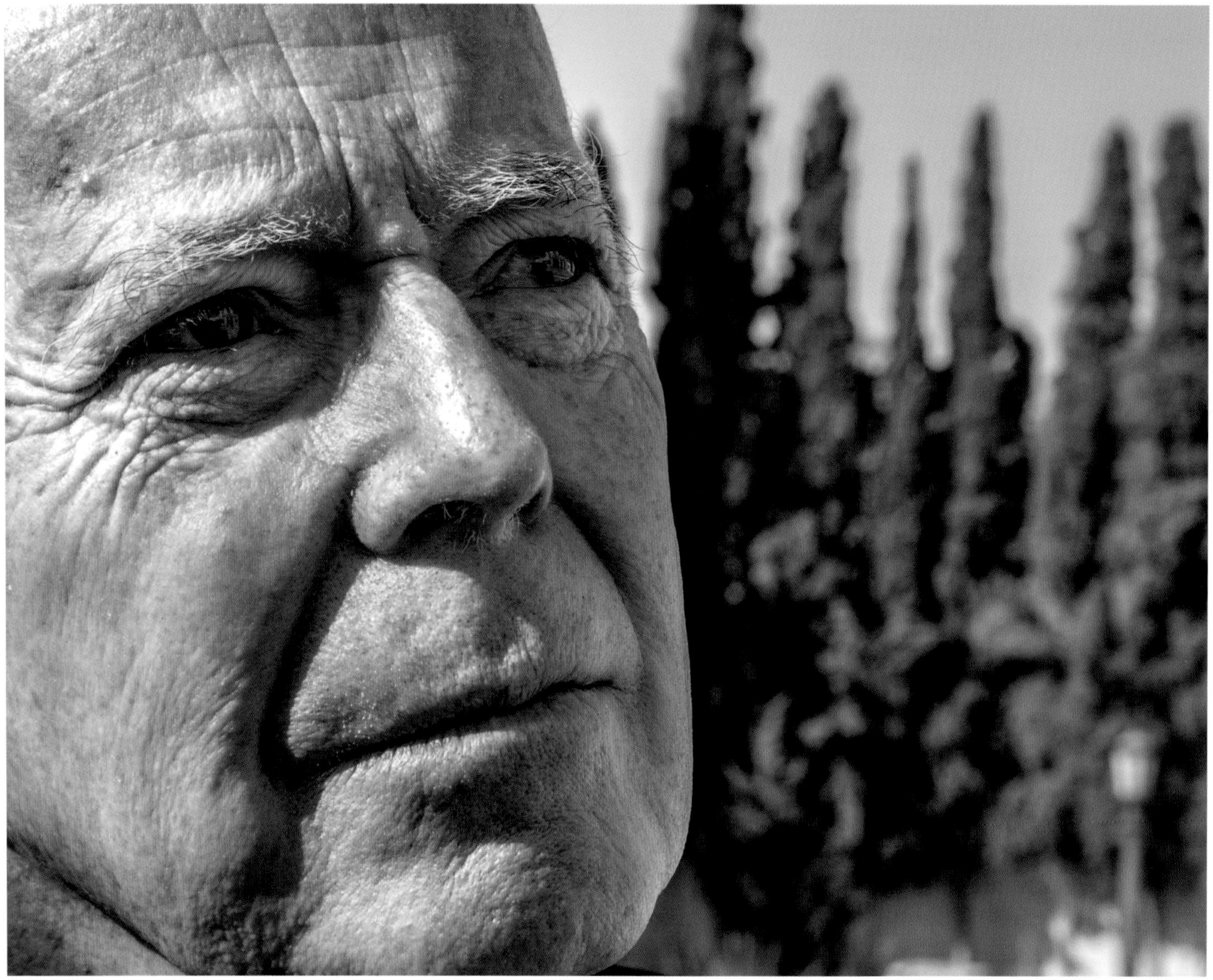

I always was the first aid guy on the high school hockey team, but I never thought of it as a potential profession. I became interested in medicine during college, but the dean of science told me I'd be a bad fit . . . said I was too sensitive . . . I'd care too much. I remember asking him, "Well, isn't that what it's all about?"

I spent a summer studying public health in Algeria soon after it gained independence from France. The country was still unstable and, while I was there, hundreds of people were killed in a bomb attack. This caused the government to declare martial law. I guess they saw me — a white Canadian boy, lost and running around — and thought I might be part of the rebellion. So, they threw me in jail. Fortunately, they decided to deport me to France, where I slept by the roadside and spent the rest of the summer trying to get back home.

After medical school, I went into practice in an outpost fourteen-bed hospital in the North Highlands area of Nova Scotia. It was beautiful — my ideal place. I worked alone for six months during the busy tourist season and saw every busload of American tourists. God love them . . . they were taking more pills than I had ever seen — big garbage bags full, all with American proprietary names.

We were doing a lot of house calls at the time, squeezed in between our morning and afternoon clinics. One day, I had to go see a ninety-eight-year-old lady who'd broken her hip by falling out of a plum tree. I headed down in my Jeep but didn't come back. I hit a moose and went over a cliff. When they found me four or five hours later, I was hypothermic and had a head injury that left me partially paralyzed and unable to speak. I could understand what people were saying, but I couldn't respond — just couldn't get the words out. I had wild emotional ups and downs . . . I was always bursting into tears. It was a great kerfuffle.

I was in rehab for about four months and even though I was really out of it, I could hear what people were saying. "Oh, what a shame. His life is over . . . his career is in the toilet. . . ." That talk would make me upset and crazy, so then I'd hear, "Uh oh. It looks like we need to sedate him." I'd just think, "No, you need to shut your mouth . . . that's what you need to do."

As I improved, I started using a wheelchair. Doctors would stand over me and ask questions, but I was stuck in a cervical collar and couldn't look up. I got mad enough to write an essay called "Conversations with Crotches." I finally asked, "Will you please sit down, so I can look you in the eye?" I never did publish the essay because I thought it was too bitter, but I didn't forget the experience. Later on, when I was teaching, I'd initiate every new medical student group by having them start off in wheelchairs. I'd tell them, "Don't you ever stand over a patient and talk down. I don't care if you think they're bonkers . . . or unconscious . . . you must level up and talk to everyone directly."

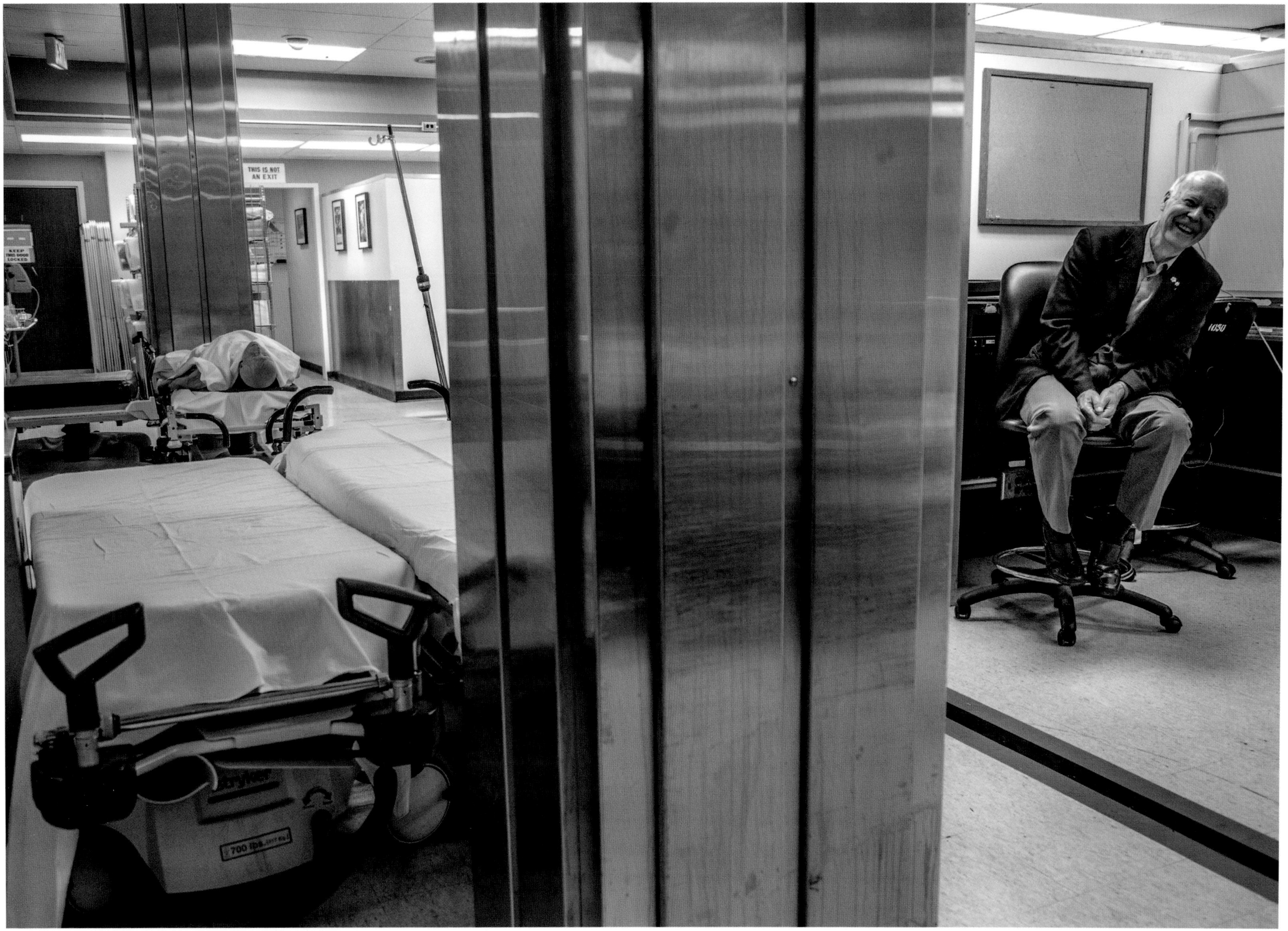
KEEP THIS DOOR LOCKED
THIS IS NOT AN EXIT

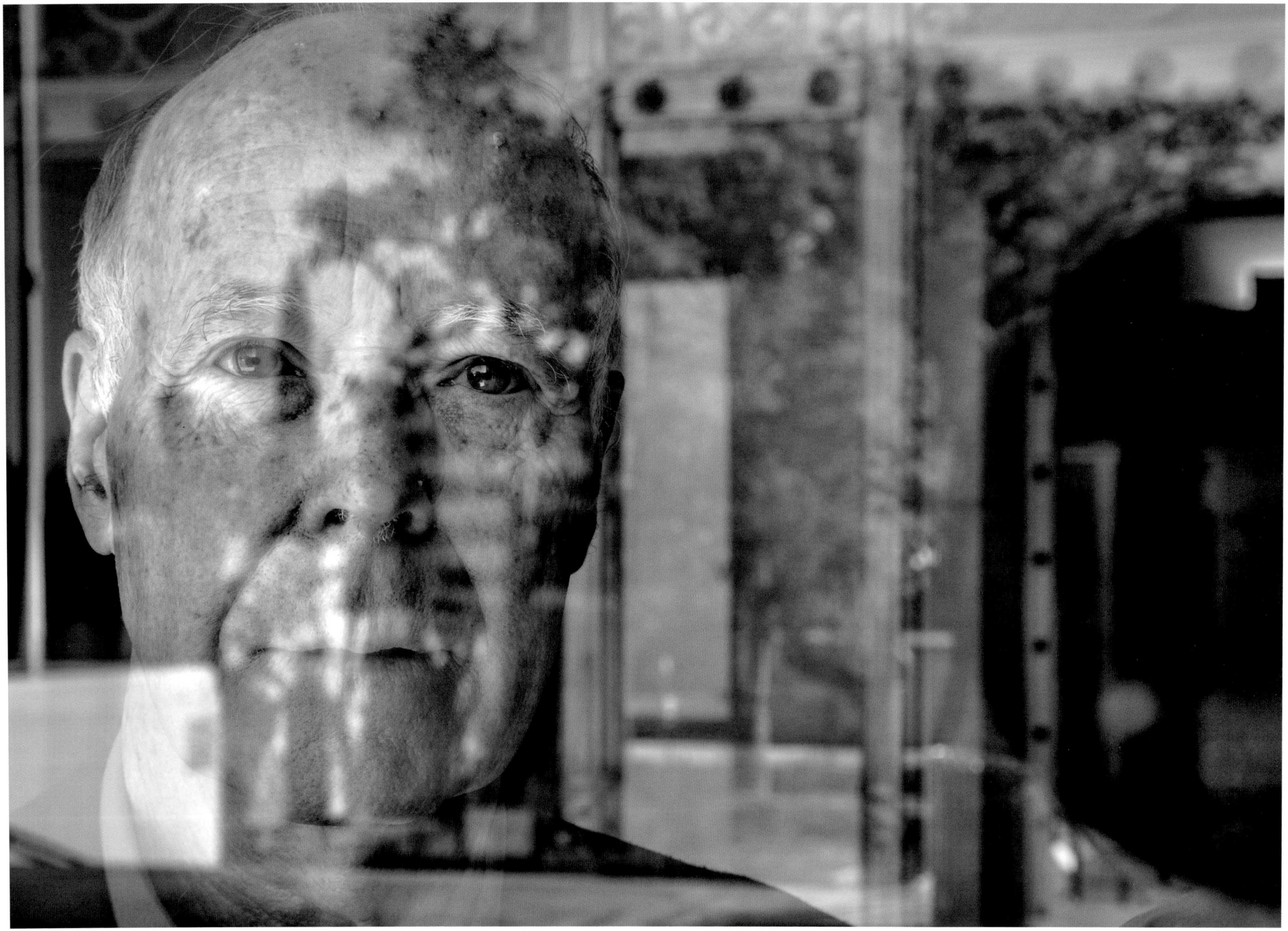

I went back to practice quicker than I should have and moved to California for more training. When I got off on Soto Street to start my new job, I turned left instead of right and found myself in the parking lot of what I thought was LA County Hospital. I got out of the car and walked up the stairs — and into a lingerie department. I asked the security guard to point me toward the emergency room, but he said, "What?! This is a Sears store!" Okay . . . I knew that, I knew that.

The accident left a huge impression on me in many ways, and it colored the way I interact with people. There are times when you're working . . . and you're exhausted because it's the sixth or seventh inning . . . and you'll get a patient who's not very nice to you. You know, some lady in a fur wrap who's just a little too smart for her own good. You want to say, "Listen, it's 3 o'clock in the morning, and I'm just trying to survive." But I was never able to do that. I'd just take it on the chin and think about how fortunate I was to be there.

In my little hospital back home, we saw about one thousand patients per year, but in Los Angeles, we saw one thousand per *day*. Even so, the biggest surprise for me was not the volume but the pathology . . . the illness that came through the door was wild. I had never seen a gunshot wound before. I'd never seen a stab wound. Trauma was not a Canadian disease. Drug problems . . . jail inmates . . . I'd never had those experiences.

One Friday night, a couple of gangs got into a brouhaha after a high school football game . . . and then out came the guns and knives. We had five or six patients show up at once — two of whom were critically injured. One of the kids died, so we pulled the family aside to deliver the bad news. This, of course, enraged the gang members and they started shooting . . . right there in the hospital. Security came running . . . people were fleeing . . . it was horrendous. I dove under a stretcher and bagged a patient while lying on the floor. I had no idea what was going on, but I knew I should just keep squeezing that bag . . . that was my job . . . keep squeezing. . . .

Three weeks after I reported to a new job in Pittsburgh, I was called to an incident on an old bridge over the Monongahela River. An iron worker had become trapped when the bridge collapsed — just like scissors — and caught his legs below the knee. The drama was broadcast on live television for about three hours. The firemen were able to free the patient's left leg by melting the metal struts with an acetylene torch, but the engineers radioed up and said, "Dr. Stewart, the bridge just shifted five inches . . . we can't guarantee it's going to stay up. You've got five minutes to get down."

That's when we made the decision to amputate his other leg at the scene. We got him out of there in about forty seconds. The patient did well, but he sued everyone. He sued the bridge commission. He sued the transportation commission. He sued the city government. But he never sued any of the physicians or paramedics.

I was schooled in the French philosophical approach. It might be a little iffy, but it works for me. In *Candide*, Voltaire wrote, "We must cultivate our own garden." That's what we do in emergency medicine. That's the only thing we *can* do. In this world, there's very little one individual can do to effect sudden change. We must all do our parts . . . and if we do them well, we may make a difference, together. ✚

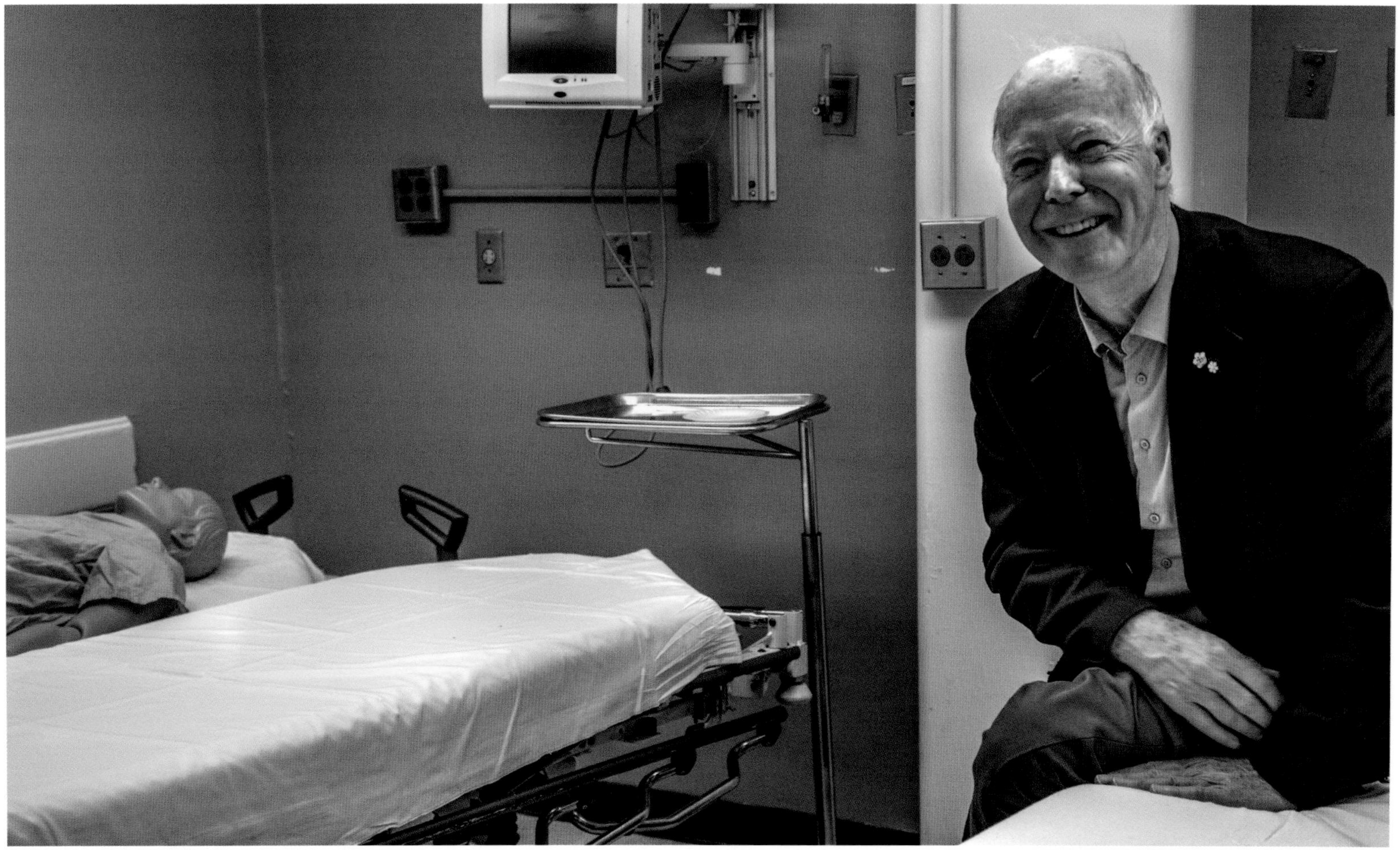

Emanuel Rivers, MD

Emergency & Critical Care Physician
Sepsis Researcher
Detroit, Michigan

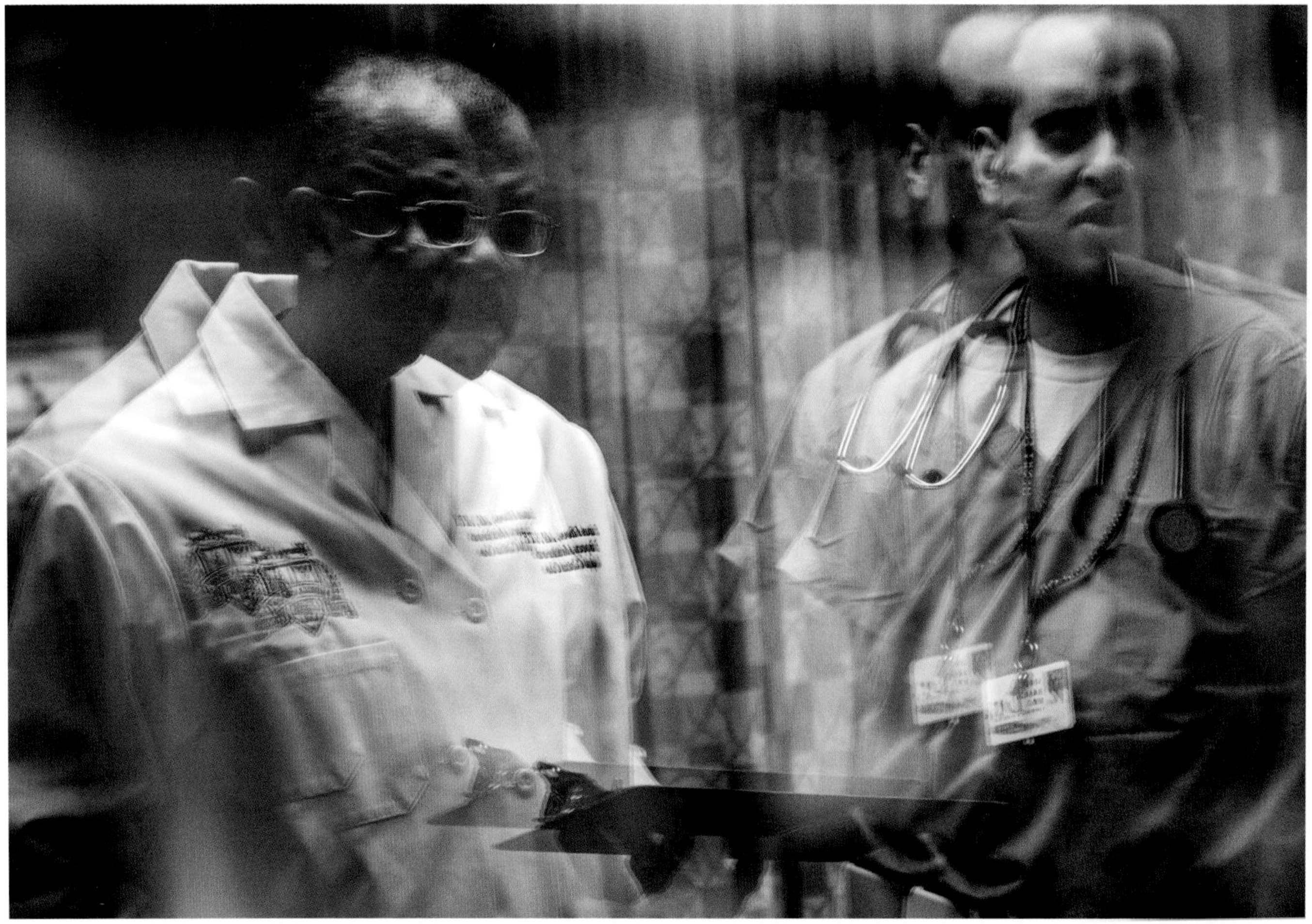

The '67 Detroit riots started right in front of this hospital. The city was plagued by so much social anxiety; racial tensions boiled over and the whole place went up in flames. Black patients were segregated in the basement . . . put in a special unit for the treatment of "undesirable problems." Things gradually changed but, still to this day, some of our older patients come in with a palpable angst. You can sense the history in them.

When my dad came here from Alabama, he could barely read or write. He got a job at Ford Motor Company and was able to raise nine kids; we never saw poverty. He'd take us down south in the summer and make us pick cotton from 6 am until the sun went down. He wanted to show us what life would be like without an education.

Detroit was a proud industrial city back then, but things gradually changed. Once the car industry started to teeter, the local economy just crumbled — it wasn't diversified enough and people couldn't find jobs. That's my sense of why things got out of control — people began to lose hope. Maybe the youth had been spoiled, or perhaps they didn't understand how much work it had taken to build the community, but we lost focus. The illicit activity — the drugs — just took over.

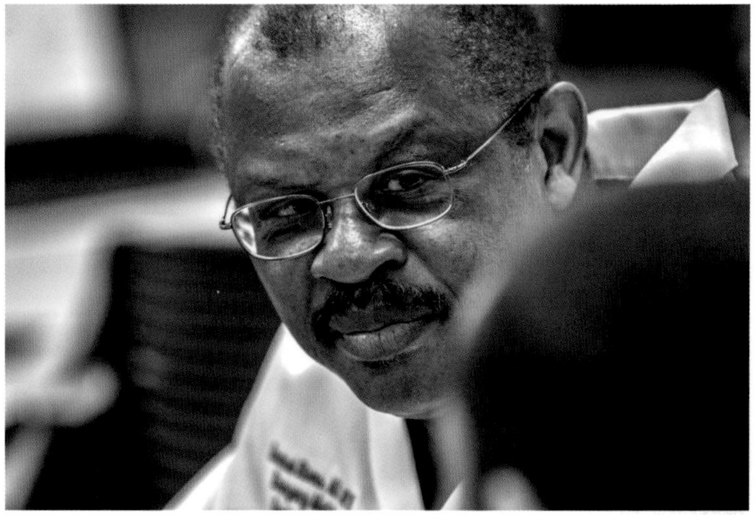

Patients would come in, they'd be drunk, high — just not doing what they're supposed to be doing. I would write them prescriptions for two grams of pride, P-R-I-D-E. The nurses would come back and say, "We don't have that drug." I'd say, "Just tell the patient that you've got to have some pride." I could probably get into trouble for that nowadays, but I don't know . . . I felt empowered to do it because these people were my neighbors. I cared about what happened to them.

I became addicted to the ER in med school. It was like Dante's Inferno — a place where you could see the landscape of human suffering. The mortality rate in Detroit was so bad in those days. About 99.9 percent of the patients who came to the ER in cardiac arrest died. The city didn't seem to value emergency medical services. Paramedics would go out on calls without any medications; they had nothing. That's the truth. No major city in the United States had that kind of mortality, so we knew we had a problem. People were just dying.

I got lucky, though — those problems made the city a playground for research. I was in the right place at the right time. I immersed myself in acute care. I saw patients with heart attacks, strokes, sepsis, you name it. I was on call twenty-four hours a day. I would resuscitate a patient any chance I got. From death to life — I saw it so many times it became a religious experience. I could tell when their spirits left their bodies.

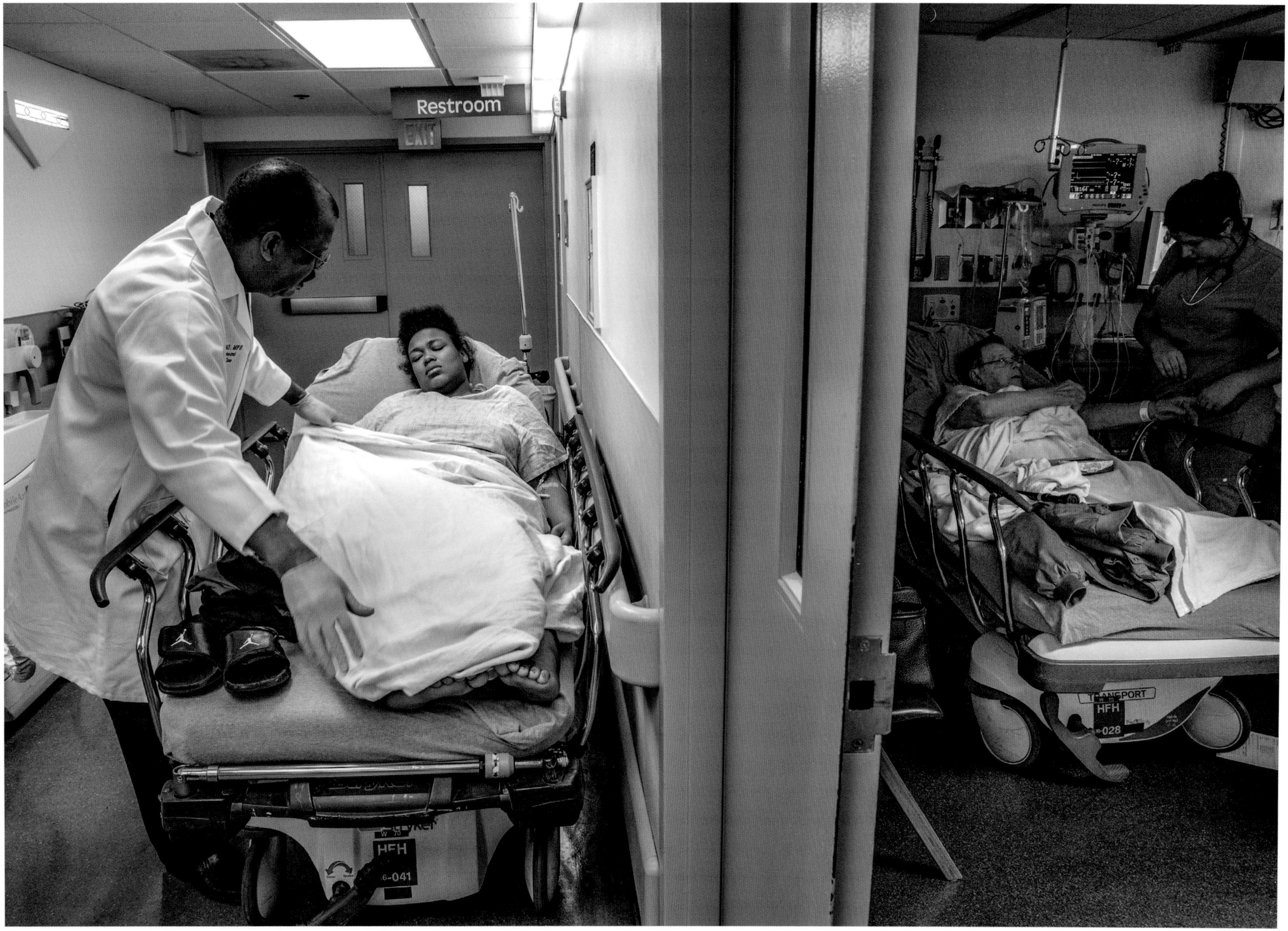
Restroom
EXIT
HFH
TRANSPORT
HFH
-028
HFH
6-041

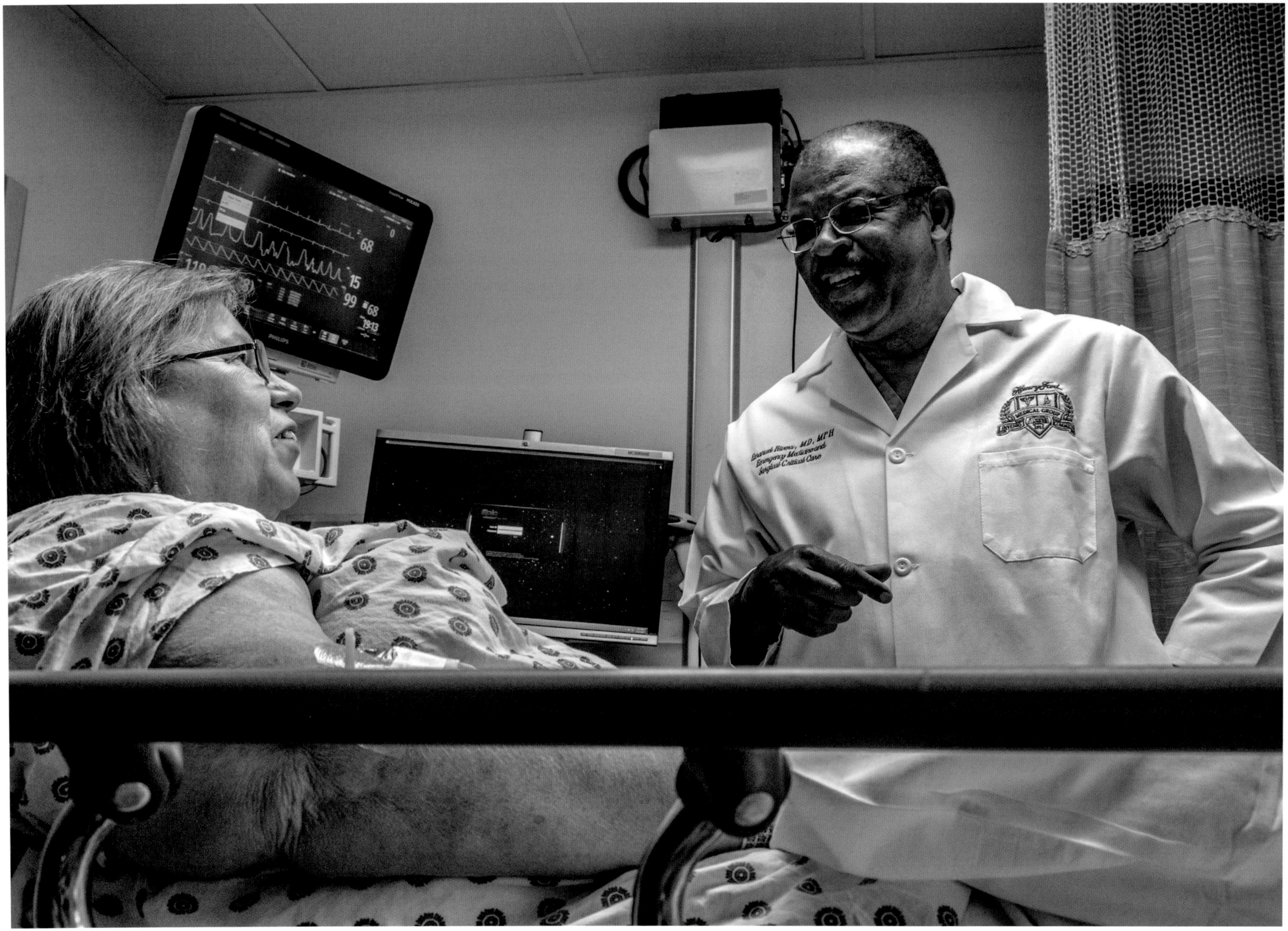

We started looking deeper into what we were doing wrong and developed new methods for the treatment and early detection of sepsis — a recipe that totally revolutionized the care of critically ill patients. When my study got published in the *New England Journal of Medicine*, everyone asked, "Who in hell is this guy from Detroit?"

I always think about Ignaz Semmelweis, the Hungarian researcher. He studied two groups of physicians. Half were told to wash their hands before they delivered a baby and half were told not to. The guys who didn't wash their hands — 50 percent of the babies and mothers died. So, in 1865, he presents his data at a national scientific meeting, and everyone thinks he's crazy, everyone. People just hate his guts. So, they throw him in a cell, lock him in a straitjacket, and beat him . . . and he dies of septic shock. I mean, this is what you get for inventing *hand washing*?

When you push for change, there will always be people who are resentful — people who just can't believe you did it. That's just the nature of the beast. Humans are something else, man. They'll hate themselves if you allow them to. ✚

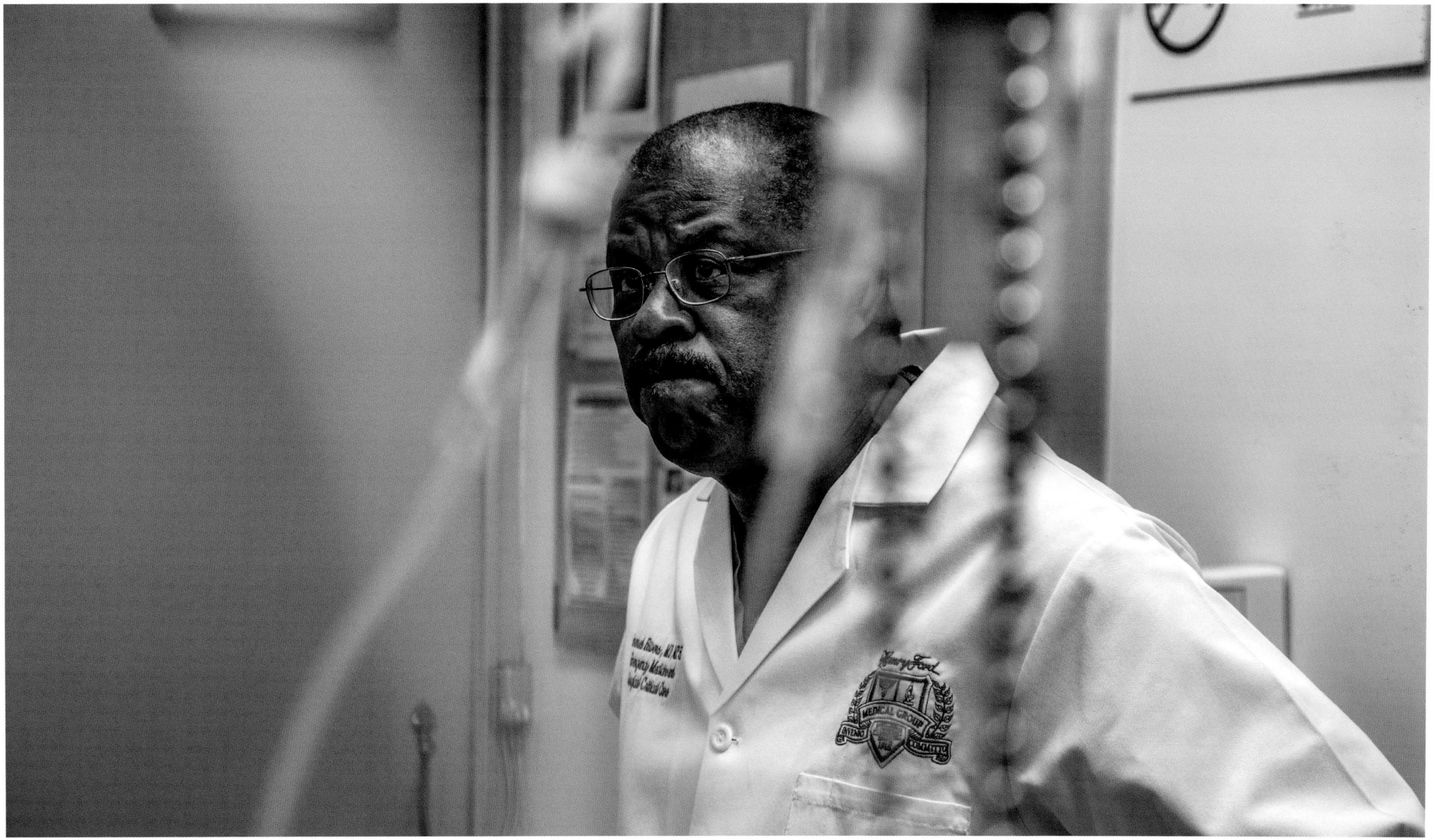

Carl Chudnofsky, MD

Emergency Physician & Emergency Department Chair
Los Angeles, California

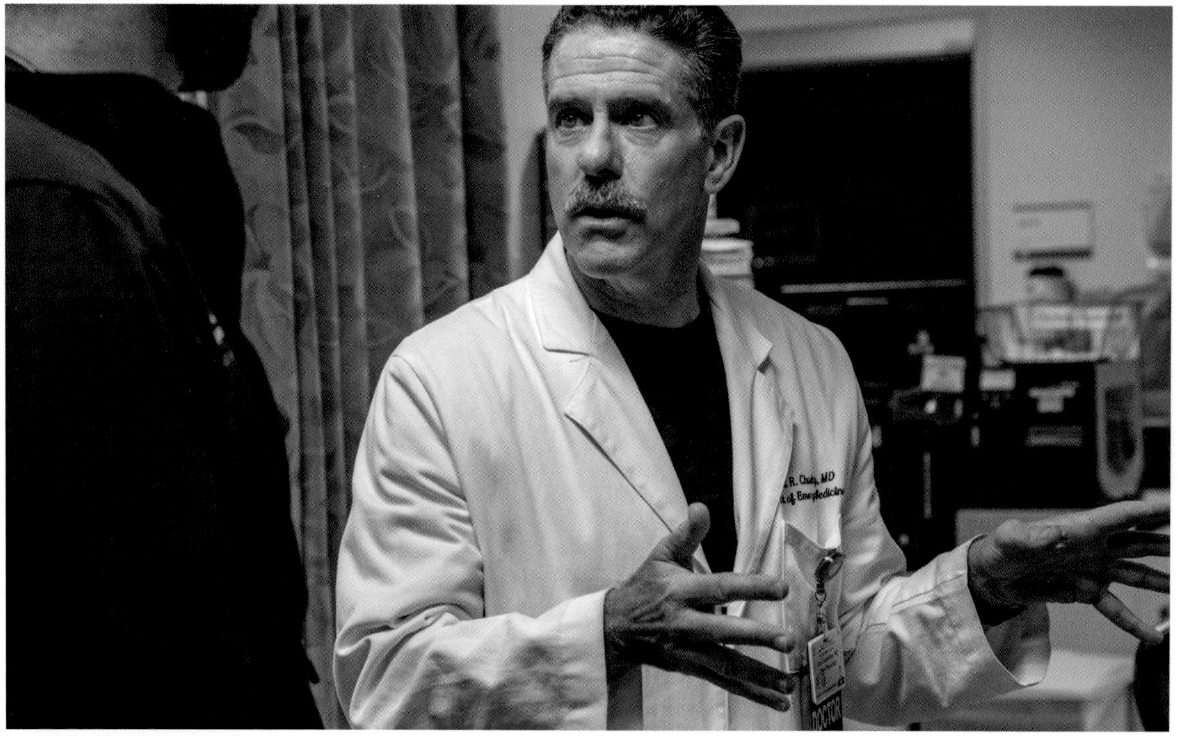

When I was seventeen, I lied about my age so I could become an EMT. It felt like destiny . . . I thought it was the most incredible job anyone could ever have. I made $5 an hour working for a local ambulance service and loved every minute of it. I did EMS work all through college, but the more I went into hospitals, the more I noticed the ER docs. I was just amazed by how cool they were . . . how much they seemed to know. It was enough to convince me. A few years later, I found myself in medical school. I figured I was going to be like Marcus Welby . . . the real deal.

My interest in emergency medicine continued to grow in med school. I recognized how special it was to be there during a patient's most vulnerable moment. But I'll never forget the conversation I had with the dean during my fourth year. When I told him I wanted to work in the ER, his smile faded. He stopped, put his pen down, looked me in the eye, and said, "No, no, no. You can moonlight anytime. What do you want to *do* . . . what kind of *doctor* do you want to be?" Even as recently as the '80s, emergency medicine didn't command much respect. But I can't complain . . . he wrote me a nice recommendation letter, and here I am.

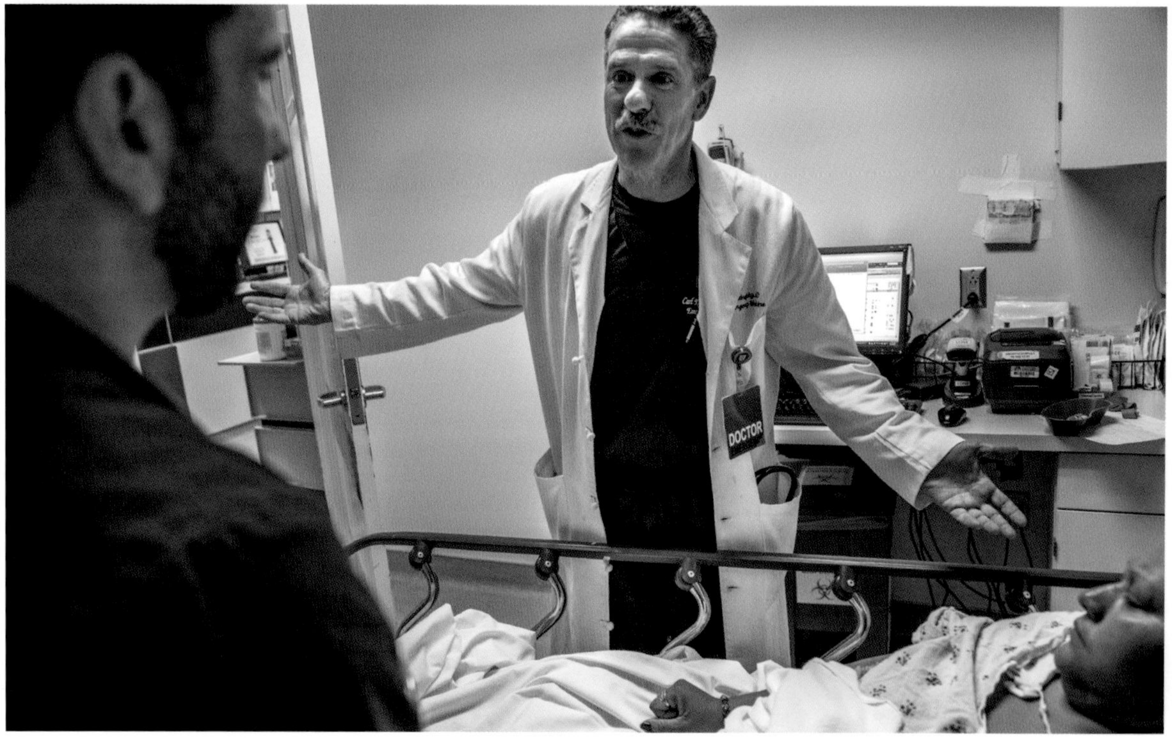

This specialty really is all about *stories*. Patients have theirs, and we all have ours. It's a cliché, but you just can't make this stuff up. Some of the things you see leave you shaking your head; *there's no way that could have happened*. Yet it did. As a clinician, you're faced with a problem and only have a few minutes — or even seconds — to do the right thing. You must make a decision — and live with it. You have the life of a complete stranger in your hands.

That gestalt is one of the hardest things for young docs to wrap their heads around . . . that gut feeling that tells you when a patient is really sick. Some of that knack is instinct, but most of it comes with clinical experience. You can't underestimate the value of having "seen that before." Sometimes a brand-new intern will be in a room, methodically examining a patient for thirty minutes, and the senior nurse will run up to me and say, "Hey, we don't have time for this. The patient needs intervention *now* . . . you better get in there." You know what? More often than not, the nurse is correct.

But I couldn't run this place without the residents. Their idealism is contagious, and their passion and intense desire to positively impact the world keep me young. There's no doubt teaching has made me into a better doctor. The gratification I get from watching a new graduate transform from a timid intern into a confident physician is hard to put into words — and even harder to match. I love when they ask questions. I love to see them learn.

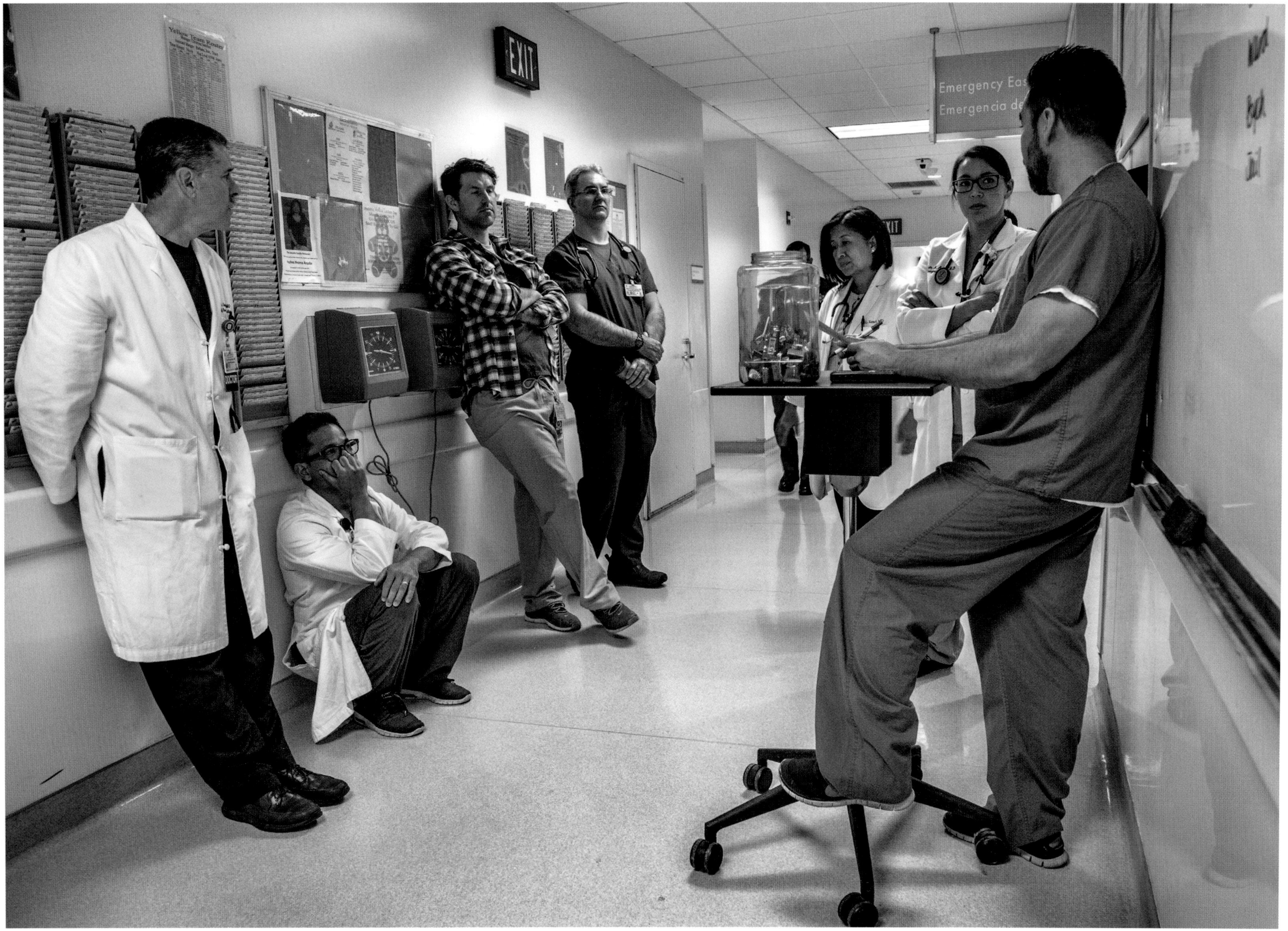
EXIT
Emergency
Emergencia

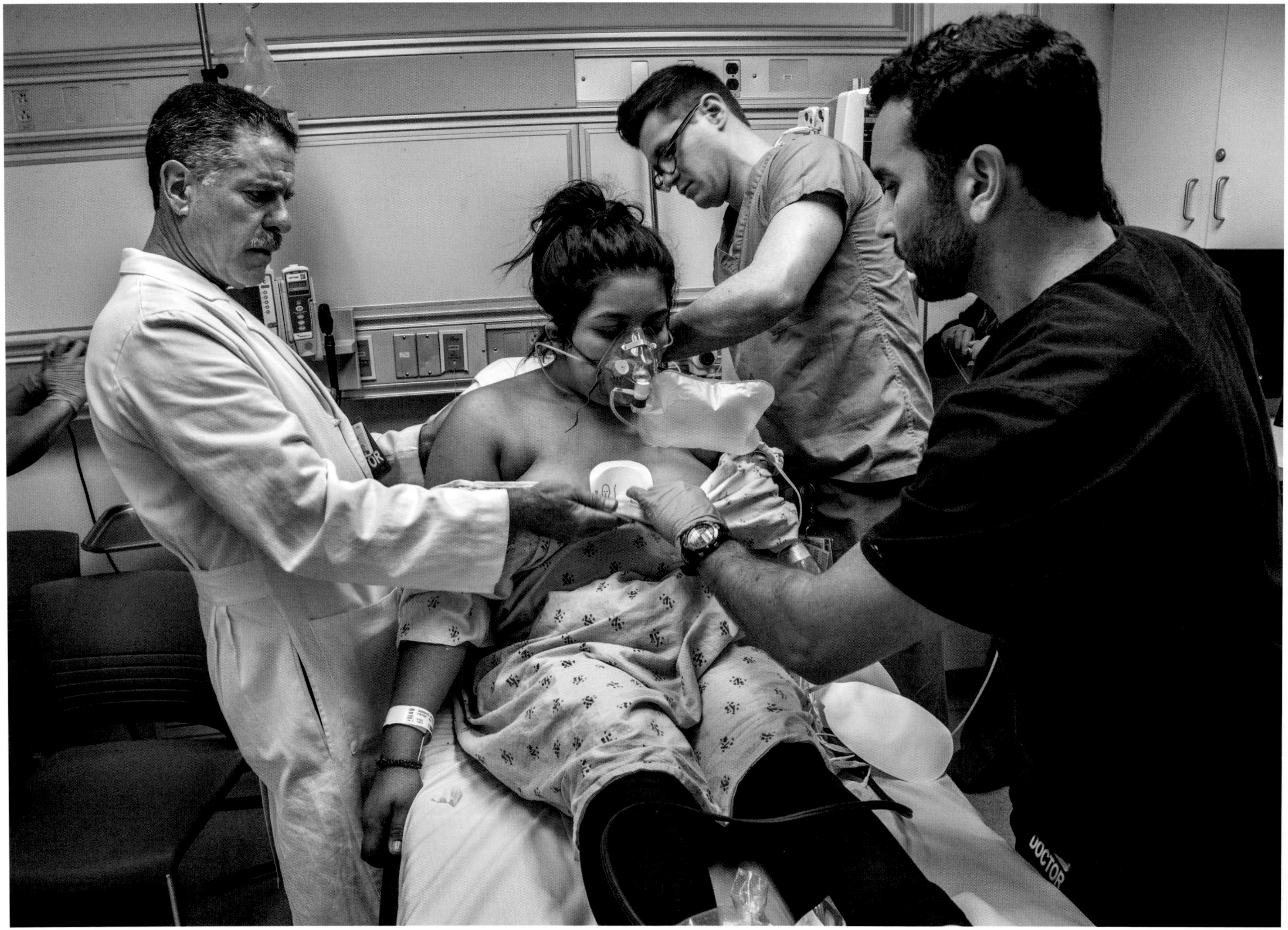

These young docs don't do it for the money. They do it because they love what they are doing . . . we all do. I've had a few residents over the years who took a wrong turn — latched onto a job because the money was so good. But they never lasted more than a year. I always counsel them to love the work first. *Is this the right fit for you?* If the answer is yes, *then* you can worry about making enough to survive.

Emergency medicine takes a special kind of person . . . we're a different breed. I'll remind my residents that some days are hard. It's tough to manage the exhaustion . . . the sadness . . . the stress. Oh, but the rewards are phenomenal. Nothing compares to working in the ER, amidst the broad, beautiful array of humanity. ✚

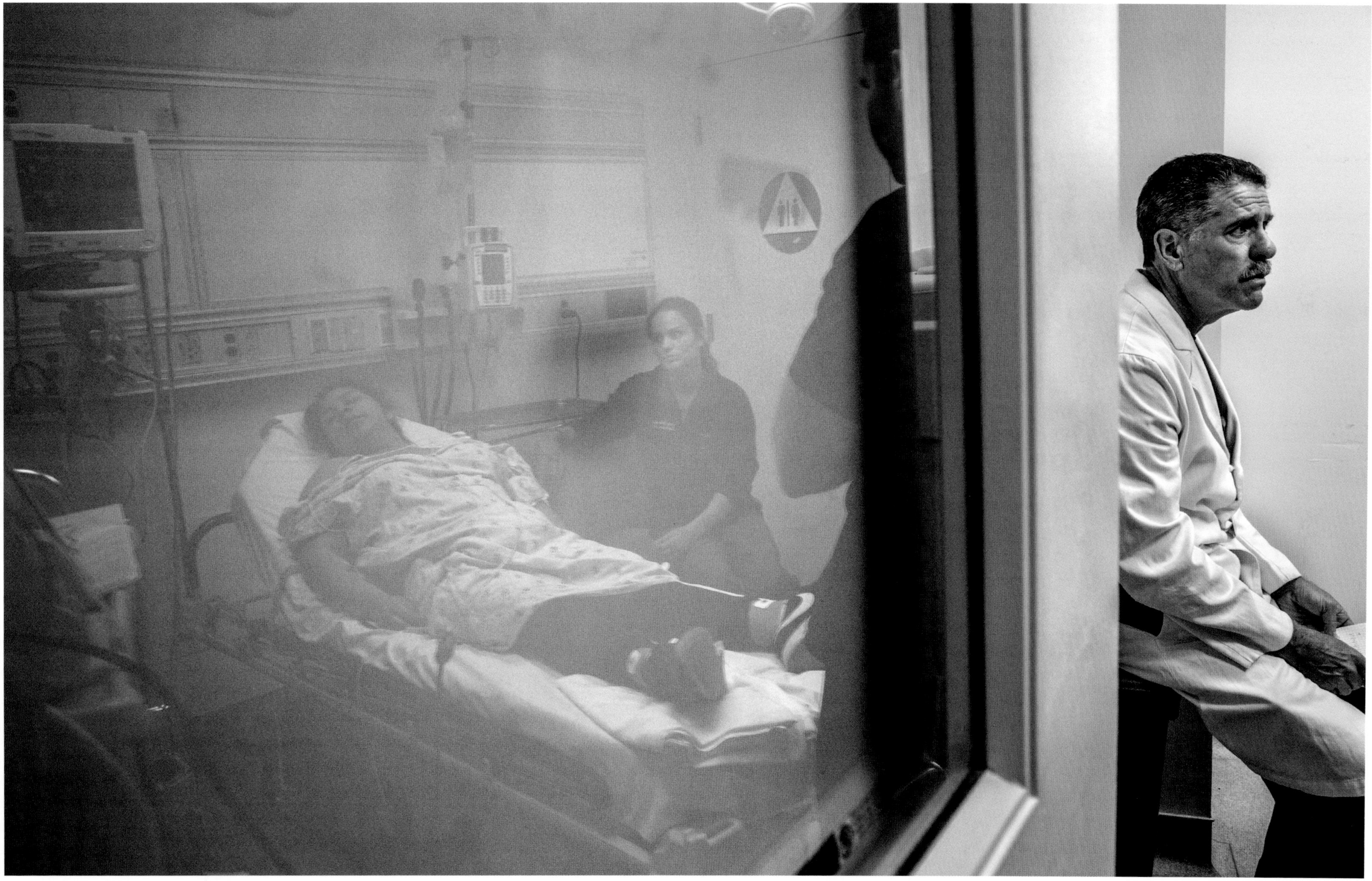

Amy Bastman

Paramedic & Firefighter
Los Angeles, California

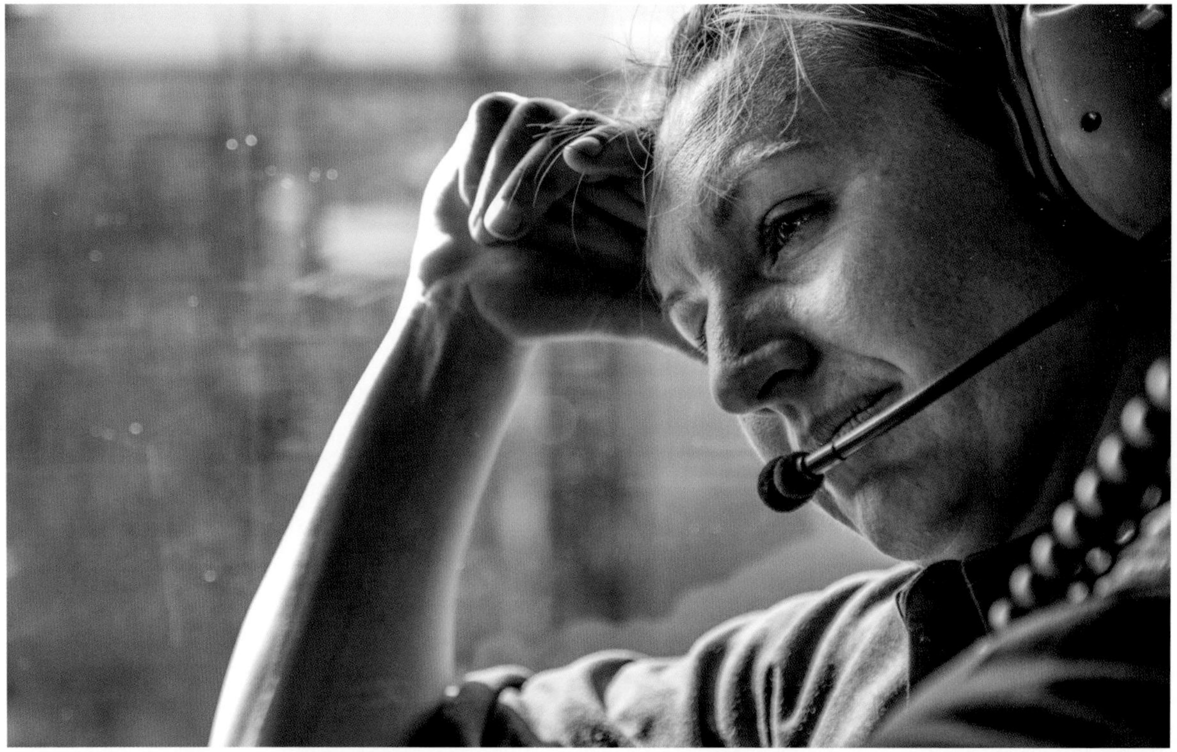

I've been out on almost 10,000 calls and have been in several situations where I thought, "Well, this could be it!" It's dangerous work but I know I'm there to do the best job I can . . . whatever happens, happens. We'll hear gunshots from time to time, so I've learned how to duck and cover. Gang violence, drugs and alcohol . . . I can't tell you how many dead bodies I've seen.

But I'm here because I want to be. During training in the drill tower they'll tell you — and it's true — there are 100,000 people waiting for your job; if you don't appreciate it, do something else. It doesn't matter if it's dangerous or hard, or the equipment is heavy, or it's just a bad day, we all love the work. We're not stuck in a cubicle; we get to do something different every day.

I'm very lucky in my own marriage, but firefighters have a very high divorce rate — somewhere around 50 percent. The stretches of time away from home . . . it's easy to lose the connection, end up living separate lives. It's also hard to leave all that competitiveness and intensity back at the fire station. Not everyone can handle the stress. For a lot of families, it just doesn't work. A successful relationship requires a lot of communication, a lot of understanding. You have to be mindful of that or one day you might go home to nothing.

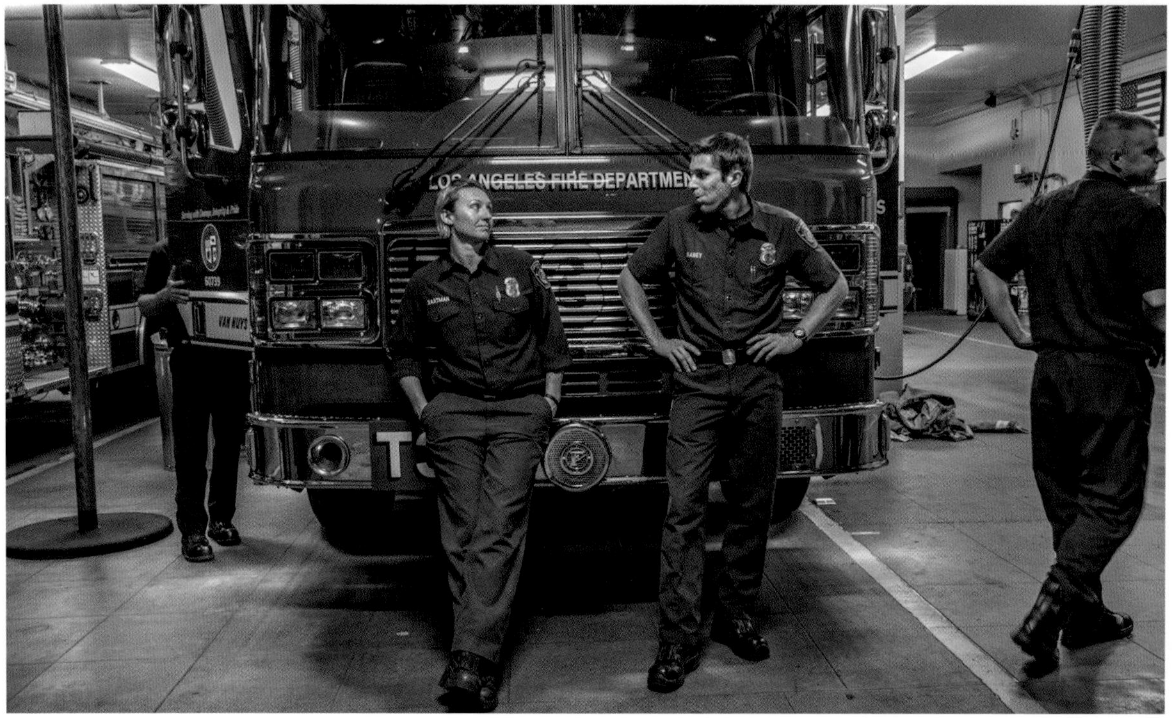

Work hard, play hard — that's always been my philosophy. I love extreme sports — riding dirt bikes, surfing, snowboarding. I've done heli-skiing in Alaska and Canada. After college, I spent a lot of time in the mountains and took a class in outdoor emergency care, which allowed me to be a volunteer ski patroller. That's how I got introduced to EMS.

Nowadays, I keep working until I crash out, but I go to bed prepared to get up in the middle of the night. My mind stays preoccupied with a certain level of readiness. My wife and I have two teenagers and a ten-month-old baby girl, and I work at one of the busiest fire stations in Los Angeles. I can't even remember the last time I got eight hours of sleep. Just as I'm shutting my eyes, I'll get a run. I've been doing it for so many years, though, I think I've just gotten used to it.

When we're out on calls, other women will sneak me a thumbs up, or a wink, or a "You go, girl," and they'll pump their fists in excitement. Little girls wave when they see me in the back of the fire truck or with my head near the window. Their faces just light up. All of a sudden, they imagine the possibility of something they never thought they could ever do . . . there's a woman, right in front of them, doing it. ✚

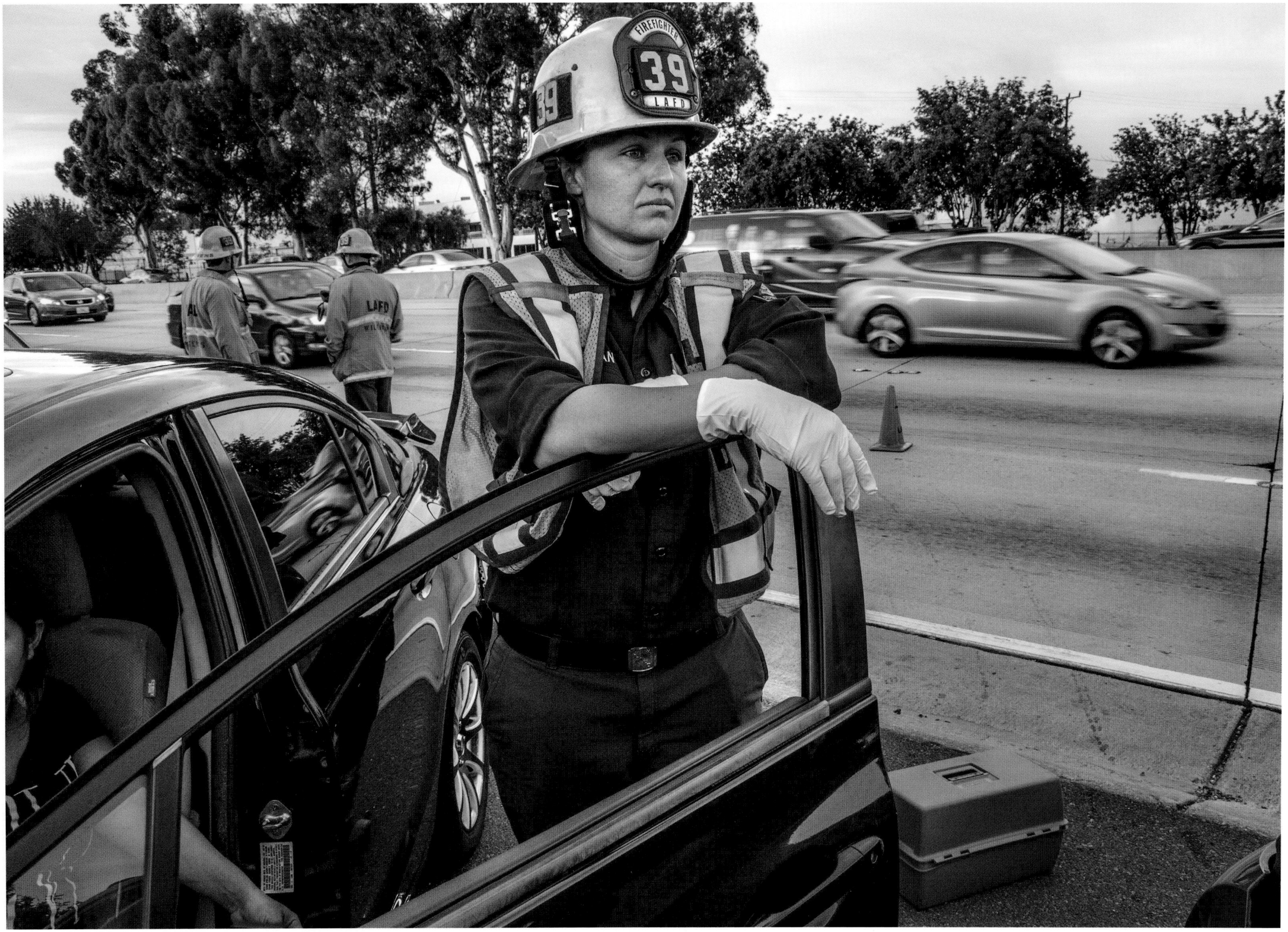
FIREFIGHTER
39
LAFD

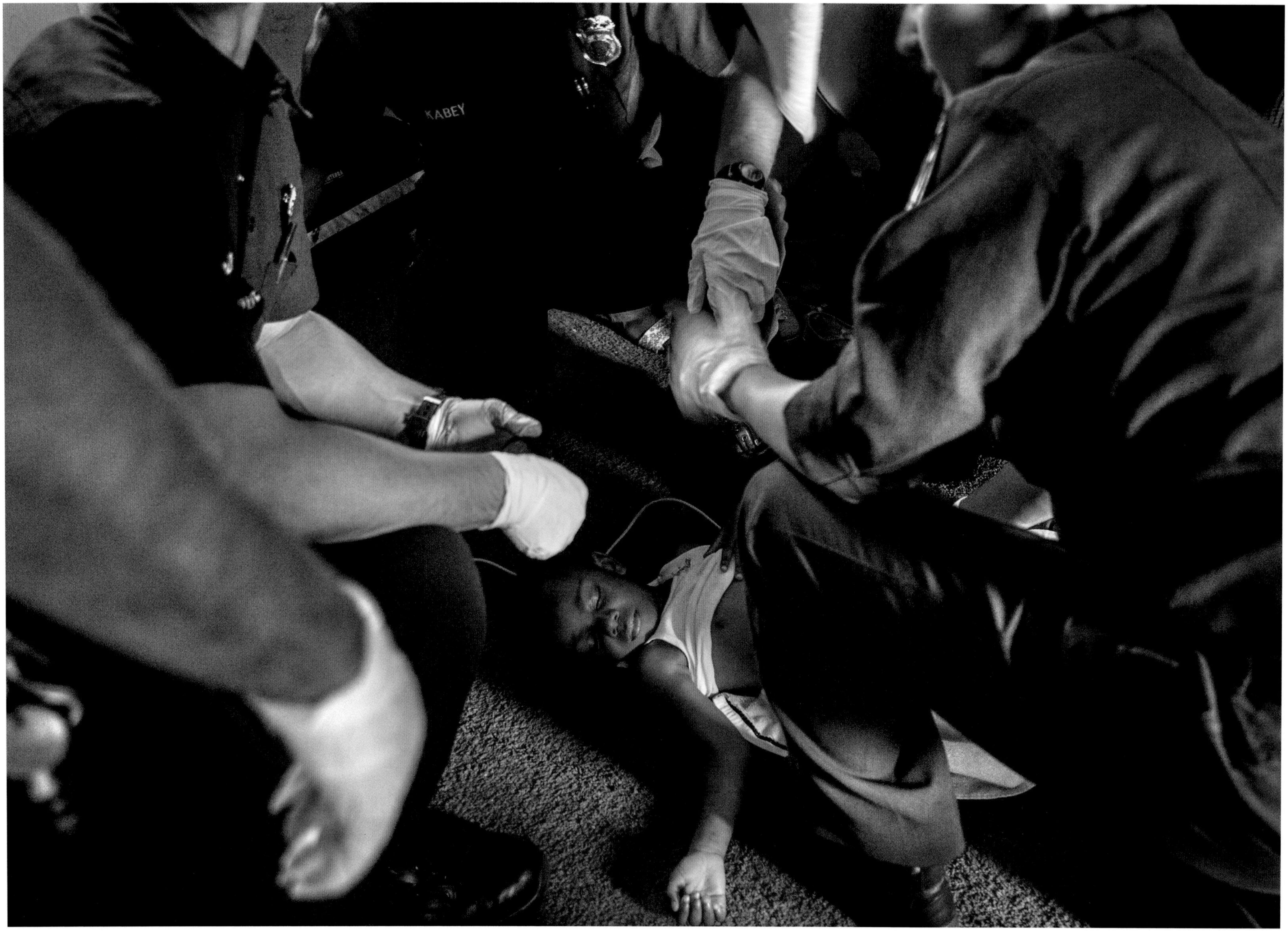

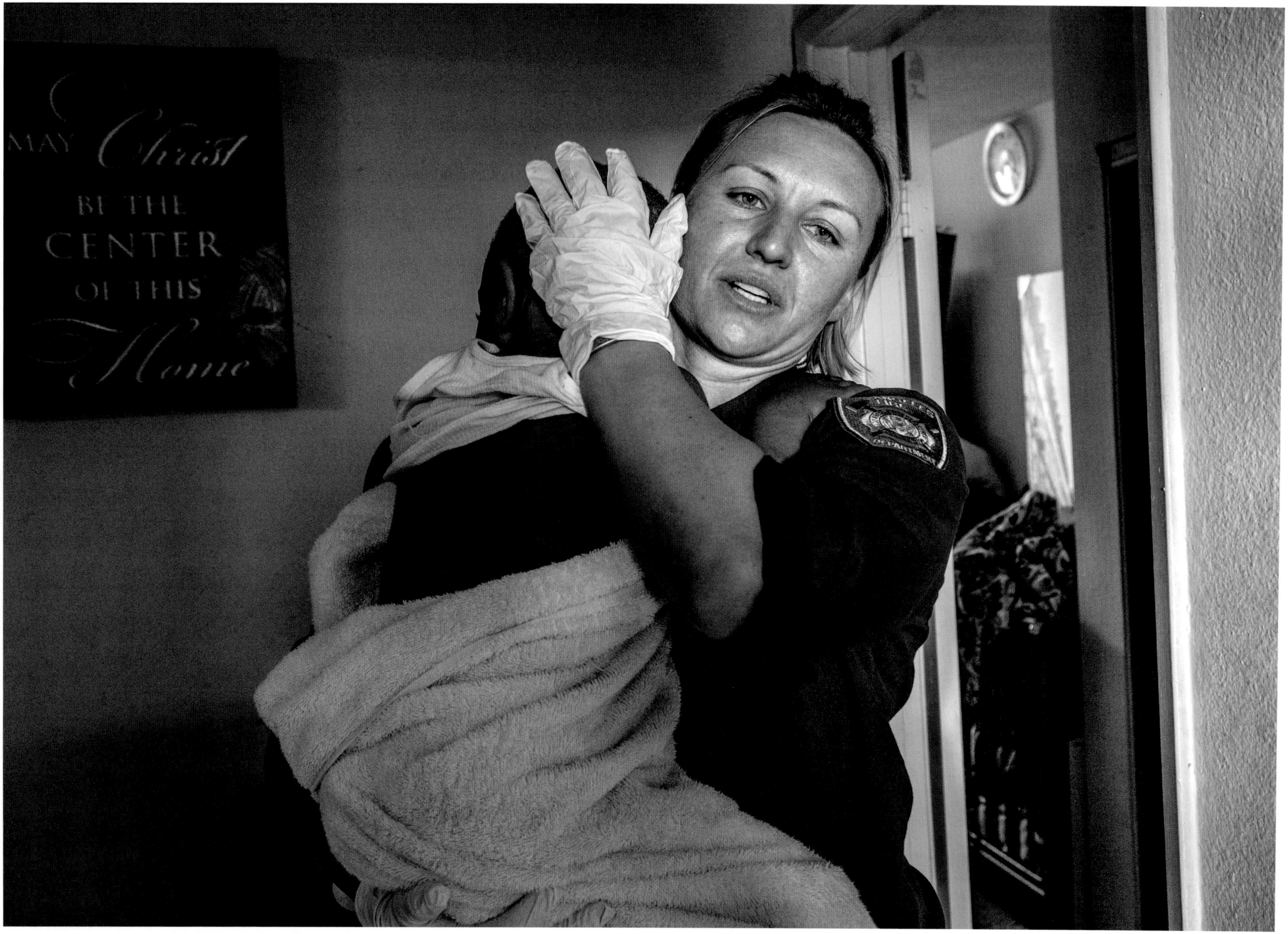
MAY Christ
BE THE
CENTER
OF THIS
Home

Crystal Brown, MD

Emergency Medicine Resident
Los Angeles, California

I look young. I mean, I *am* young. *Yes, sir. I get your Doogie Howser joke. Can we get past the age thing? Good. Now let's continue*. Yeah, I understand I could pass for a teenager but ultimately, I hope my patients leave feeling they were treated by a competent physician, who was compassionate and spoke to them with respect.

Residency is all about exploration and self-discovery. For a lot of us, the first year is one of total uncertainty. Medical school is over, and now you've got to jump in and learn how to be a clinician — a *real* physician — for the first time. You have this new title behind your name, but you really don't know what to do with it. But I blinked, and I'm now in my fourth — and final — year. When you're constantly moving, you don't realize how quickly the time has passed.

I think one of the reasons I love working in the resuscitation area is it gives you the opportunity to make a really sick patient feel better. Someone will come in, looking terrible . . . so you do your interventions . . . and they perk up. That's what excites me; it's a great feeling. But, no, I never really envisioned some of this. The soiled patient covered in stool . . . the combative patients who are intoxicated or high . . . the smells . . . people at their lowest. I've just learned how to bring a different energy to those situations. You have to let your compassion take over and decompress through humor.

I'm wired when I leave a shift. Every now and then, I'll stop at my parents' house before I head to my place. They'll tell me I'm talking a million miles a minute — just full of adrenaline, buzzing.

I've never been the greatest sleeper but nowadays, forget it. If I feel I've fallen short in any capacity, the guilt gives me insomnia. I think we all have a natural inclination to strive . . . we want to do the right thing . . . want to be the best.

But even if you've done everything right, this is an unpredictable place. ✚

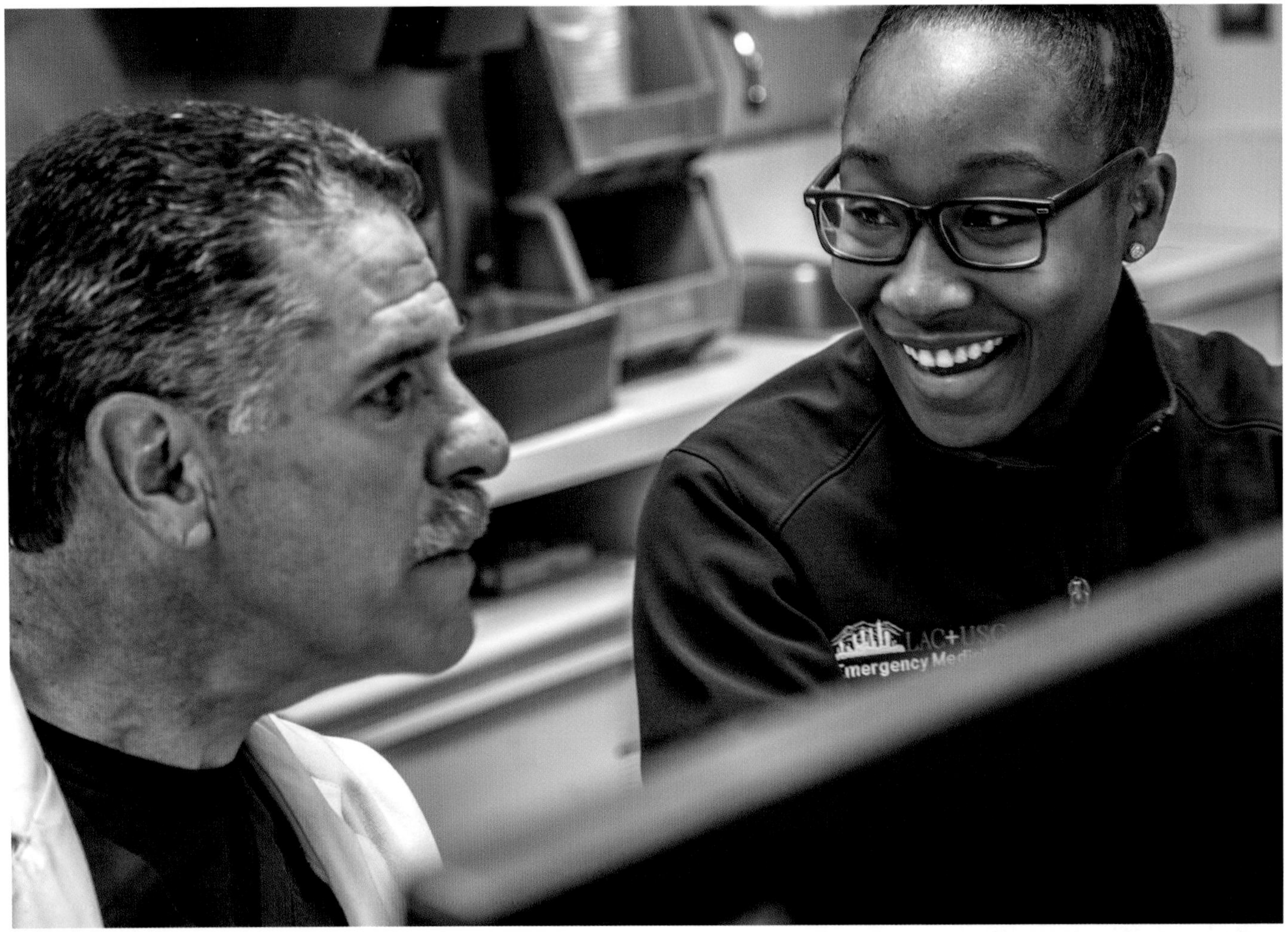

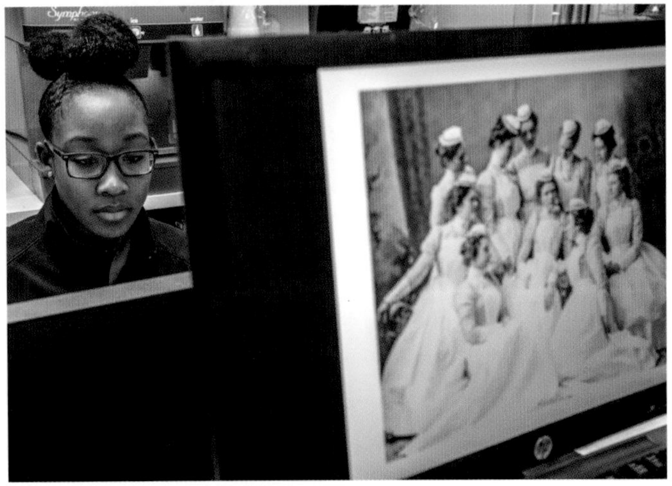

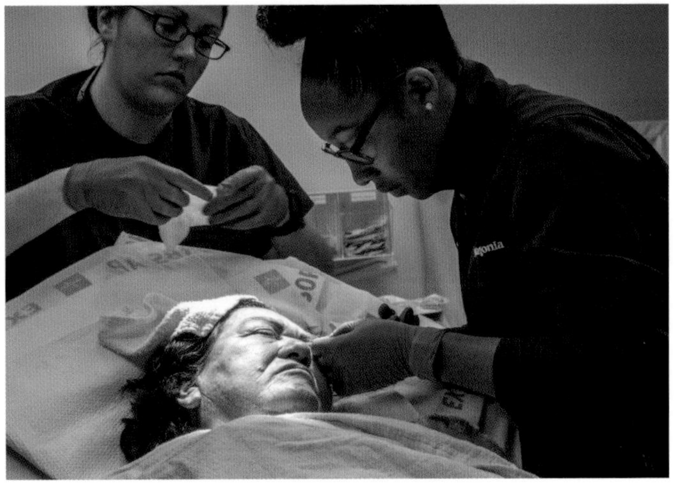

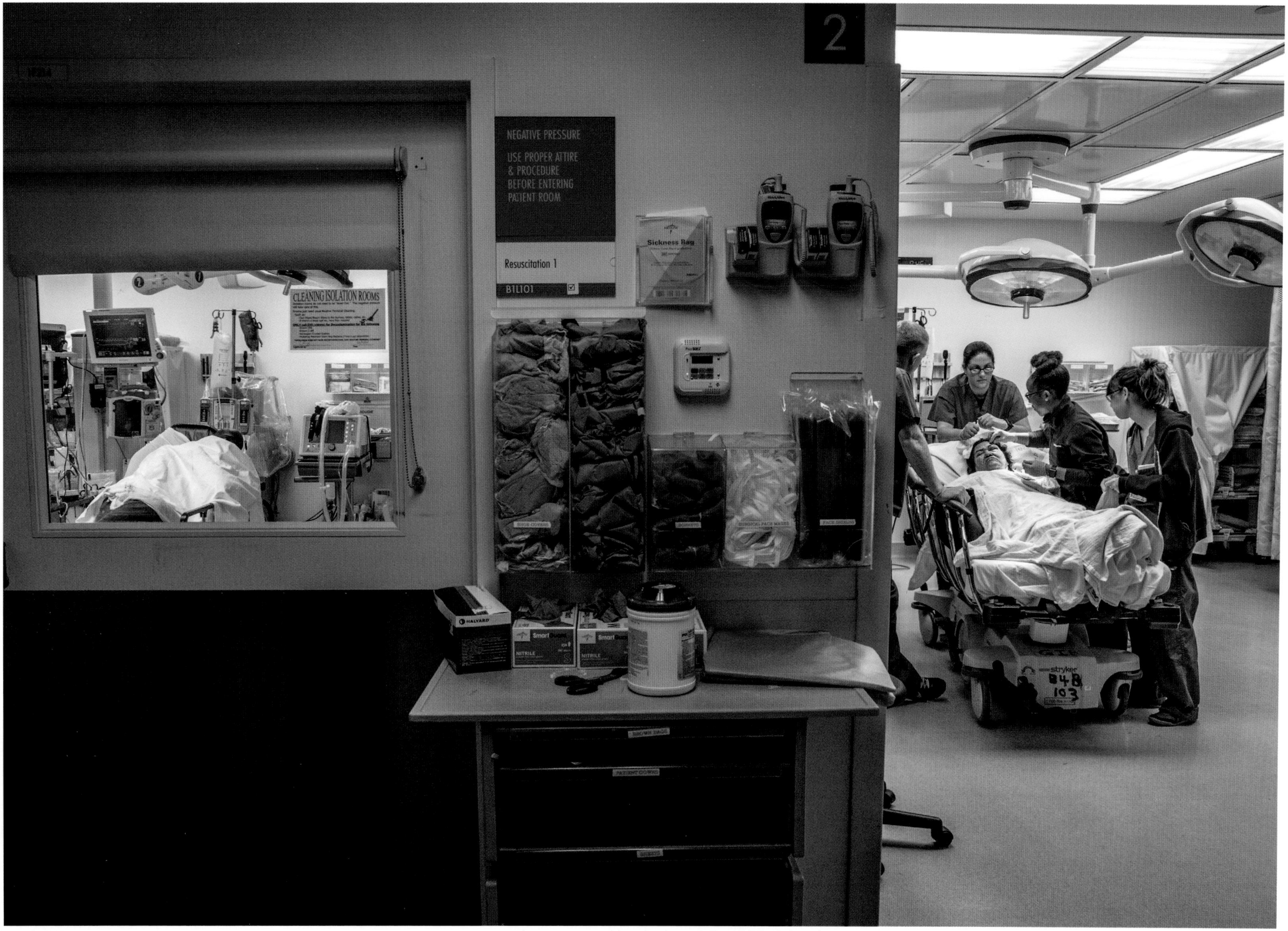
2
NEGATIVE PRESSURE
USE PROPER ATTIRE
& PROCEDURE
BEFORE ENTERING
PATIENT ROOM
Resuscitation 1
B1L101
Sickness Bag
CLEANING ISOLATION ROOMS
HALYARD
NITRILE
NITRILE
stryker
B48
103

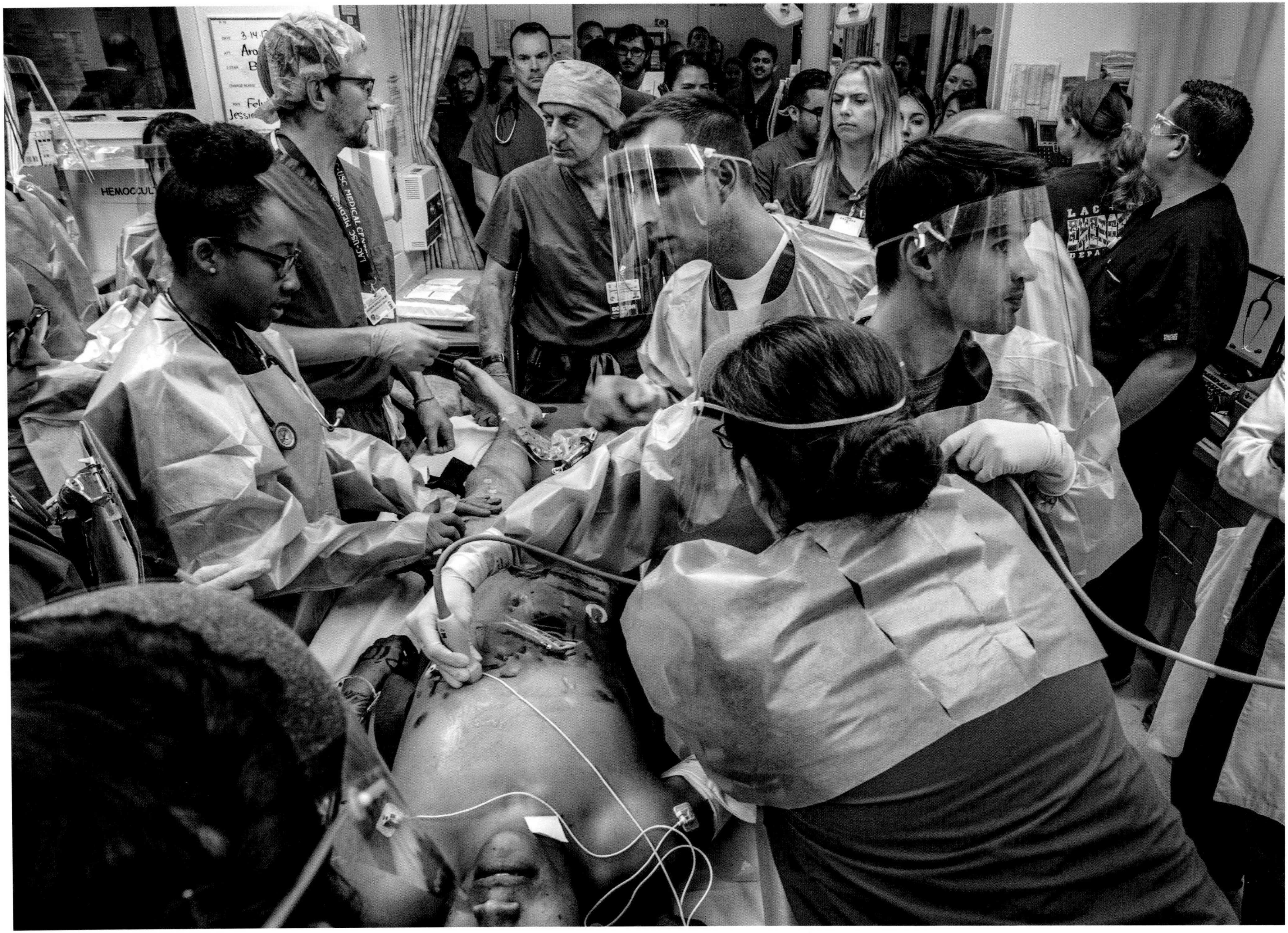

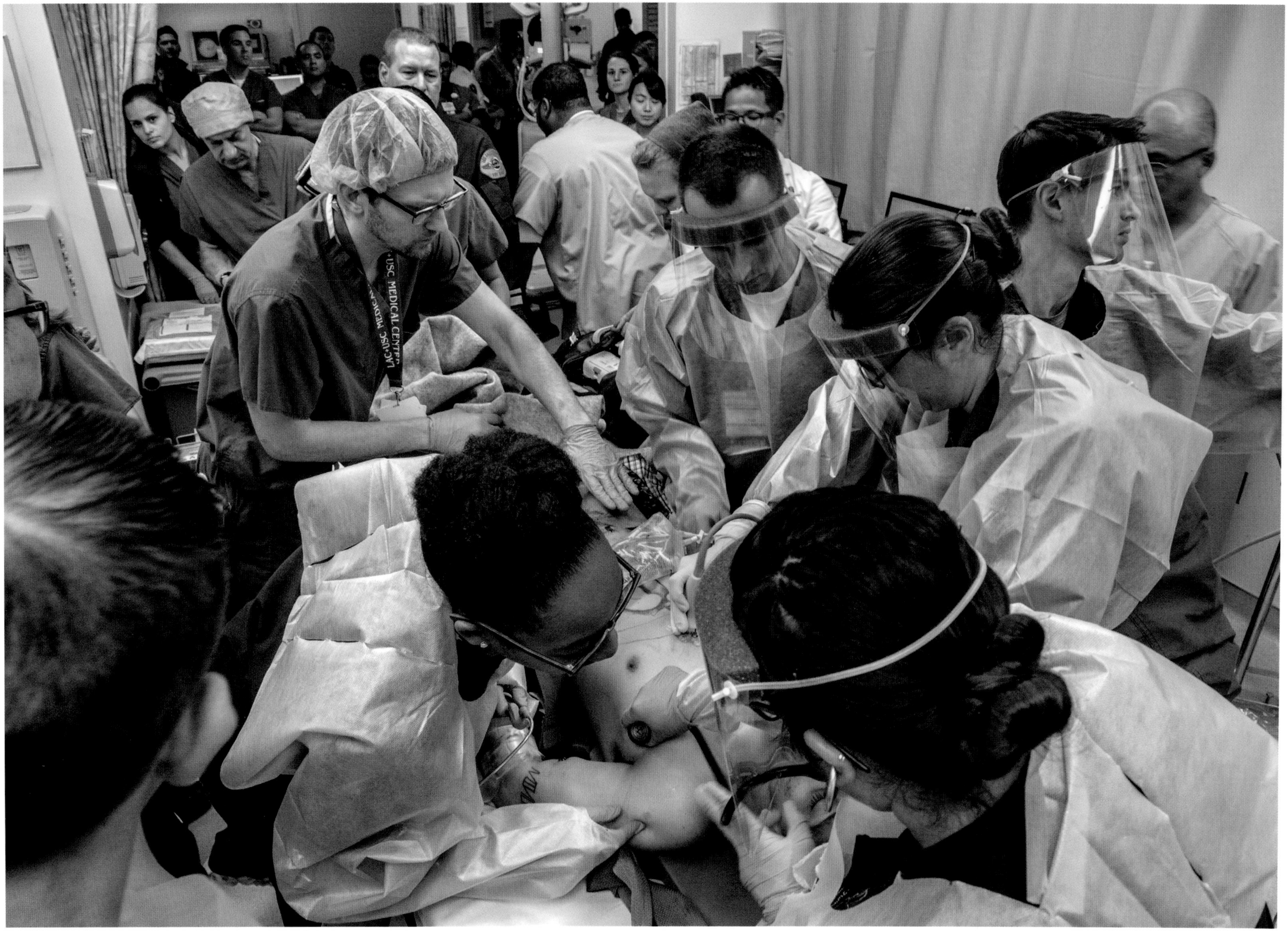

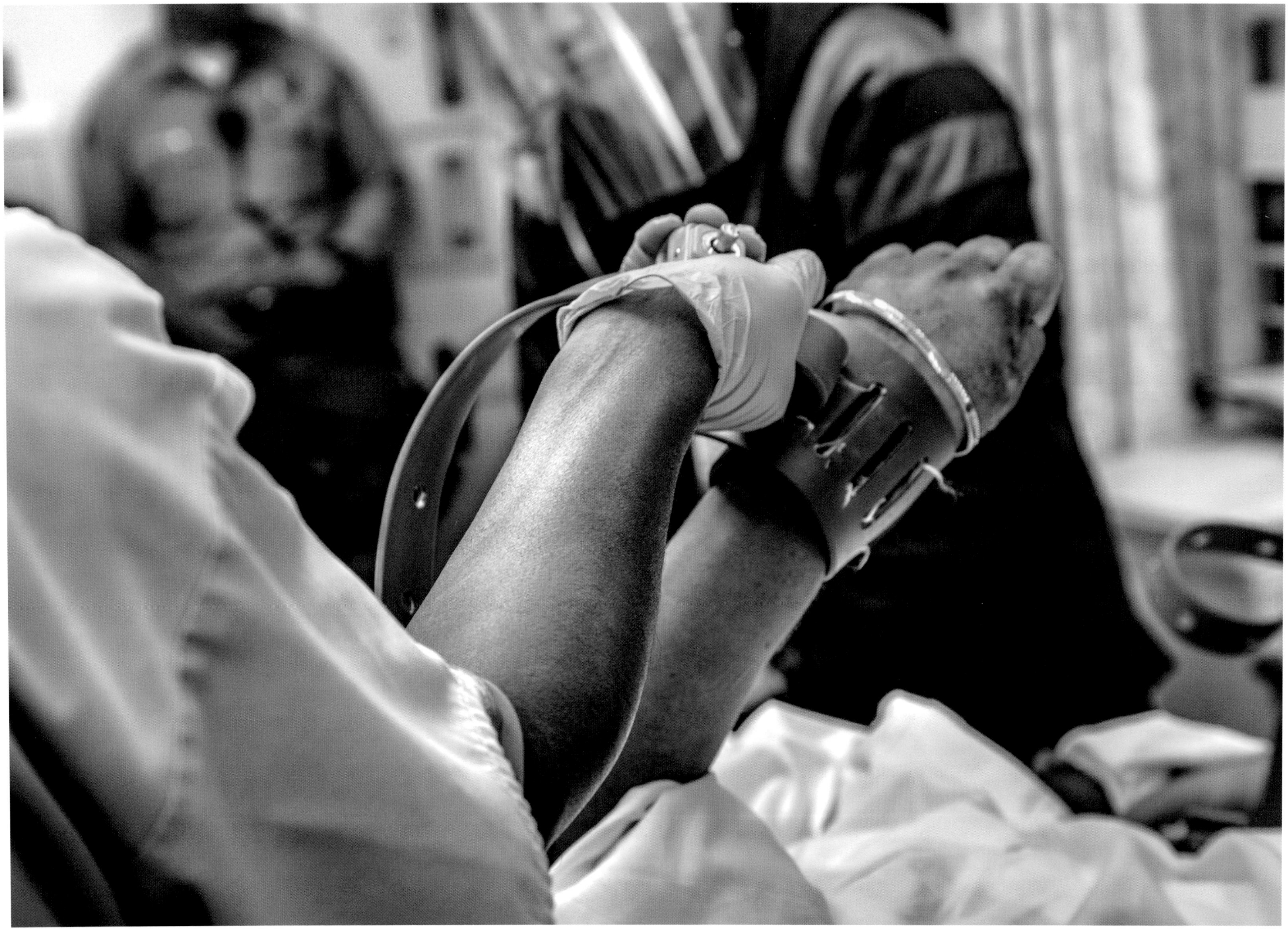

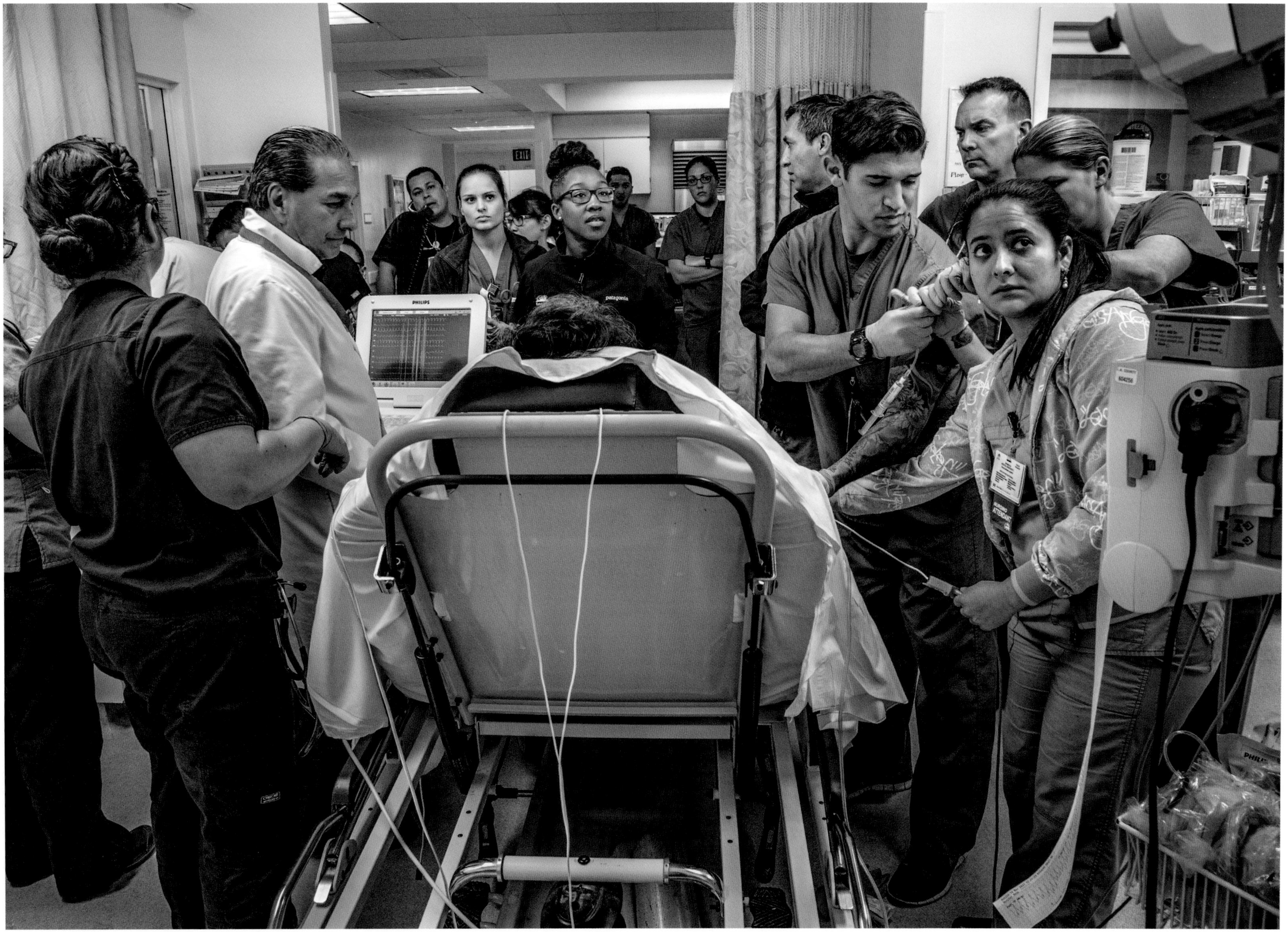
PHILIPS
patagonia

Gregory Hays, MD | Julia Hays, MD

Emergency Physicians
Detroit, Michigan

Julia: I could hear him speaking on the other side of the curtain . . . he was explaining to a family what was happening to their loved one and what we could do to help. It was the first time I felt like I had been paired with somebody who cared about patients the way I did. He taught his residents to treat them like human beings, not just charts.

Gregory: I knew she came from a very conservative environment, but she never backed down from anybody — not even the toughest guys from the streets of downtown Detroit. At the same time, she treated every patient like family and I really admired that.

Julia: We worked midnight shifts and would take the residents out for breakfast in the morning. We'd talk. Those breakfasts started to include fewer and fewer residents and pretty soon, it was just the two of us. One day he said, "You realize that this is a date, right?" I didn't think he dated coworkers. It never crossed my mind. Still, we were married within the year. I admired and adored everything about him.

Gregory: Yeah, I thought she was a nice person and a great doctor. But she was quite a hot number, too.

Julia: Stop it!

Gregory: We've been married seventeen years and we're never apart. It's unbelievable. We drive in together . . . work the same shifts. We know each other's moods, and I very much depend on her expertise. If there's a patient that's better suited for her or I get overwhelmed, I can just pick up the phone. She can do the same thing. We mobilize our resources to help each other out.

Julia: One advantage of living outside the city is the drive. It allows us to de-stress on the way home. After forty-five minutes, we hit farm country. Then it's just, "Ahhhhhh, the sunflowers are out today." We take in the visual beauty and relax. One of our favorite things to do is take a walk at sunset. The colors of the trees . . . the different greens . . . the light as it plays on the pond. . . .

Gregory: It's a perfect counterbalance to work. We usually plant crops in the summer. We have an asparagus patch that grew naturally next to the road. We can leave the hospital behind . . .

Julia: . . . and be totally different people. ✚

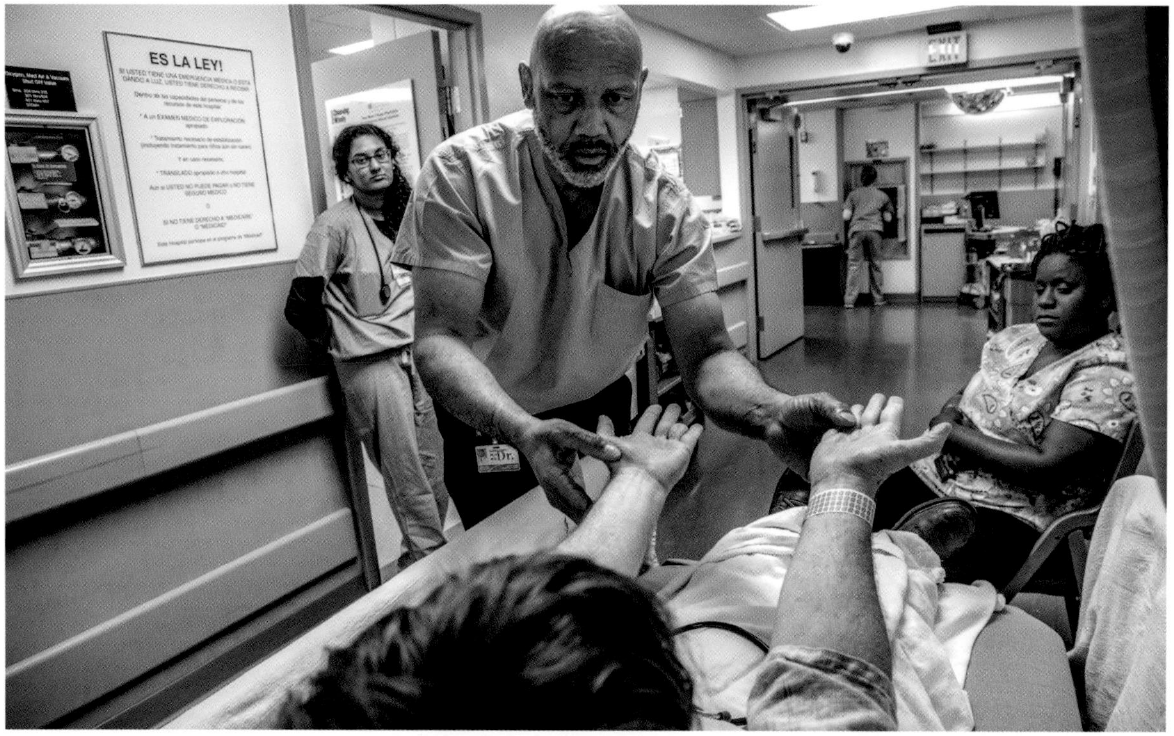

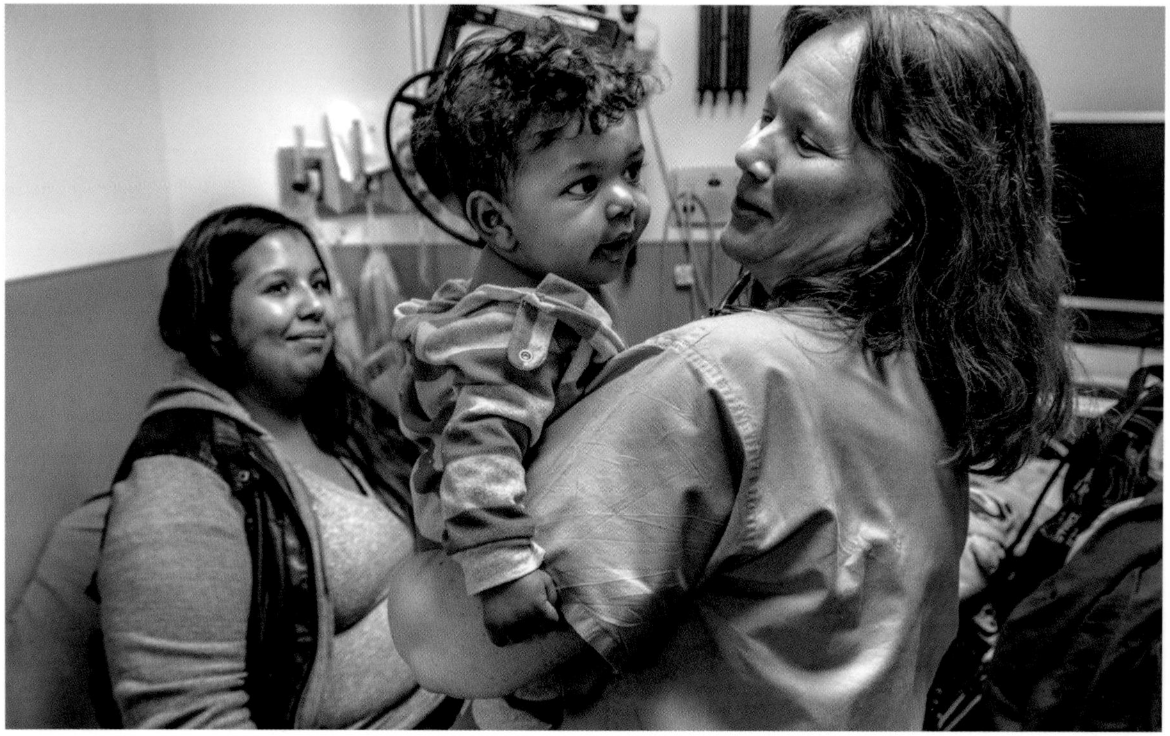

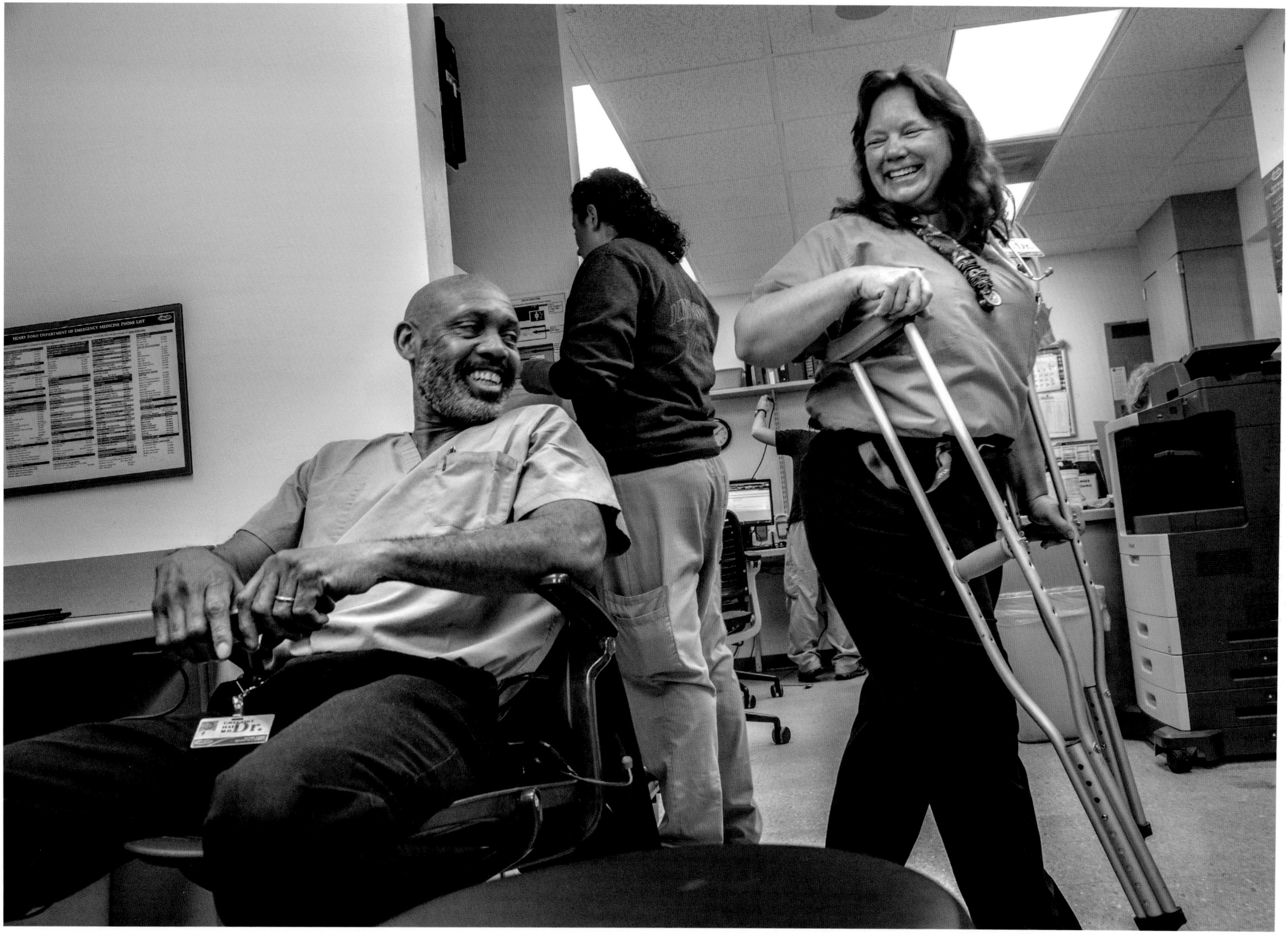
Henry Ford Department of Emergency Medicine Phone List
Dr.

Christopher Lewandowski, MD

Emergency Physician
Detroit, Michigan

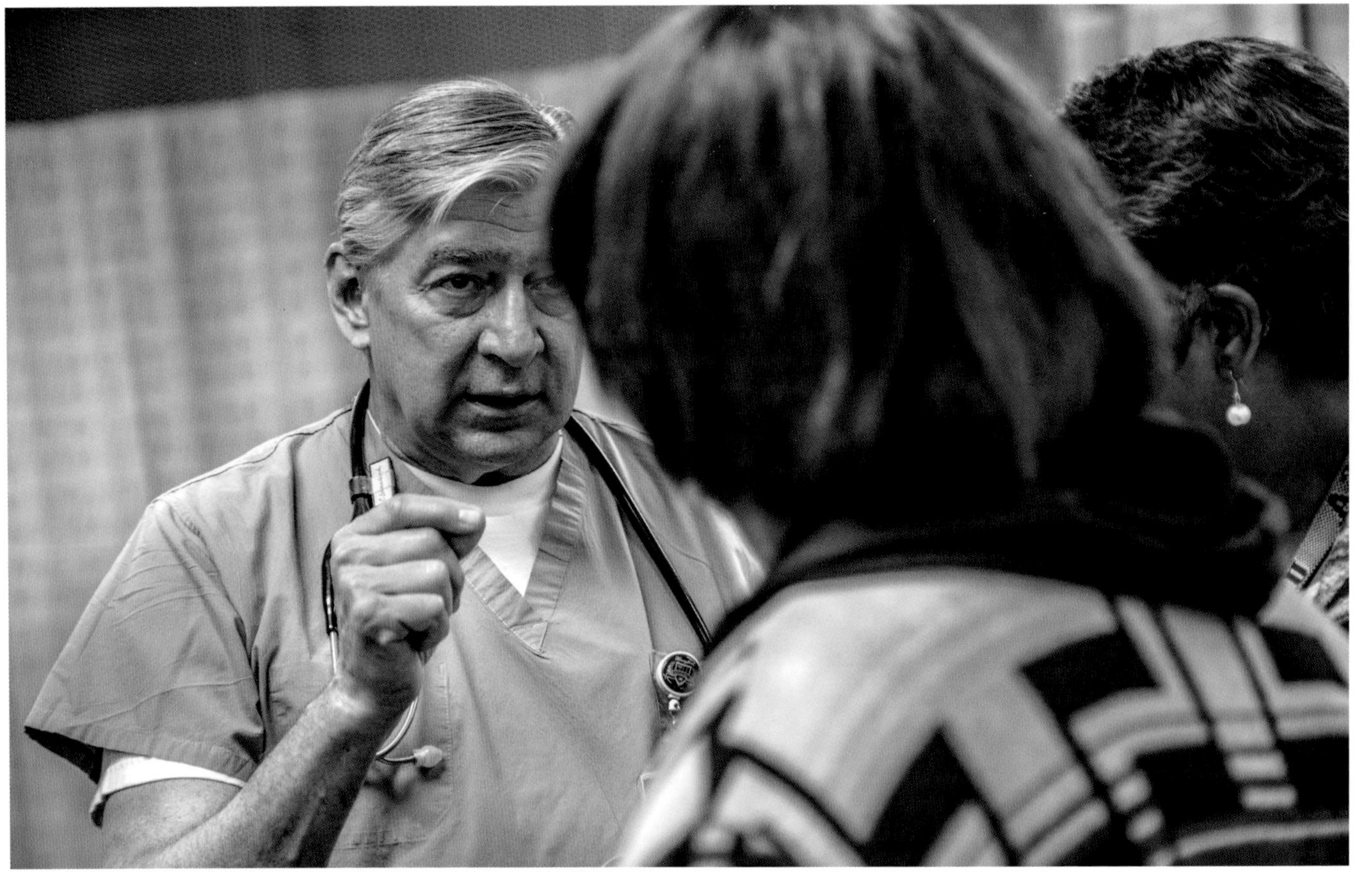

You just go about your day-to-day work, and the time slips by. It's like in the movie *Grumpy Old Men*; one day you turn around and you're not eighty-five anymore. That's how it goes.

During my second and third year of college, I spent a summer working in a Milwaukee cardboard factory for $5.50 an hour. We'd load these huge rolls of paper onto a corrugator that converted them into cardboard. The machine gave off steam, so the entire factory stayed at 102 degrees year-round, and the cardboard created a fine paper dust that would linger in the humid air.

I ended up with paper cuts up and down my arms from carrying stacks of freshly minted, flat boxes. The guys who'd been working there for a long time were immune because their skin was so calloused. You couldn't wear a long-sleeve shirt because it was too damn hot. The whole place was filled with immigrants, who would bust their balls on ten-hour shifts just to send their money home. Those boys had the best attitudes . . . they were grateful as hell to have a job, and they raised the rest of us up. They taught me a lot about work ethic that — even now — I carry with me.

I became interested in stroke research fairly early. When I was a resident and a young staffer, there was very little we could do for stroke patients, and most never went home again. Those cases always stuck with me. In the early '90s, tPA (tissue plasminogen activator) was being used as a clot-busting drug for the treatment of heart attacks, but researchers across the country were starting to look at it for strokes. I worked on a tPA study for the first five or six years of my career. I would run to the hospital to see anyone who'd had a stroke, hoping they would be eligible for the drug. We eventually published a landmark paper that helped tPA gain FDA approval, and I spent the next twenty years trying to educate people about how to use it. The payoff has been restoring normalcy in stroke patients . . . getting them back home and functional.

When my dad had a stroke, the local ER refused to give him tPA. It's one of my big regrets. I called his doctor from home and specifically requested he get the drug. The guy reassured me my dad's symptoms were resolving on their own, and I believed him. I jumped in the car and drove to the hospital as fast as I could, but when I got there, it was clear his symptoms were still there. The doctor just didn't want to use the medication — it's that simple — and his bad decision affected the rest of my dad's life.

Here I'd done all this freaking work . . . dedicated years to stroke research . . . and for what? I couldn't even help my own dad — this guy who'd fought both the Germans and the Russians in World War II and survived a German POW camp. After the stroke, he had difficulty walking and speaking . . . he couldn't use his right arm . . . he needed help dressing. It was bad. But, in the end, not all was lost. He lived until he was ninety.

I still love the freedom that comes with making a diagnosis and instituting treatment . . . the ability to really solve problems and take care of people who need you.

I remember moonlighting in a little rural town in Illinois many years ago. A farmer brought in his beautiful little five-year-old girl on Christmas Day. She'd gotten a new bike and had mangled her hand in the gears . . . it was a huge mess. I didn't have any backup . . . no hand surgeons or anything . . . so I did what I could. I spent probably three or four hours sewing up her wounds. The father brought her back about a month later to show me how well she'd healed and handed me his brand-new Pioneer corn seed cap. Apparently, those hats are a pretty big deal in the farming community. I'll never forget it. He gave me his best. ✚

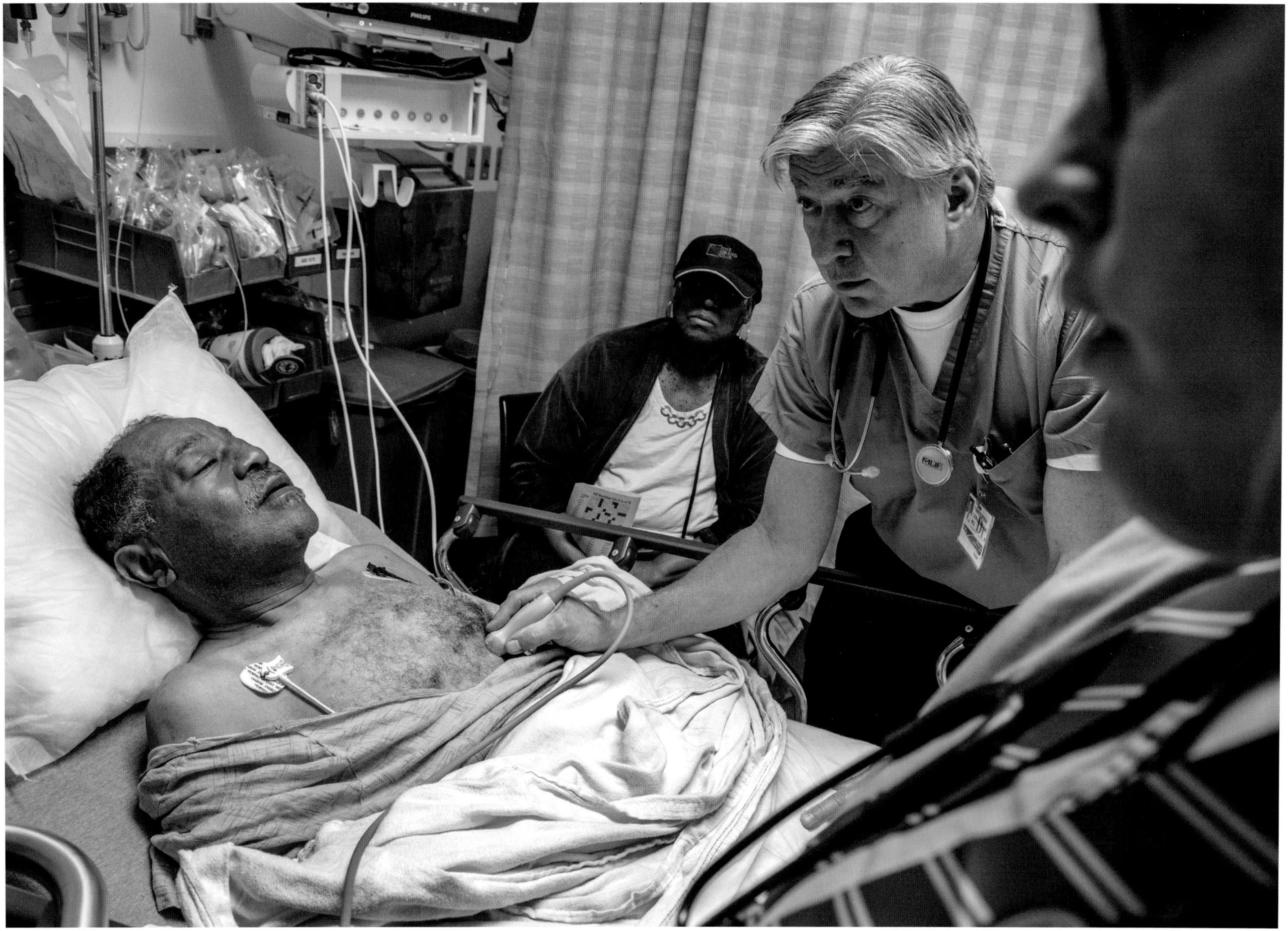

Elijah "Trey" Robinson III, MD

Emergency Medicine Resident
Cleveland, Ohio

I wanted to be the president of the United States . . . just like Abraham Lincoln. He unified a nation that was divided, and I wanted to be special like that. But then I learned more about politics. . . .

There are a lot of childhood pictures of me pulling things out of the fridge. I loved mixing stuff together to see what I could create. I had a passion for the physical sciences. *What's gravity? Why was it raining?* I wanted answers. I later learned I also really liked community service . . . liked talking to people. That's how I got into medicine . . . there was only one option for me.

I'll never forget my very first shift in the ED. There was so much going on, but I could see how quickly you could make a difference. The second patient we received was a gunshot victim with a wound to the left ventricle of his heart. It was incredible to witness this team effort among surgery — the emergency physicians, and the nursing staff — all working together to save this guy.

The patient woke up at one point but lost consciousness again. I remember his eyes . . . they looked scared. He became cold while still holding my hand. I was flooded with mixed emotions . . . I didn't sleep that night. I was haunted by the screams that came from the waiting room when his family was given the news. Yet, I was energized with questions . . . eager to learn more about emergency medicine. *What could we have done differently? Did we do everything possible?* I showed up the next day ready to go . . . ready to save as many lives as I could.

I've heard people say that in the Golden Age of Medicine — the 1940s and 1950s — physicians had control; whatever they said, went. You didn't question the doctor . . . it was his show. That model has changed, though. Now the doctor–patient relationship is ideally one of mutual agreement, a partnership. But, yeah, that can be frustrating. Sometimes I want to beat on the table and yell, "Please take your medications! *Please*. You don't want to end up here again." But then I take a step back and remember we all come from different backgrounds . . . we're all burdened by different circumstances.

Residents work long hours and manage a lot of patients in a very small space. This environment can push you to the limit, but it teaches you how to depend on yourself . . . how to make decisions and stick by them. After they've made a mistake, I've heard interns say, "Jeez, maybe I chose the wrong residency." Or, "Maybe I'm just not cut out for medicine." But I tell them to use the experience as a learning opportunity. We're human. Mistakes happen. All we can do is try to avoid making the same one twice. ✚

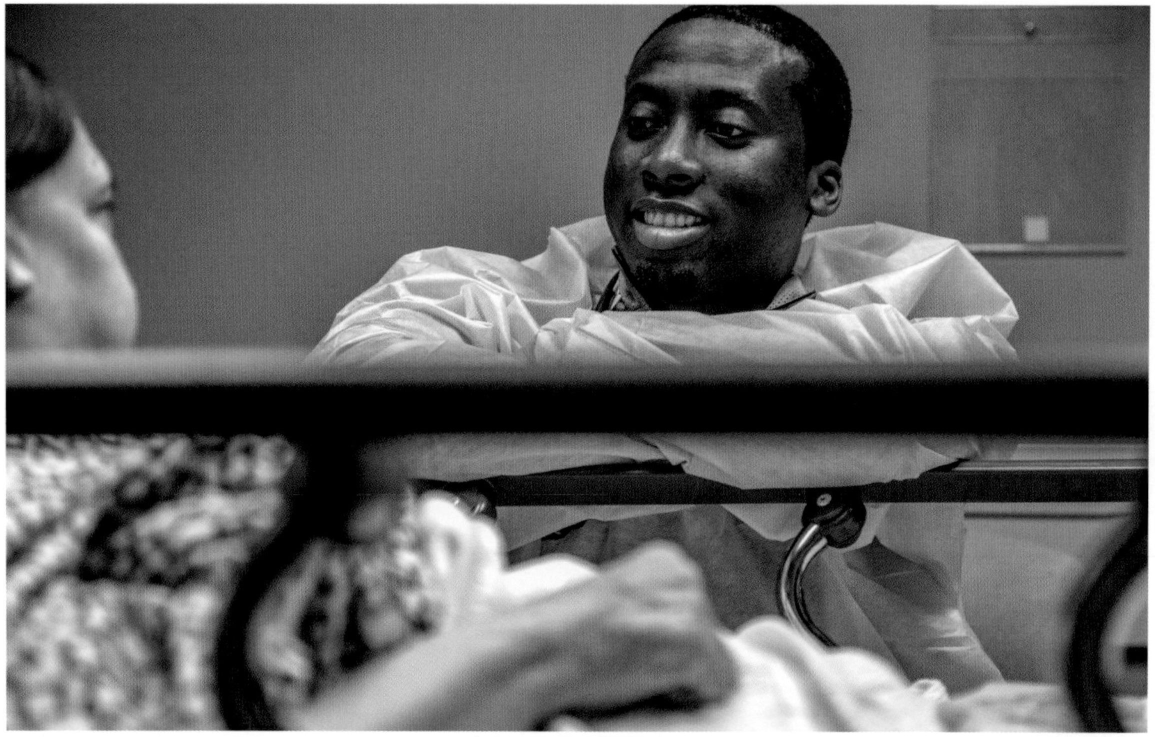

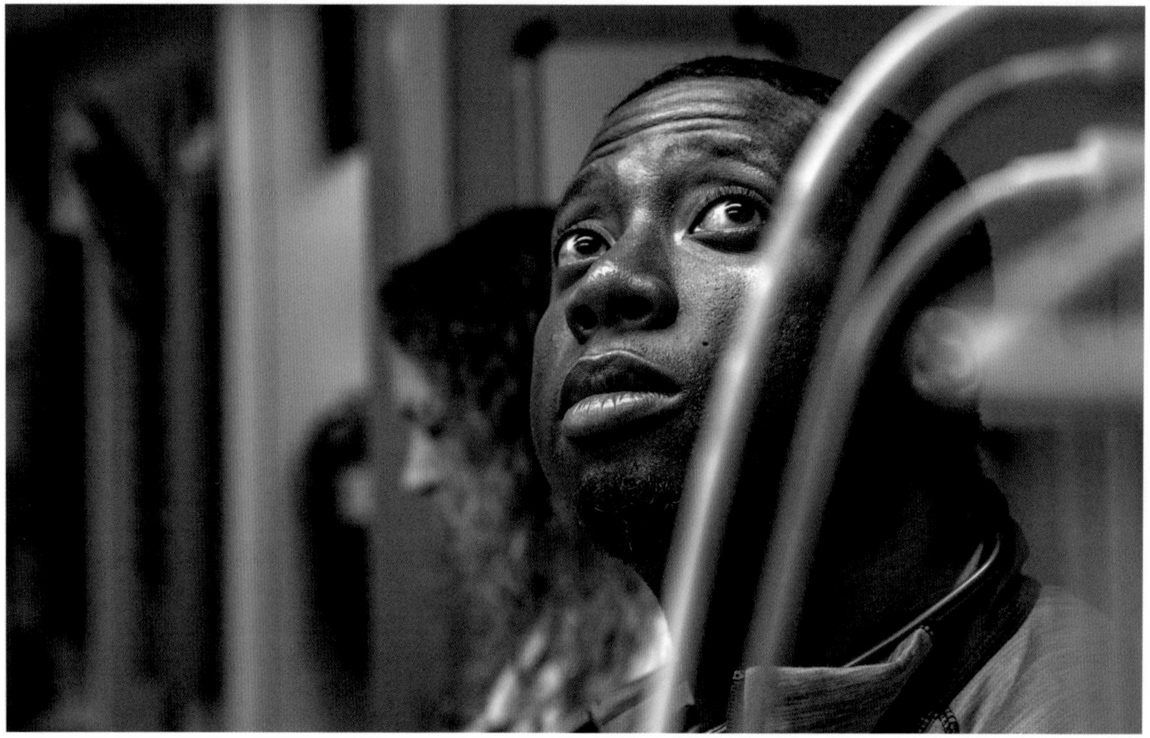

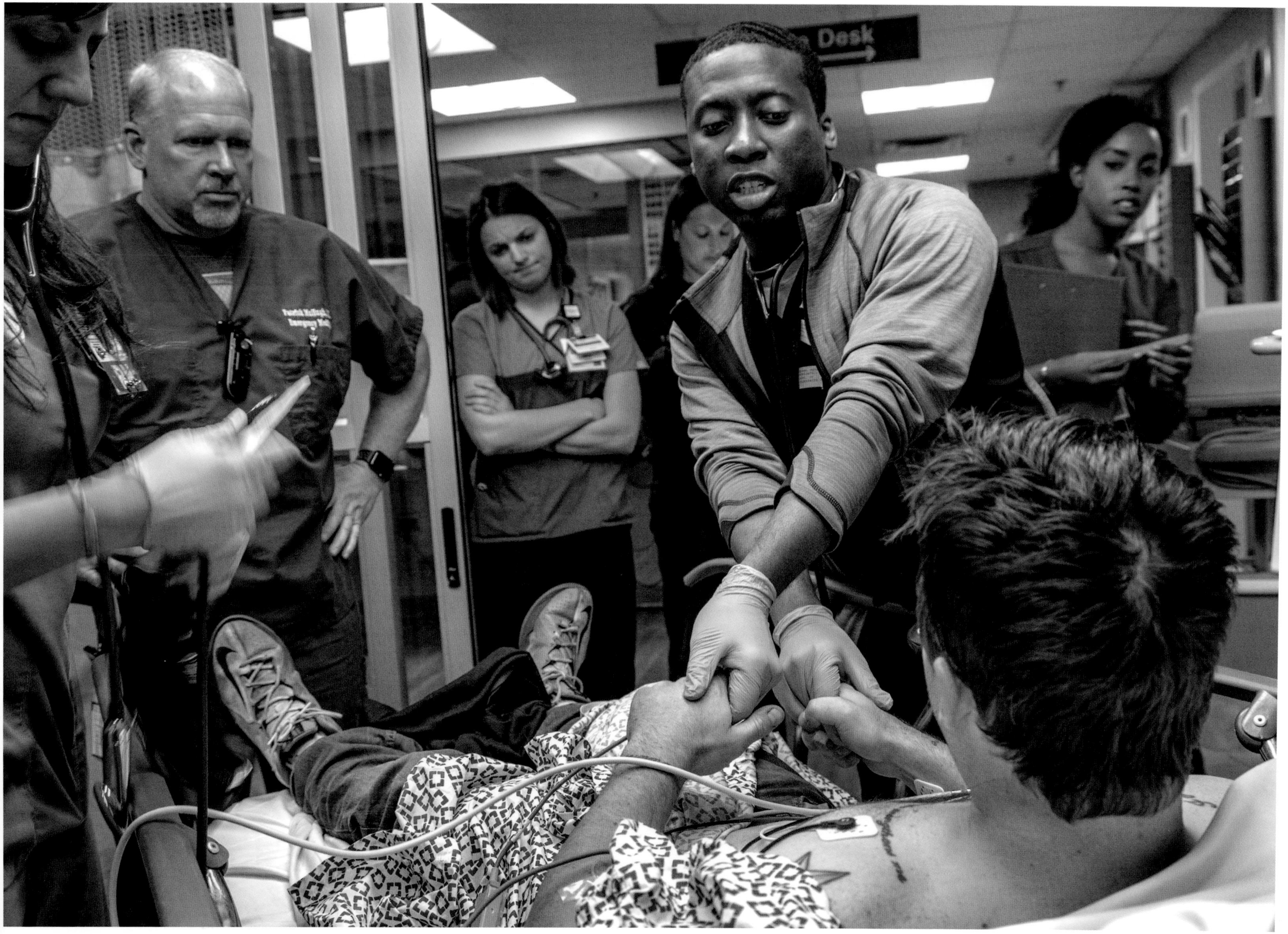
Desk

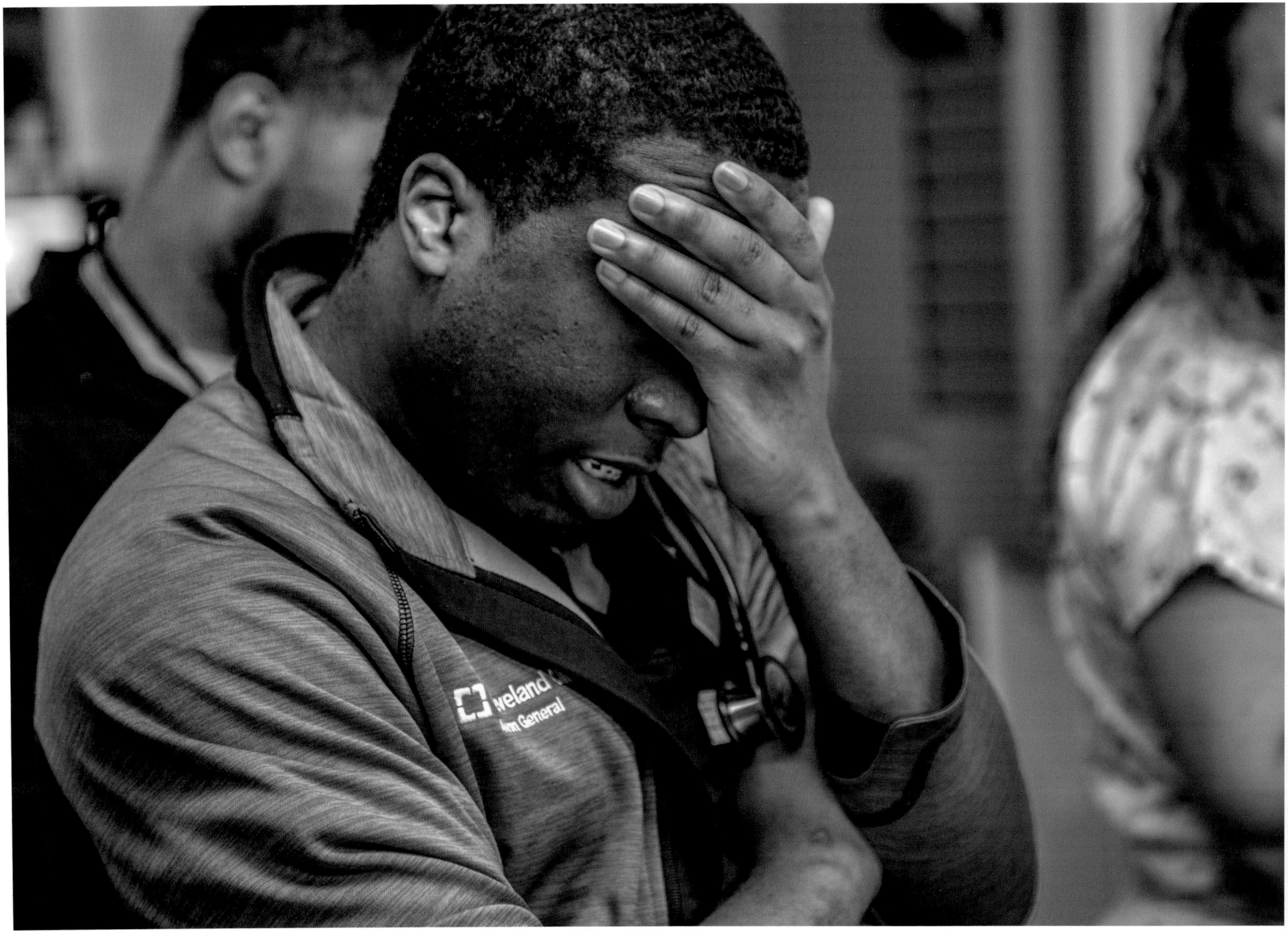

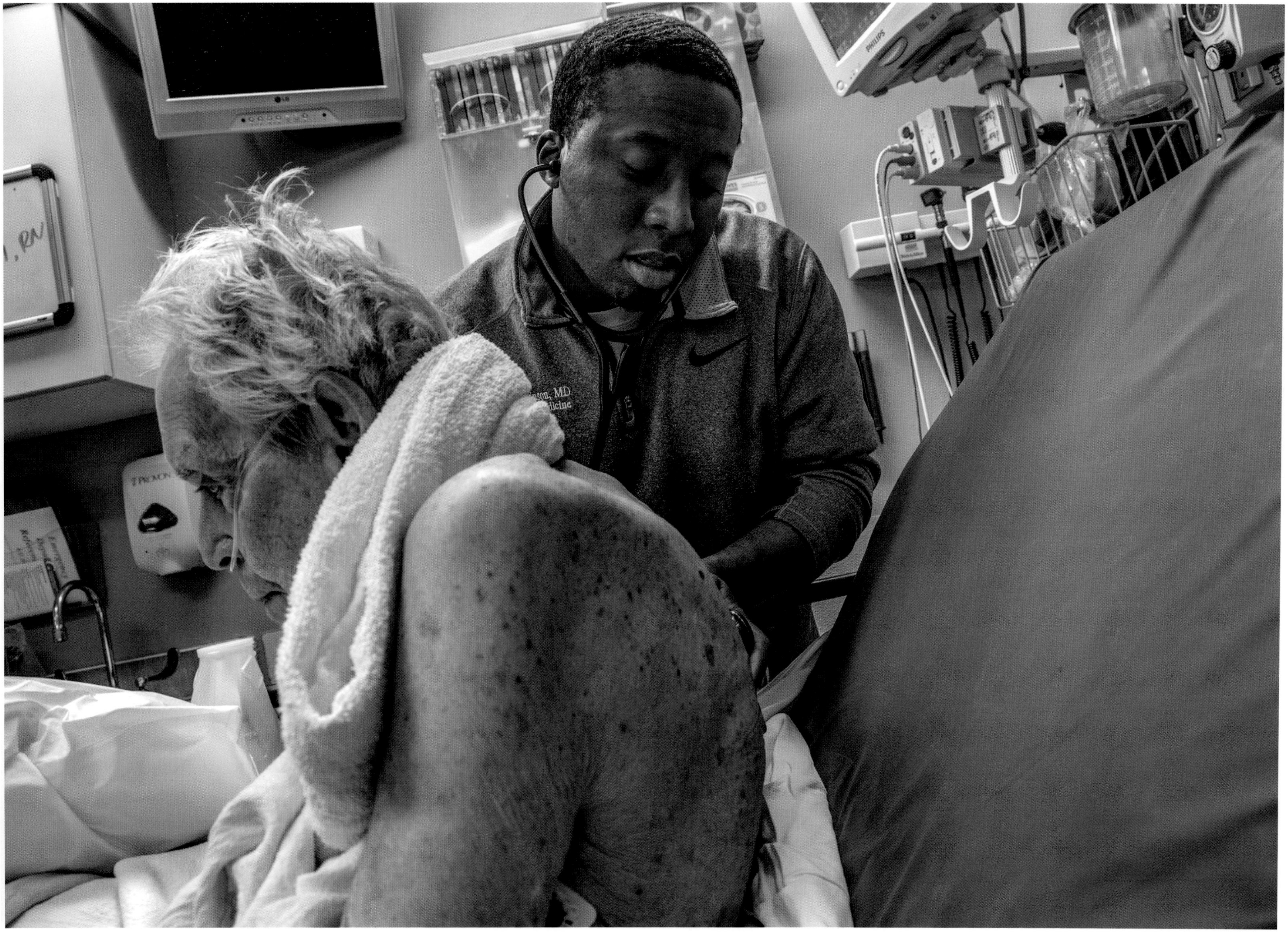

Marion Machado, RN

Emergency Nurse
New York, New York

The job of head nurse? Making sure patient care is as it should be, that standards are maintained. And being there for the staff, supporting them. Most of my nurses have been through huge difficulties in their personal lives. They've lost family, gone through divorces, things like that. It's all very well to tell them to leave it all at the door, but people are not always aware they're not coping. I've had to make the decision for them — "You need to take time off."

It's also a very special thing to help patients understand what's happening to them, help them interpret their diagnoses, give them insight when they need it. The physician will talk to the patients and their families, and the families will say *yes, yes, yes*. As soon as the doctor walks out, they'll turn around to the nurse and ask, "What did they say?"

I was born in India but grew up in England. When I was about sixteen, I decided I would do something useful, but I didn't want to be a physician like my mother . . . didn't want to study that hard. There was no "Oh, I've always wanted to help somebody." None of that. I don't know what made me go into nursing.

When I first came to the States, I worked in a private hospital in New Jersey. My first question always had to be, "Do you have insurance?" instead of, "What's wrong?" That used to drive me insane. At the time, a good friend of mine was dying of AIDS. Even with all he had to endure, he had to deal with insurance companies . . . with not being able to pay. It was inhumane.

Bellevue has always served a cross section of people, from those with true socioeconomic challenges to the terribly sick. You get a lot of car crashes, pedestrians vs. trucks, bicyclists vs. trucks . . . and subways. People jump, which is so unfair to the train drivers . . . they'll never unsee that.

When 9/11 happened, I got a page. A helicopter had gone down . . . then it changed . . . a plane had hit one of the World Trade Center towers. We turned on the radio. I stayed at the hospital for sixteen hours, went home, came back. For the next six days, we all did that . . . waiting as they dug through the rubble. We had at least eight staff for each bed — all ready to receive trauma patients. But there wasn't anyone coming in. Every time you went out of the hospital, you'd see pictures of the missing on blue boards along the walkway. All those faces.

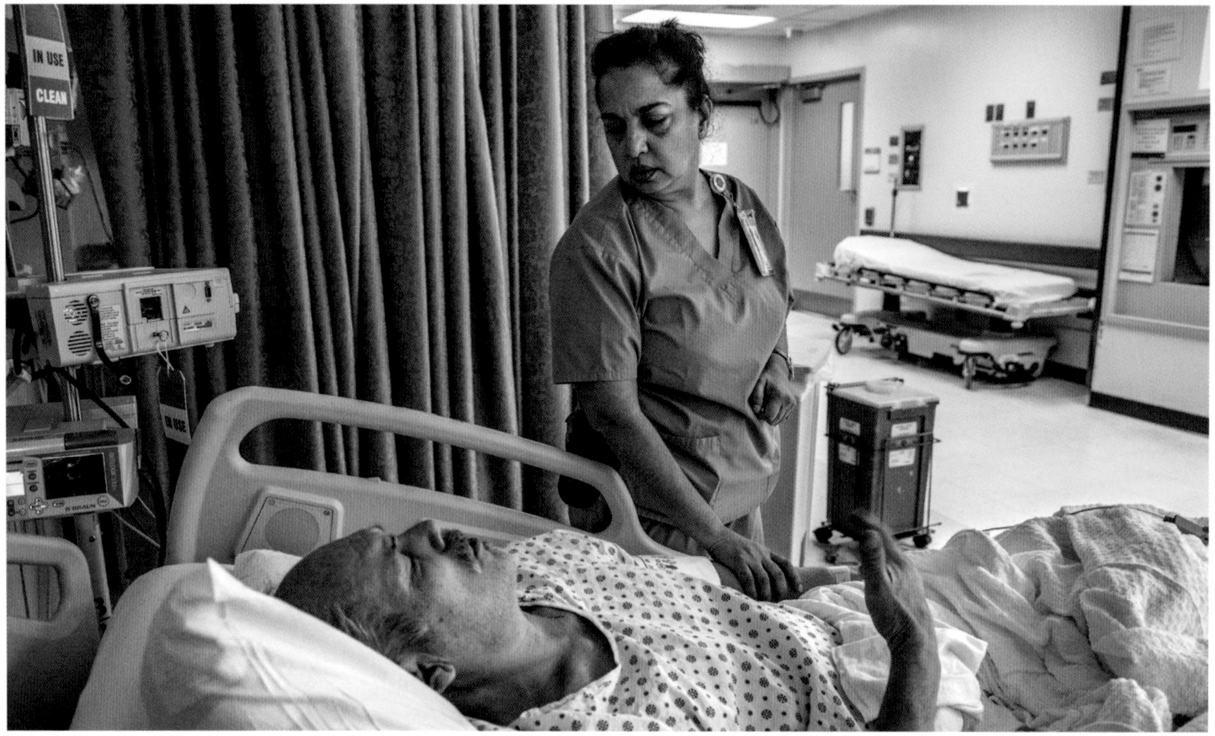

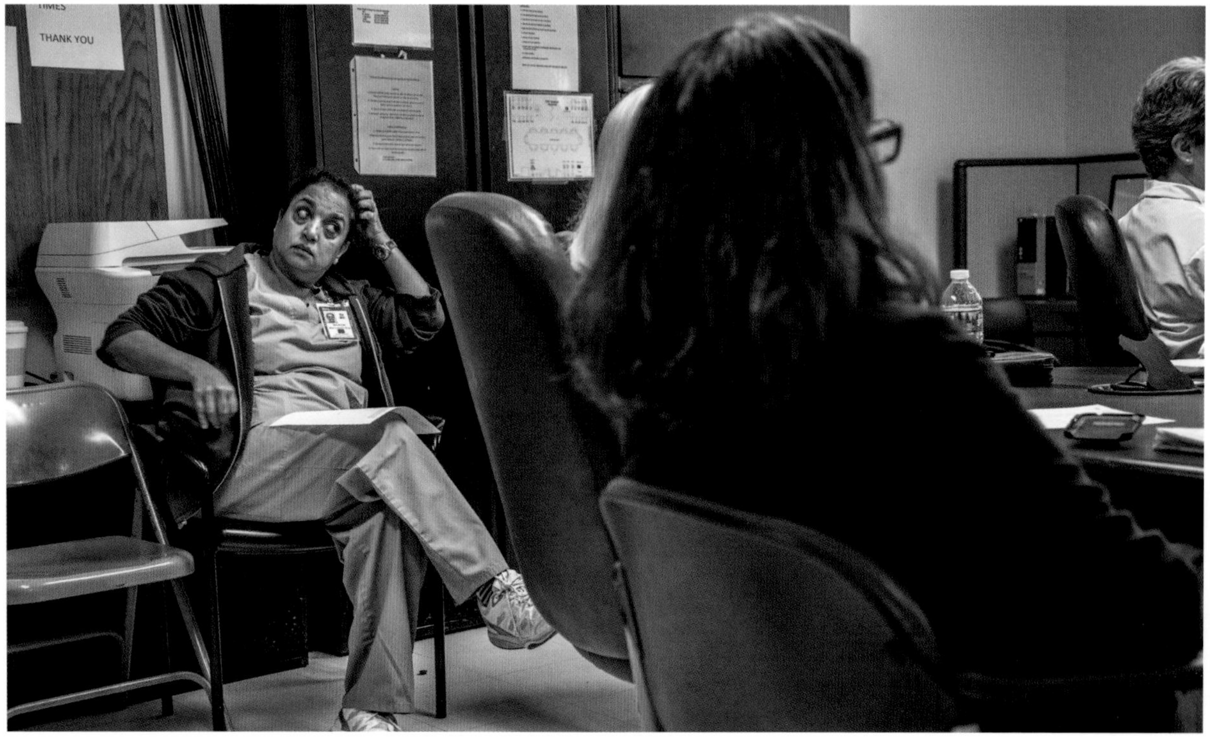

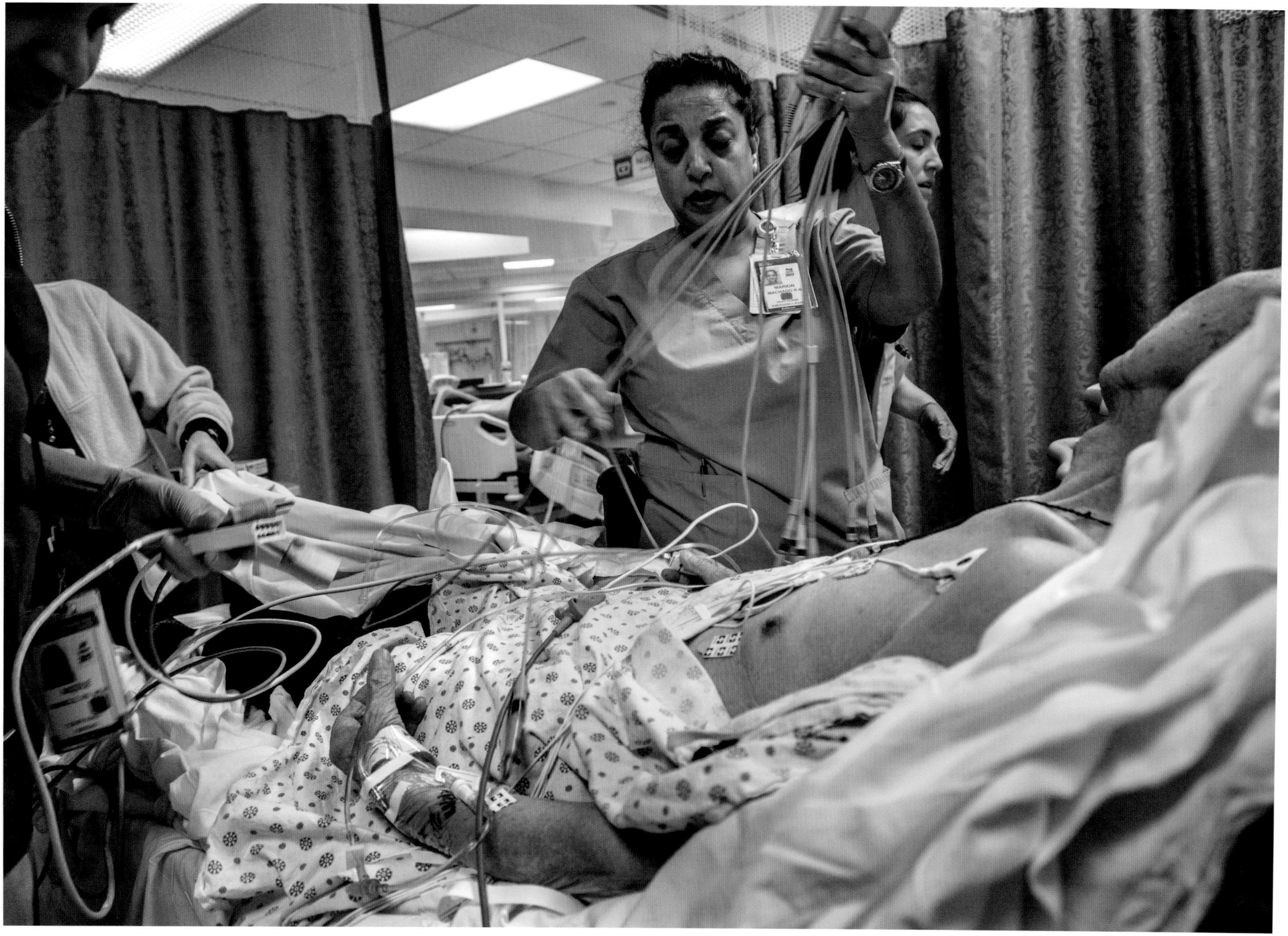

Marion Machado, RN

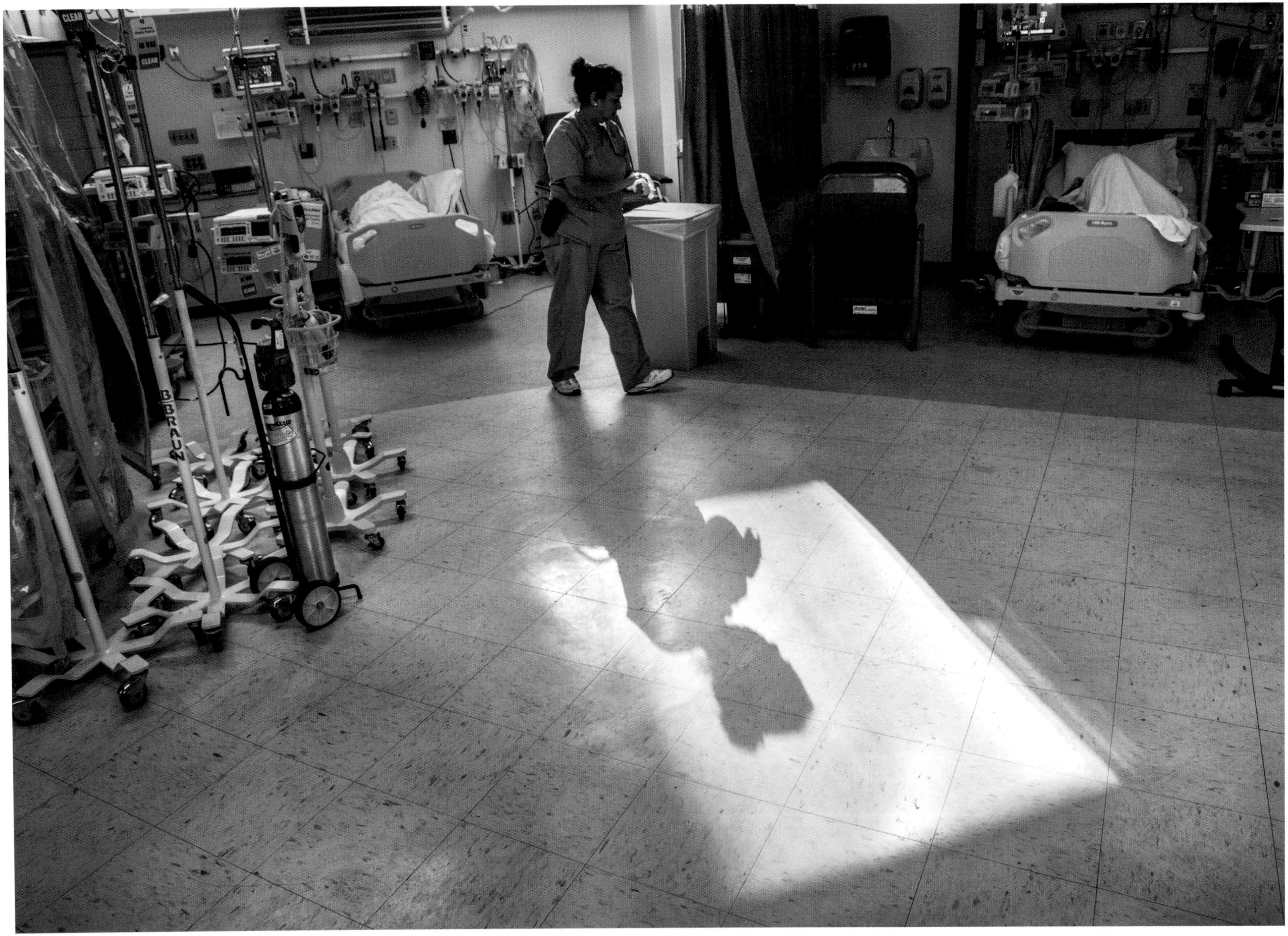
B BRAUN

We eventually went downtown to Ground Zero where we could treat the firefighters. They were covered in dust . . . I'd wash their eyes out, even though they just wanted to go straight back to work. I'd say, "You *will* sit down. You *will* let me do this correctly."

We set one area aside for the dead — a place to put the bodies found under the rubble. Still, we were always thinking we were going to have more patients. Finally, the day came when the pictures of the missing were taken down off that blue wall — when they were all gone. ✚

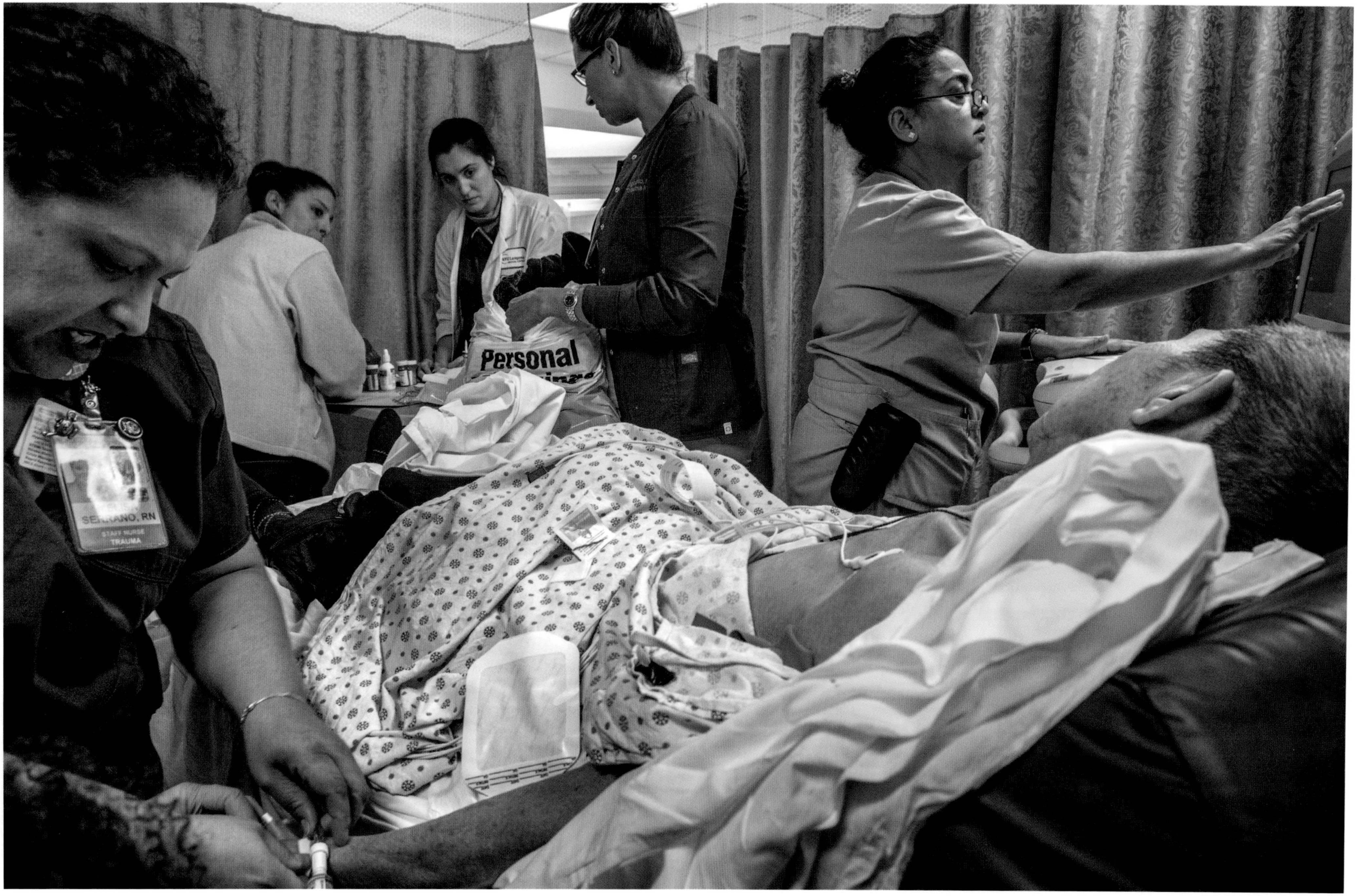

John Knight, MD

Military Emergency Physician
San Antonio, Texas

My dad left for the second time on the night before my sixteenth birthday. It threw our family for a bit of a loop. When the divorce was final, I bounced around . . . lived with friends . . . dropped out of high school . . . just did what young punk kids do when they're lost. I took the GED and got a job as a food and beverage manager at the Holiday Inn, but I could feel a weight on top of my shoulders . . . something telling me I could do more with my life.

When I was twenty-one, I wandered into a US Army National Guard office. The recruiter handed me a trifold pamphlet about special forces, which described the different specialties available to a Green Beret. I was looking for a skill that would translate to the civilian world and thought the medic job seemed interesting. That really was the first time medicine ever entered my mind. I didn't know what I was getting myself into, but a week later I was at the military entrance processing station with my right hand up.

The training was challenging, but I knew I'd found my niche. It was all me . . . nobody was telling me what to do or how to do it. I had the freedom to make my own decisions and, as corny as it sounds, I was proud to be there and loving every minute of it. Jumping out of airplanes . . . flying around in helicopters . . . trekking through the woods with a heavy backpack . . . doing reconnaissance . . . providing medical care for my team.

Eventually, I decided to go all the way — become a doctor. I took the MCAT during a deployment in Afghanistan and entered medical school at the Uniformed Services University of the Health Sciences, confident I'd chosen a profession that could extend beyond the military.

Combat and emergency medicine have a similar appeal. Both require teamwork and a tremendous amount of trust. When you're in the military, your life is in the hands of your partners. There's a camaraderie that's impossible to describe . . . a dynamic that also plays out in the emergency department. When a patient comes in on the brink of death, none of us can go it alone. Even if you're the physician directing the show, you've got to rely on the input of your staff.

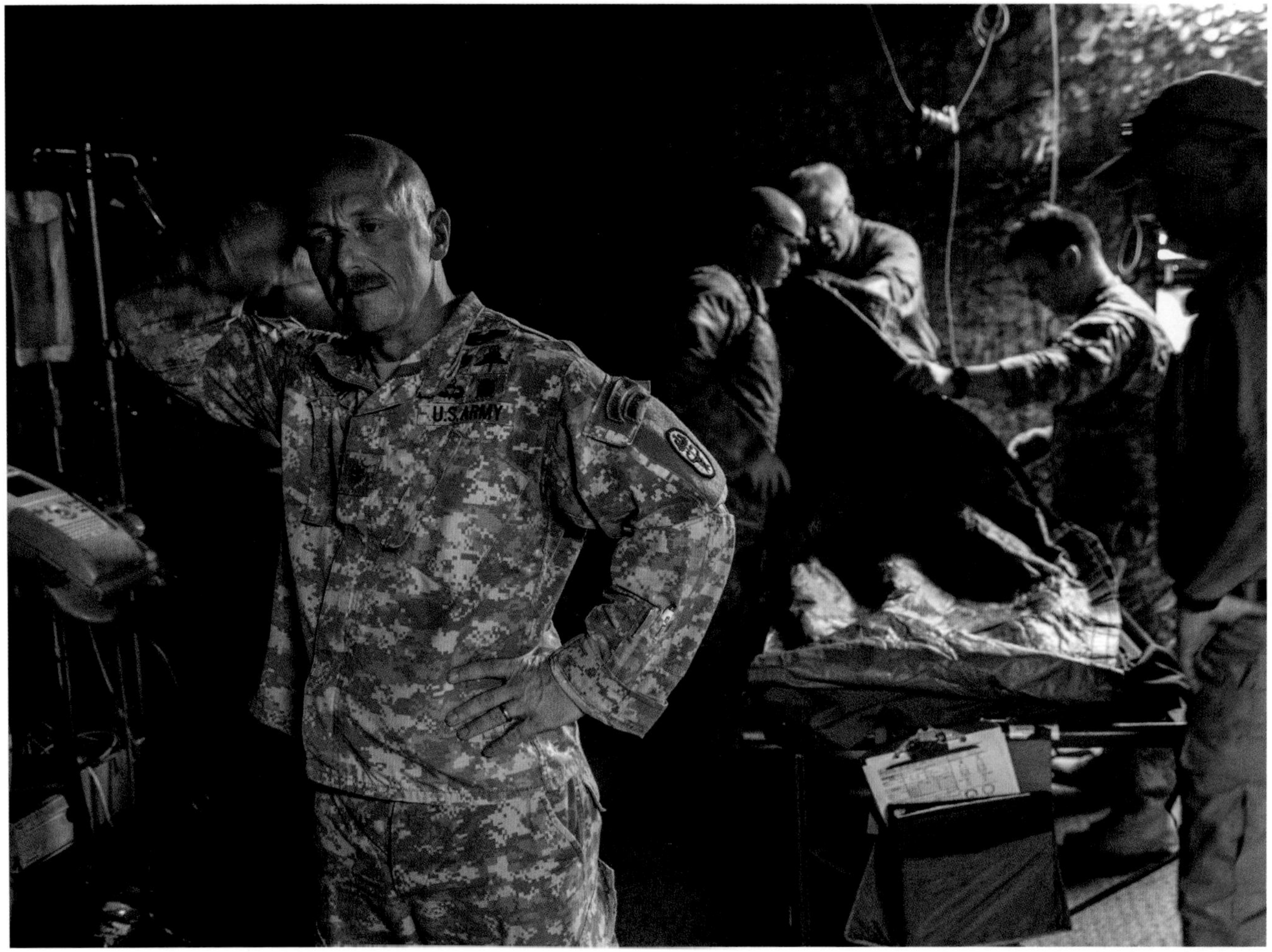

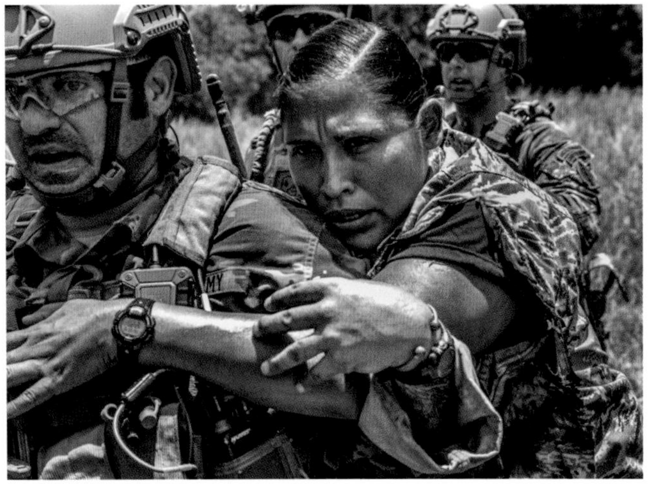
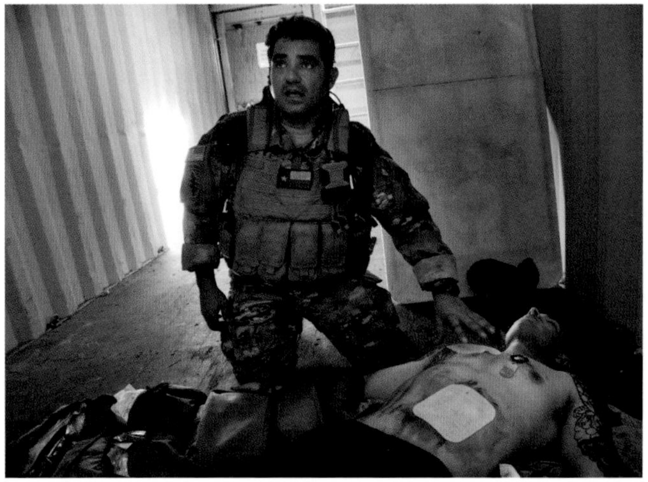

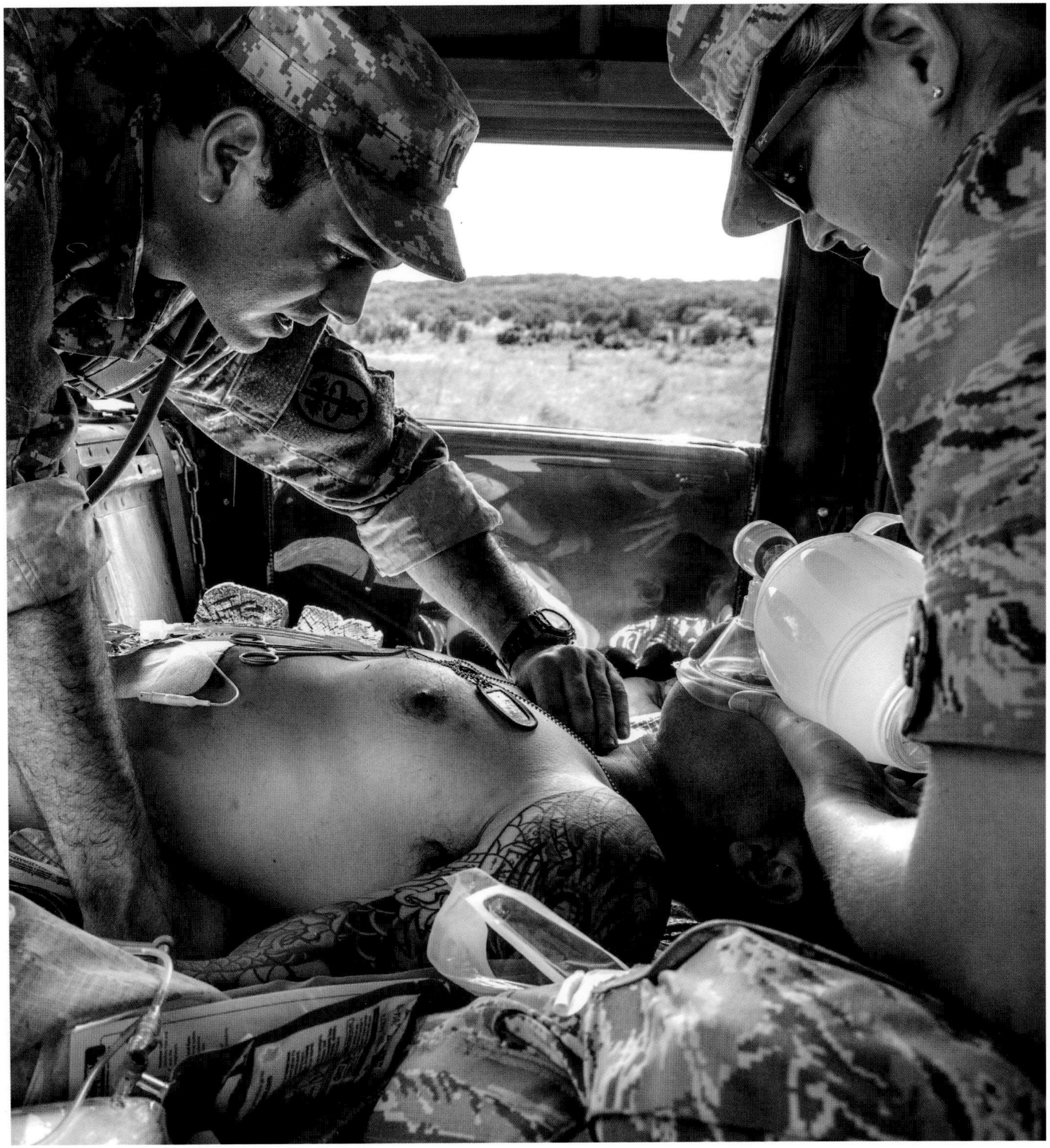

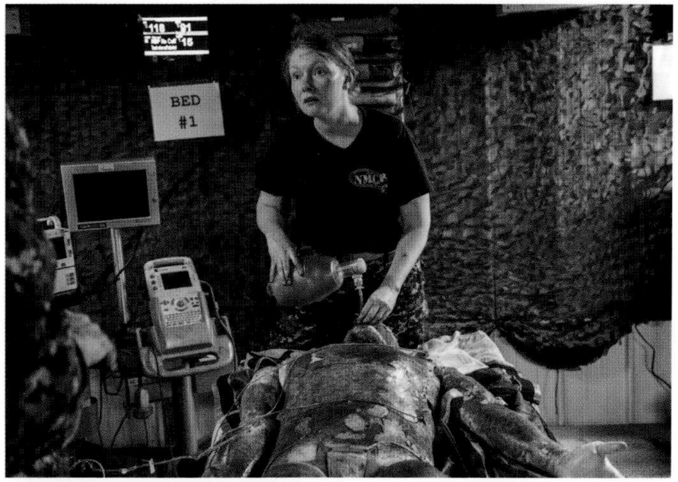
BED
#1

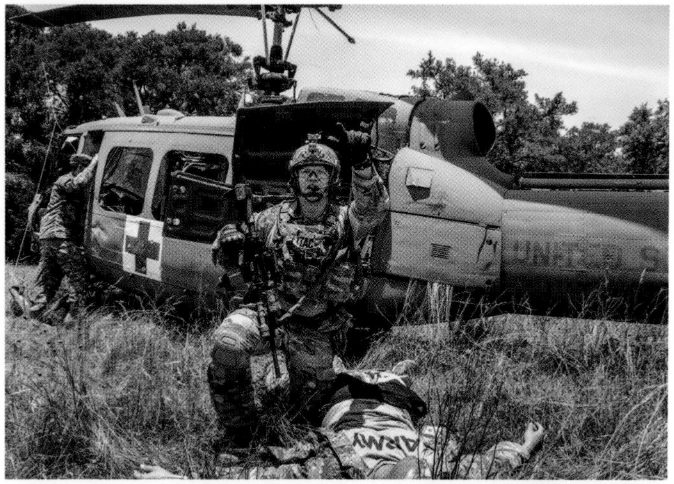

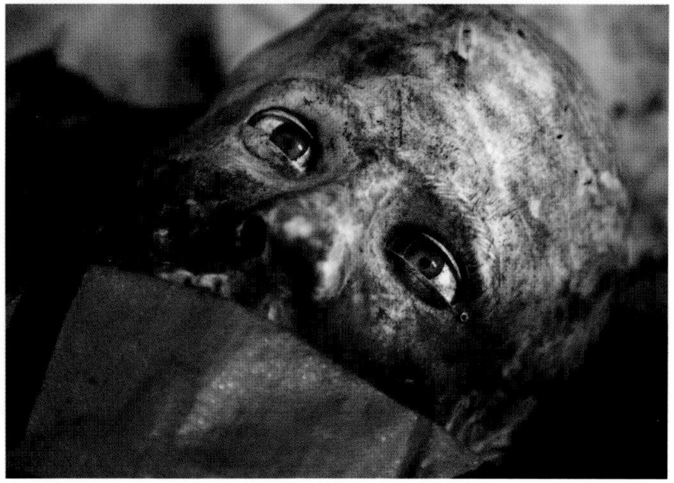

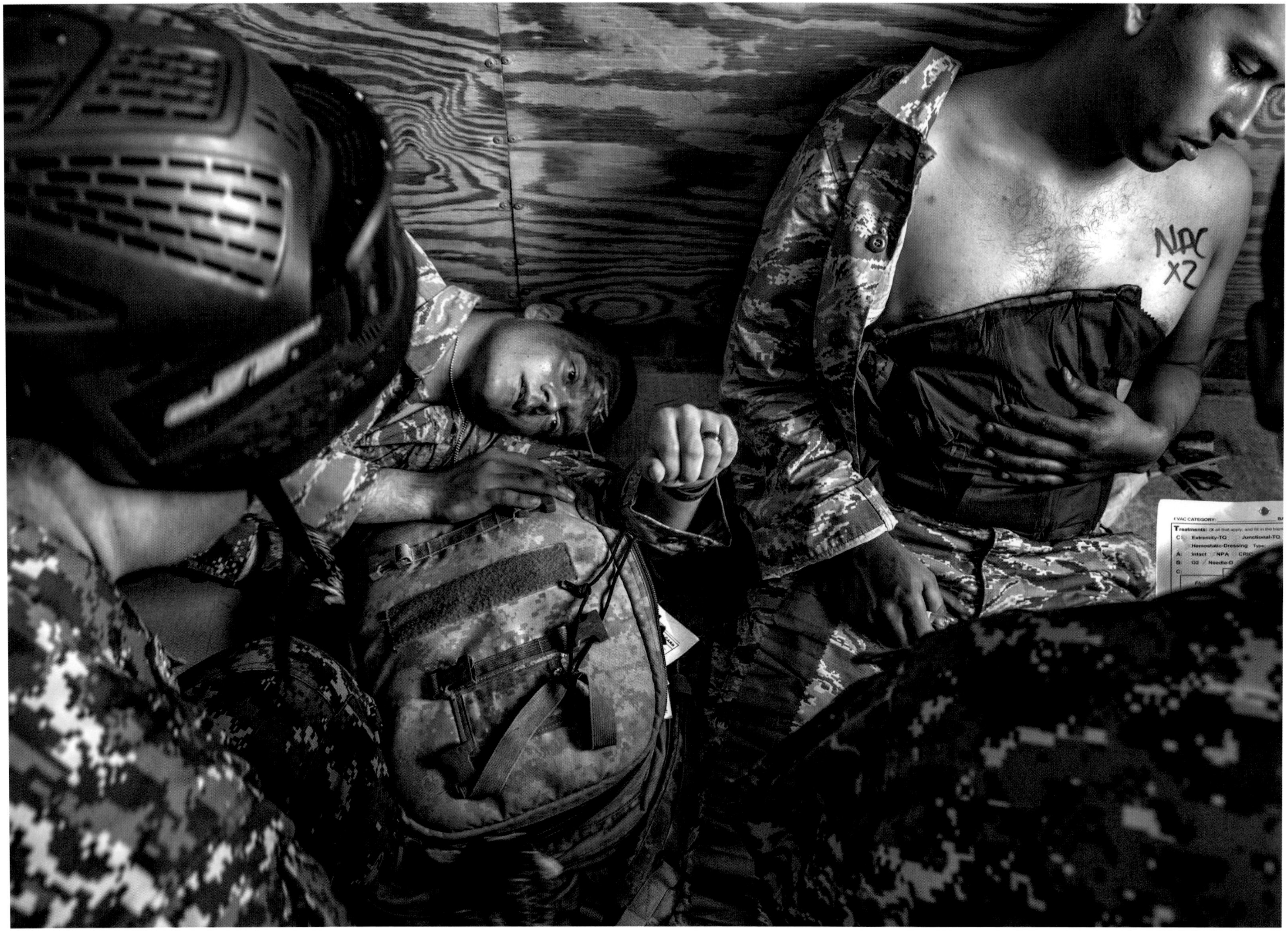
NAC
X2
EVAC CATEGORY:
Treatments:
C: Extremity-TQ Junctional-TQ
Hemostatic-Dressing Type:
A: Intact NPA CRIC
B: O2 Needle-D
C:

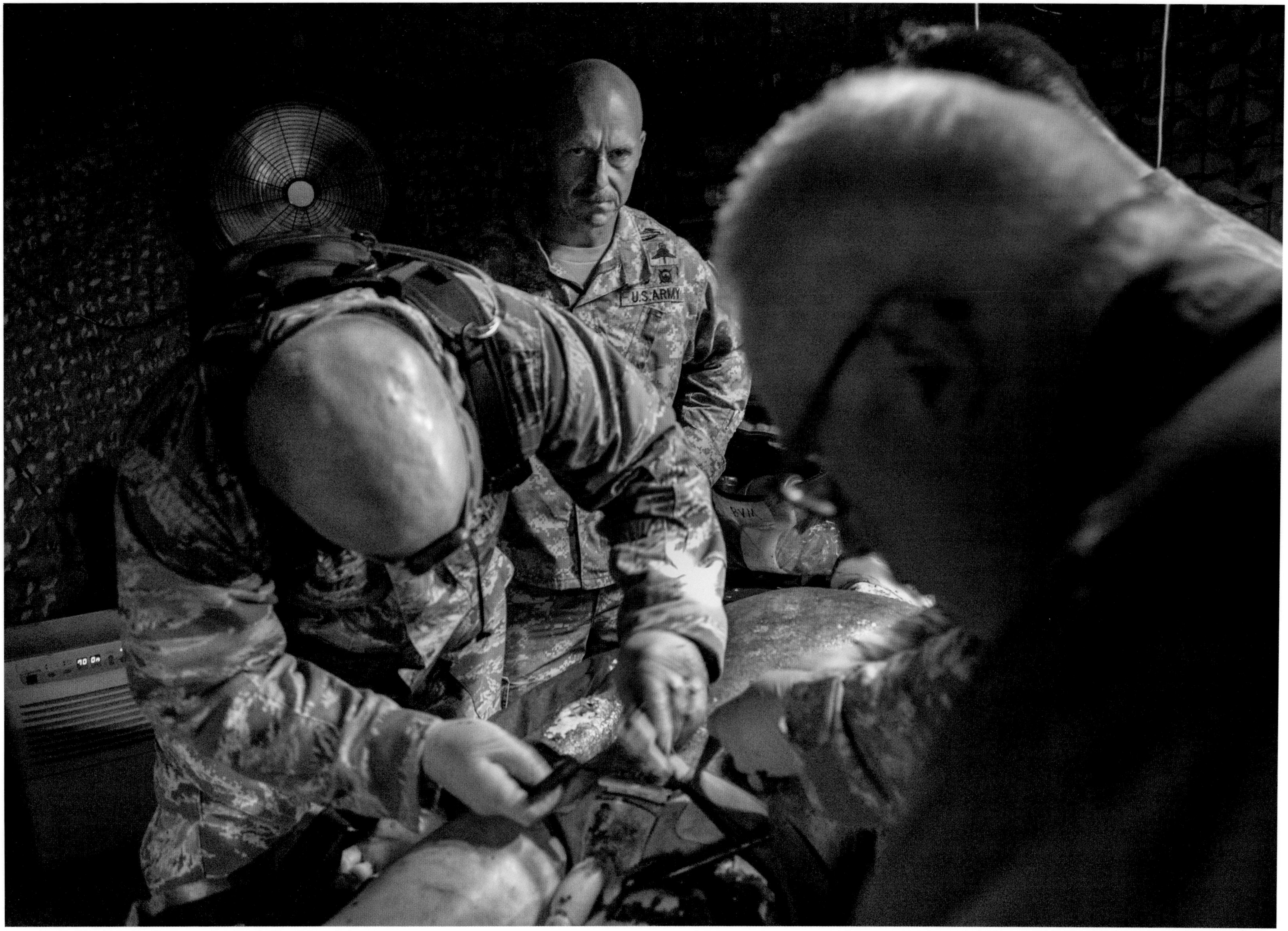
U.S. ARMY

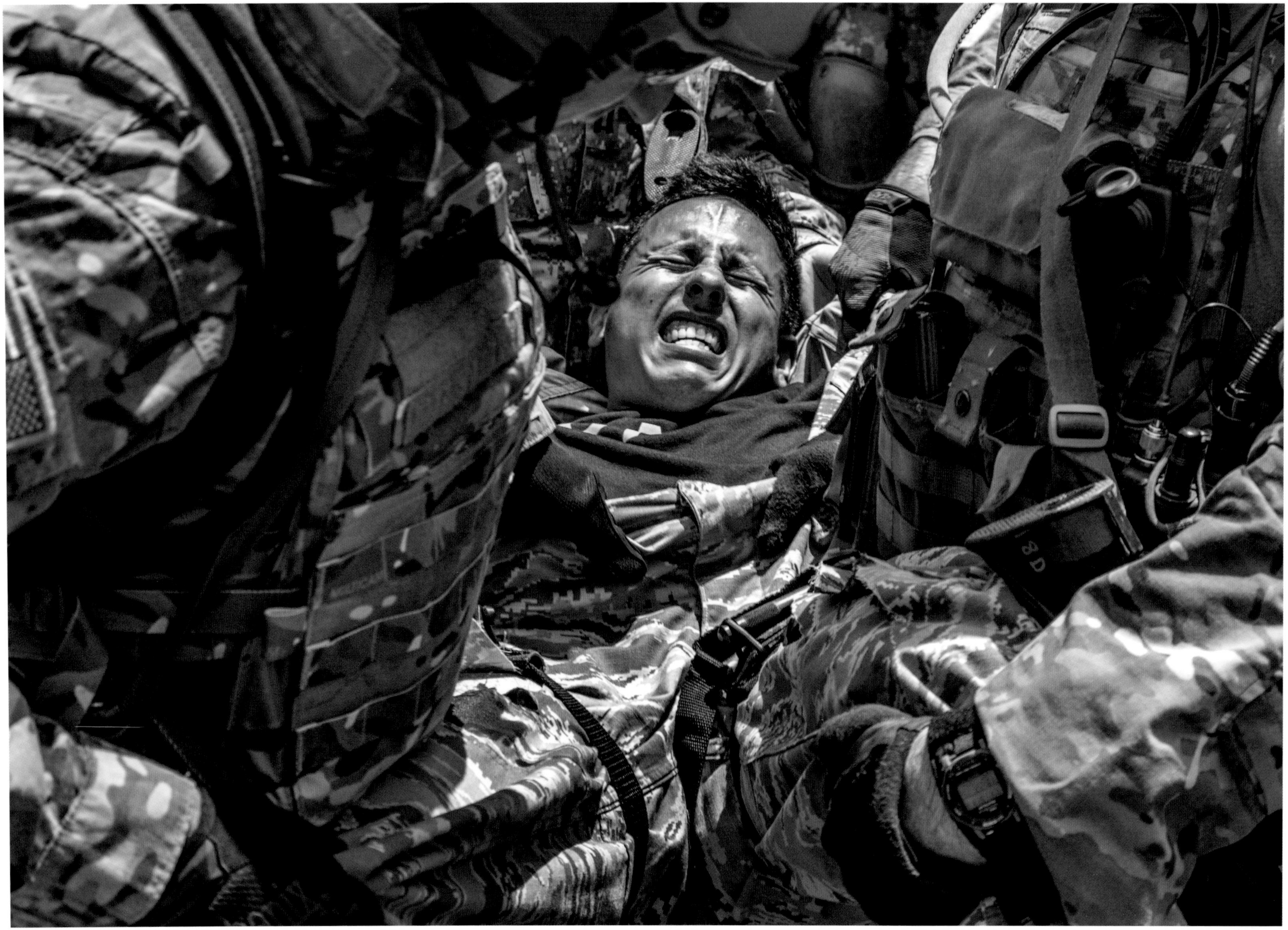

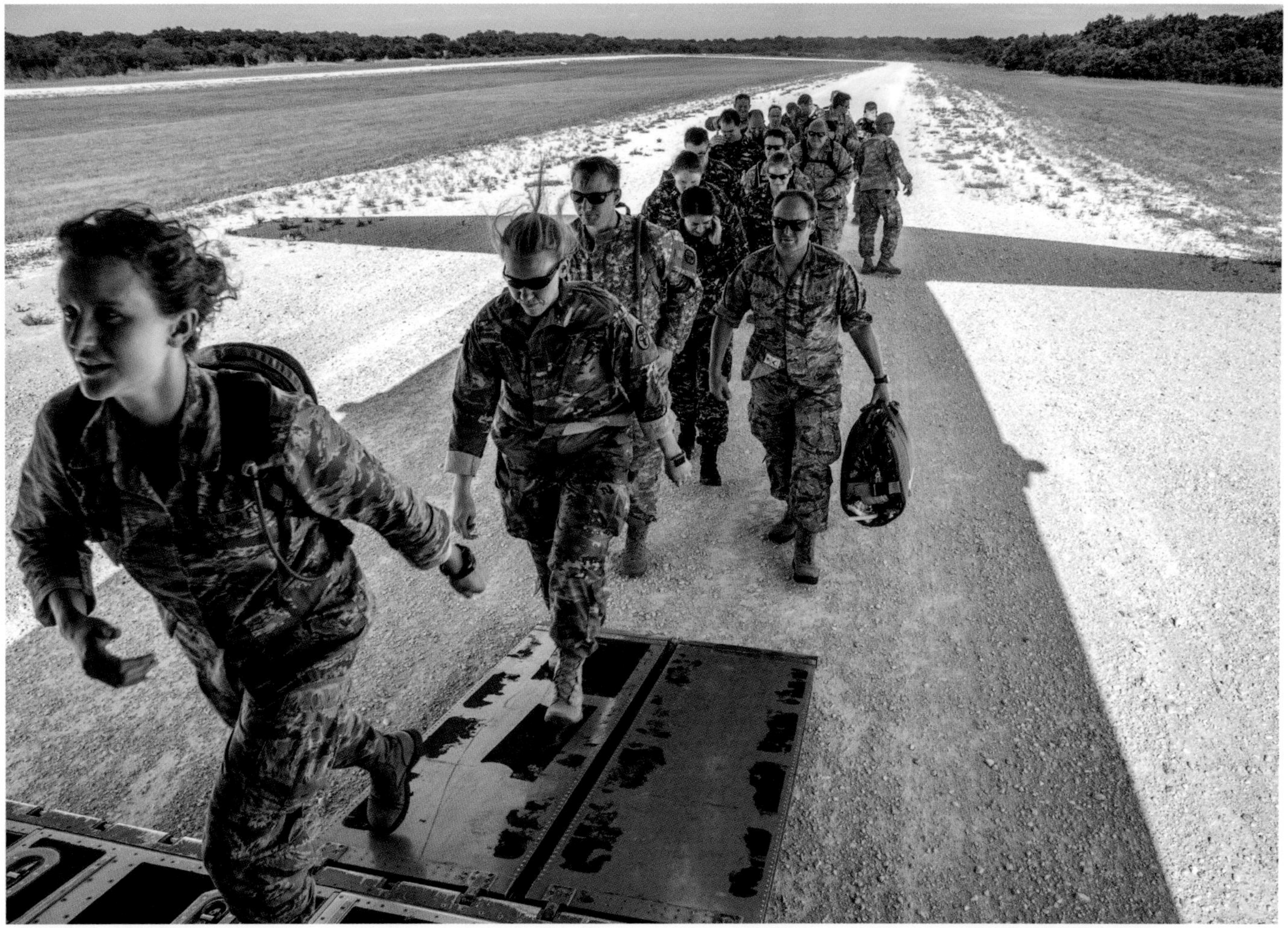

I absolutely love being an educator and am passionate about physician training. I think it's important for students to understand the full continuum of patient care from the point of injury to evacuation to a definitive treatment facility. I try to provide them with real-world experiences that mirror those of a medic on the ground . . . what it's like to treat a casualty while bullets are flying and mud's in your eyes. They need to be exposed to multiple evacuation platforms — rotary and fixed wing aircraft, ground vehicles.

Residents also need to learn how to operate in a variety of settings. When you're in the field, you won't have access to a nice big ER and a giant staff. How do you assess a broken leg without an x-ray machine? How do you diagnose a problem without lab tests? We have to make their lives a little uncomfortable so they are prepared to manage life — and their patients — down range, amidst chaos.

We used to train primarily on manikins, which were stiff . . . truly dead weight. The residents would get frustrated because the "patients" were totally non-cooperative, so they'd throw them around like the manikins they were. It was a problem because they would lose sight of the human element. We've found the training is more meaningful and productive when we get real residents to pose as patients. This way, the residents see what it's like to need medical help and, more importantly, how it feels to care for your brothers and sisters in arms. Regardless of the role each of them is playing, their uniforms speak volumes about their character. ✚

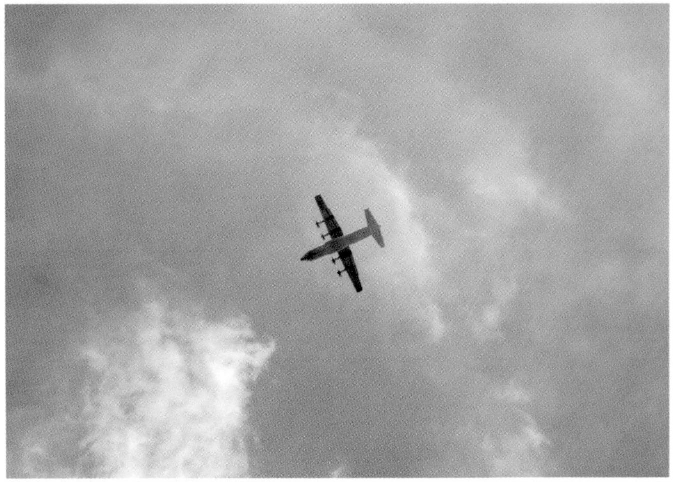

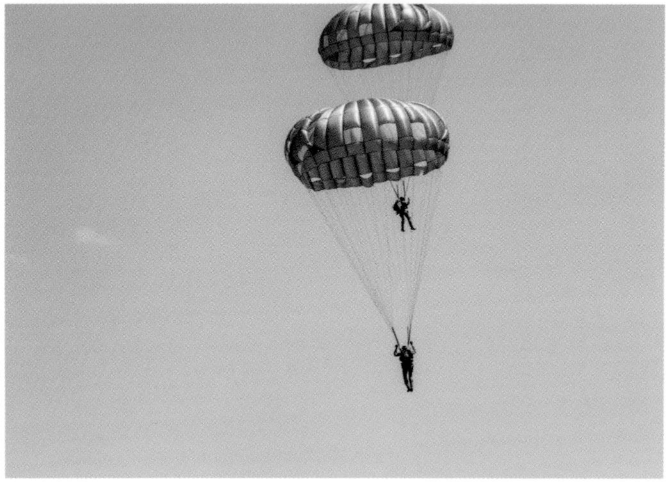

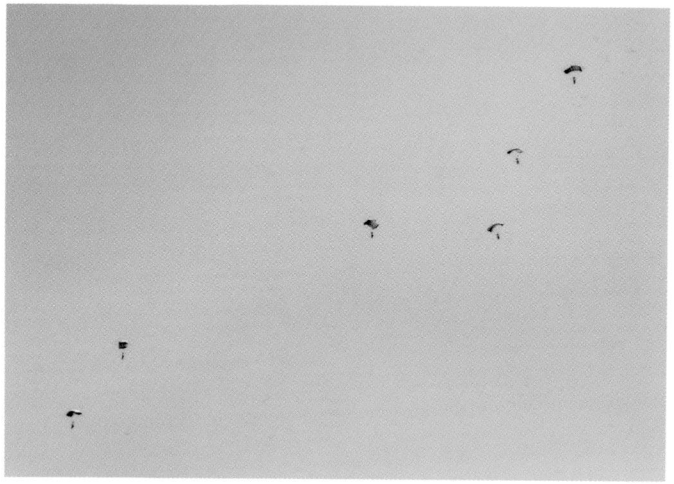

John Moorhead, MD

Emergency Medicine Pioneer
Portland, Oregon

When we started our program at OHSU in 1978, it almost felt like being part of a start-up tech company. We would come in and work, work, work all day . . . go downtown for dinner . . . and then come back and work all night. We just figured things out as we went. We functioned as a team. There was no surgical hierarchy, just a bunch of people working together to take care of patients. It was great.

I remember trying to resuscitate a patient who had overdosed before toxicology was even a field. The head of the intensive care unit said, "Somebody's got to go look up some articles about this stuff because I don't have a clue!" Someone literally ran down the hall to the library and came back with the most recent research paper they could find. We knew there was so much more to learn, but we were developing the skill set emergency medicine requires. You've got to process the information, make a decision, and move on. If you can't compartmentalize things quickly, then this probably isn't the work you should be doing.

Whatever we do, it's all about people . . . whether it's working *on* them or working *with* them. Life is about relationships . . . that's my philosophy . . . and it's a privilege to take care of patients in the scariest moments of their lives.

When we were starting out, people in other specialties would warn us that what we were trying to do was just too hard — physically, mentally. They thought we'd never be able to make emergency medicine into a real career. They'd say, "Sure, you can do this for a while, but then you're gonna burn out. Be prepared . . . you'll end up doing primary care one day." But we showed them if we trained physicians differently and appropriately . . . and they made a commitment to this job . . . they'd end up doing what I've done: practice emergency medicine for forty years. I still love every day I go to work.

I often talk to my residents about how things used to be. Nowadays, support is much more readily available. I got involved in physician education and advocacy when I joined the American College of Emergency Physicians, and we began to develop stronger training systems. We knew if you have better education, better working conditions, and a better environment, you're going to have better patient outcomes.

Doctors would complete a defined period of training and then immediately launch into a job. So, the question became, "How do we help them maintain their competency at the level necessary to be excellent for the rest of their careers?" Part of the answer was continuing education.

These programs we set up are very well intentioned, but they don't address the stress physicians face every day. Every doctor in any community in the United States is totally overwhelmed. The world has changed. These electronic medical records are awful . . . everybody's second-guessing you . . . the hospital is trying to cut your pay. I mean, how do you keep up with all that? When you keep asking doctors to do more and more, they'll eventually throw up their hands and go, "I can't do this." So, our approach needs to evolve.

Those of us who have been doing this for a long time have come to understand the way we *used* to do things probably isn't the best way for the current generation of physicians. They're expecting more . . . they want better for themselves and their patients. Young people aren't going to come to a class and just listen to somebody lecture anymore; they can get that on YouTube. They're expecting a meaningful discussion. They don't join organizations just to be members; they join to benefit society.

That's my motivation for continuing the national work I do. I'm inspired by the energy of this new generation. Through them, you can see the future. ✚

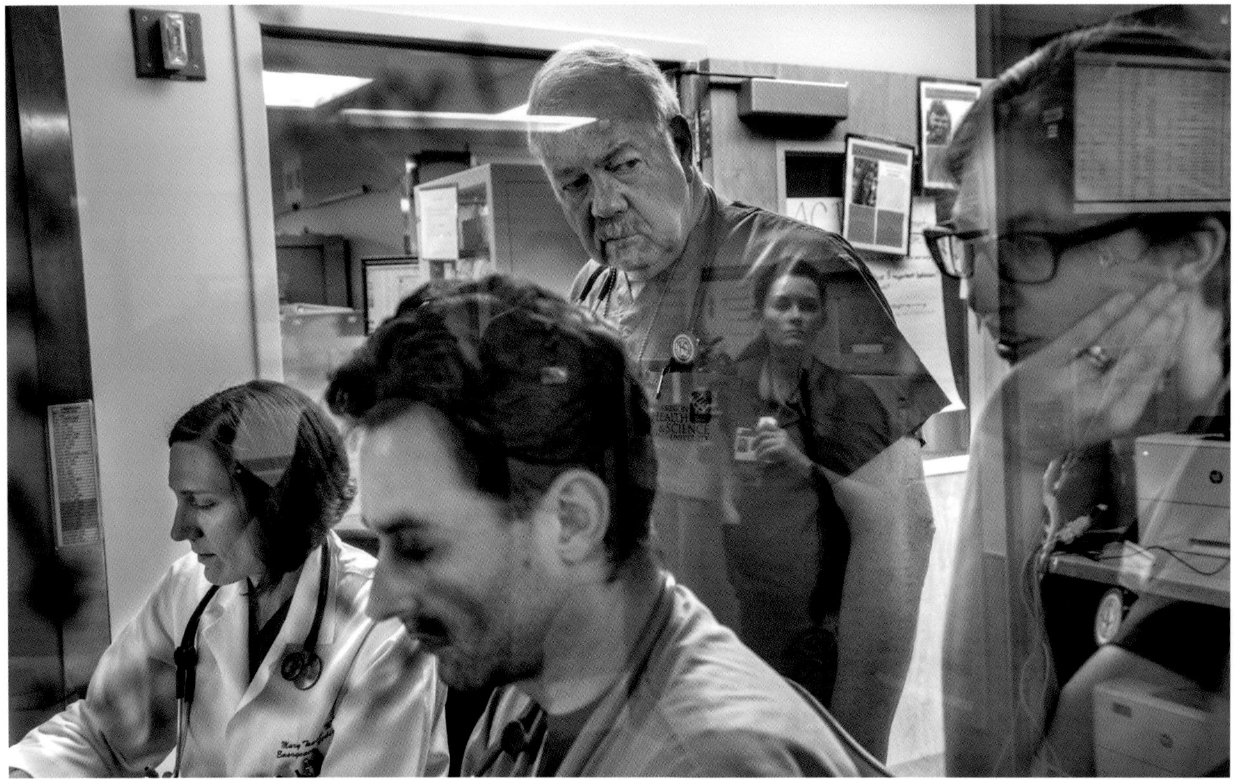

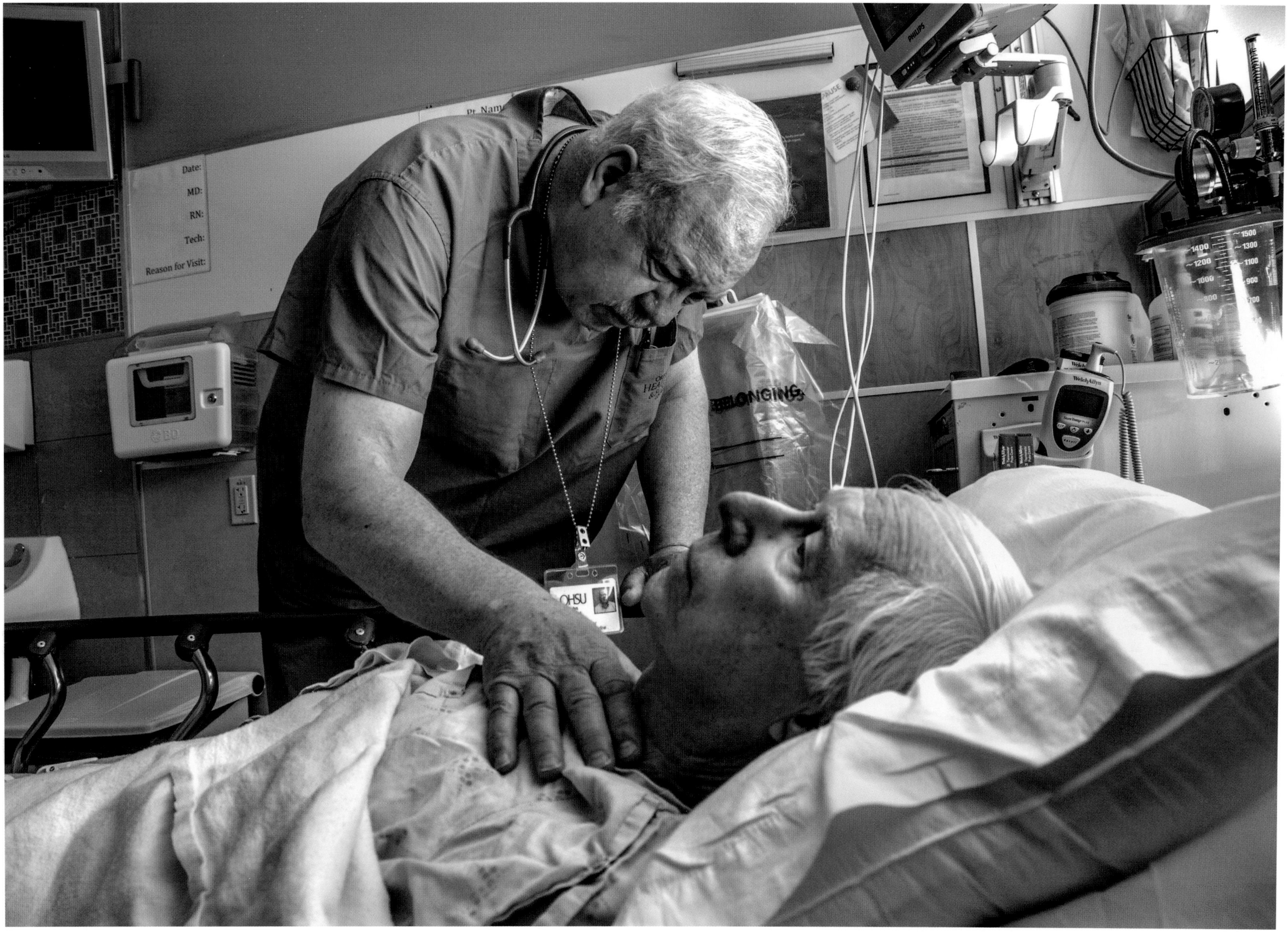

John Moorhead, MD

Patti Paris, MD

Emergency Physician
Anchorage, Alaska

The tundra is a dangerous place. Some regions are so remote, they're almost Third World. Emergency physicians talk about treating trauma during the "golden hour" but, out here, we call it the "golden twelve hours." If you fall out of a boat in Santa Barbara, you'll find tons of other boaters to help you out. If you fall out of a boat in Alaska, you're dead.

Any population that has undergone the kinds of cultural shifts Native Americans have endured will be faced with challenges. We see our fair share of domestic violence, suicide, alcohol abuse, and other social issues that plague any economically disadvantaged community. Unfortunately, there are no quick fixes for these problems, and that can be frustrating.

I'm half Penobscot Indian . . . part of a small tribe in Maine. After residency, I moved to Alaska to work for the Indian Health Service, a federally funded agency that provides medical care to American Indians and Alaska Natives, and I'm still here. When you grow up on a reservation, you don't always have access to good role models, so I'm proud when I can tell a young patient, "Yes, you can be a doctor, too." I think that's one of the reasons I went into this . . . one of the ways I find joy in my career.

This population is very interesting; most of my chronically ill patients are in their forties or fifties. Those who make it into their eighties or nineties are healthy and very seldom take medications. It's almost as if they've been "preselected" to succeed. Most of them have never had access to the little luxuries designed to help you live longer. They haven't been burdened by medicines or regular doctor appointments. It really makes you wonder if less care is more.

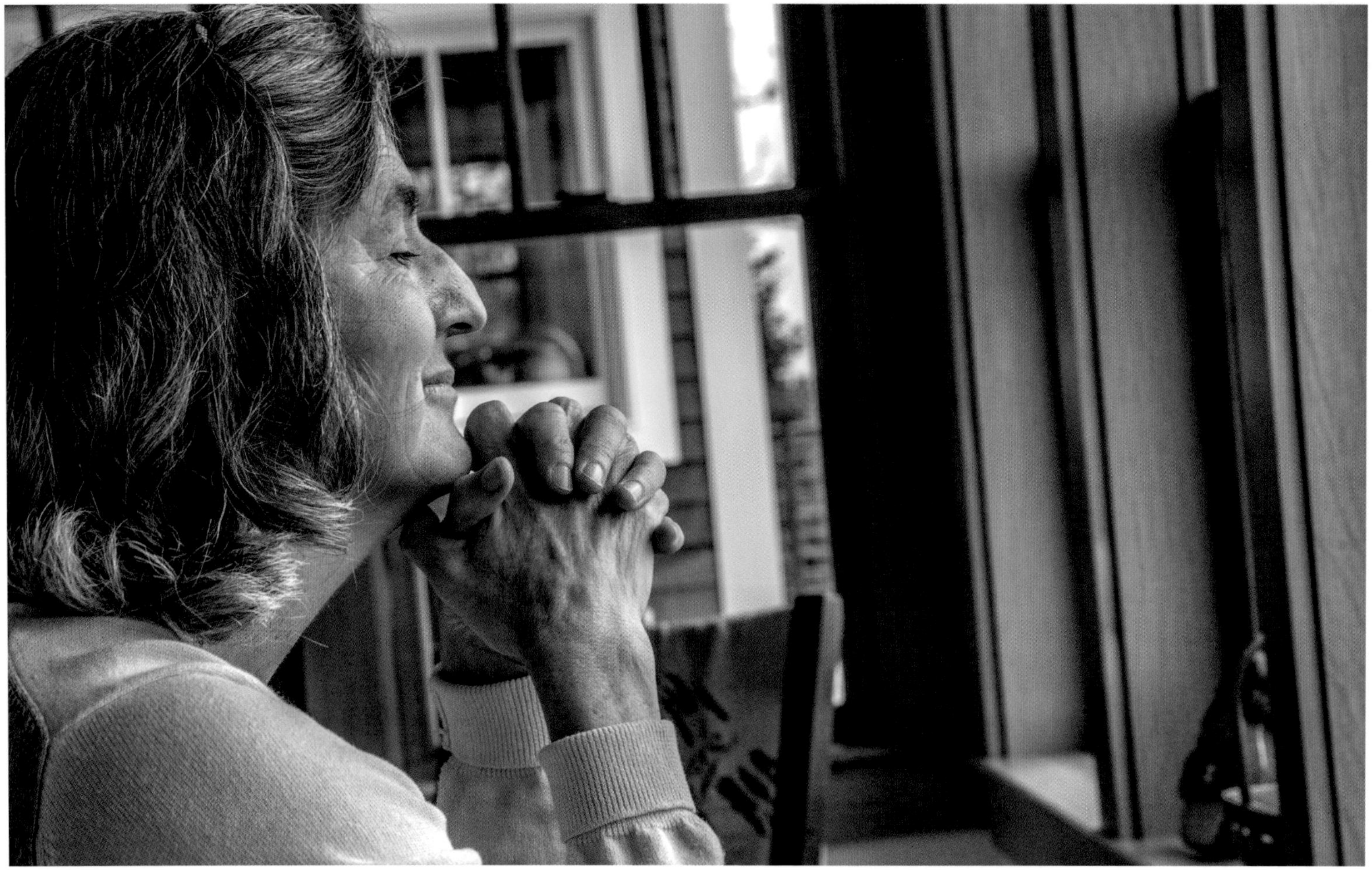

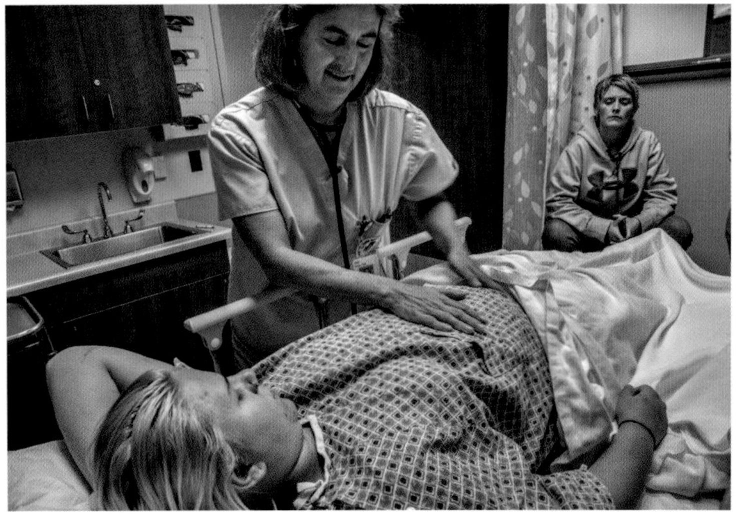

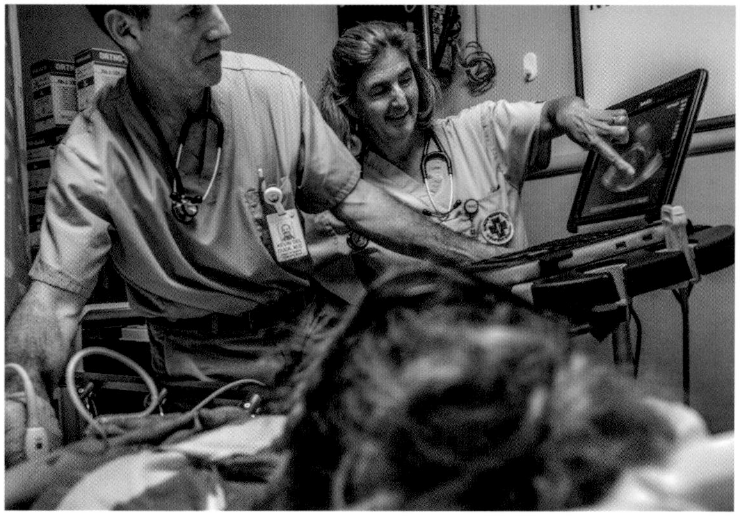

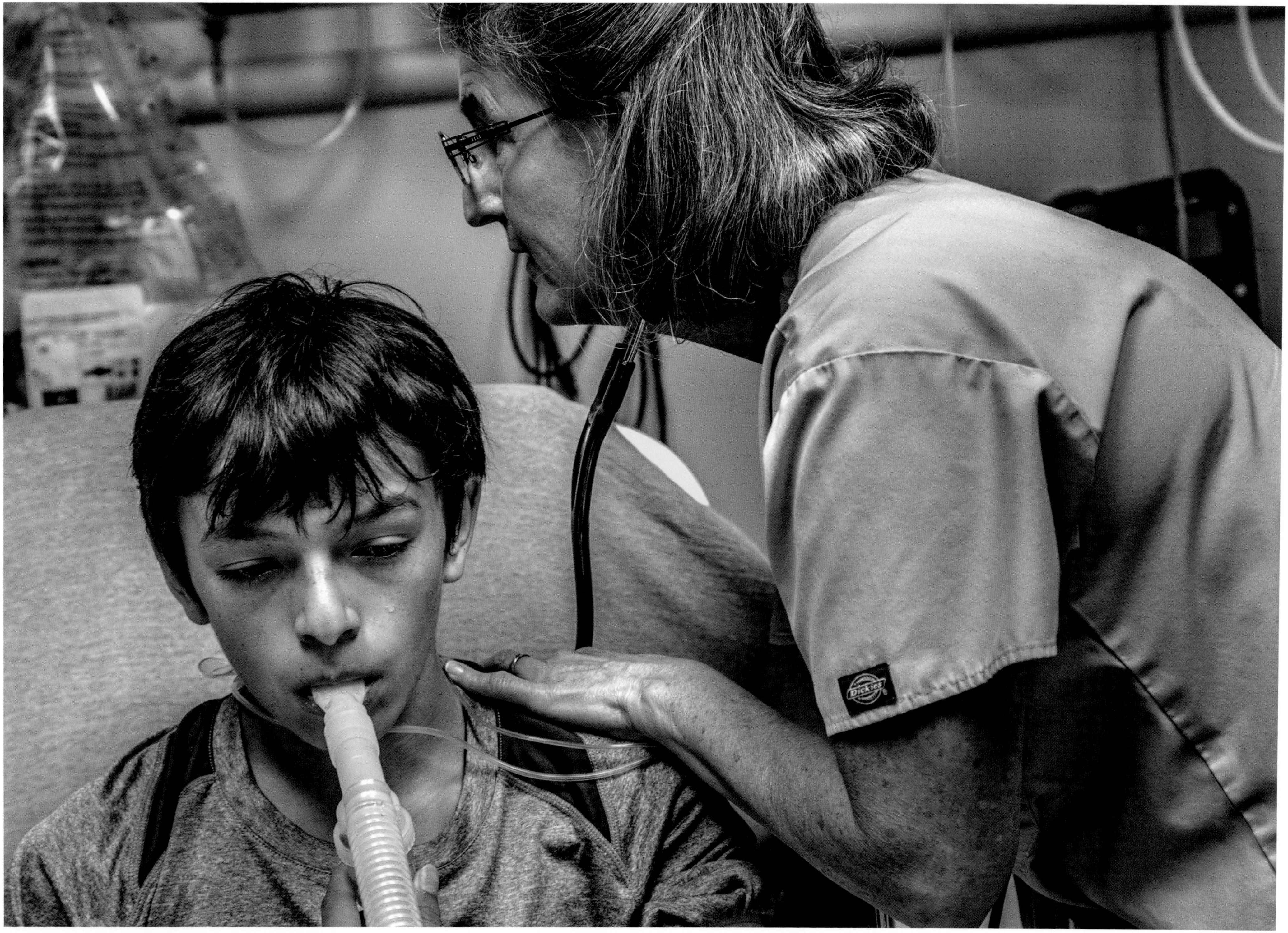
Dickies

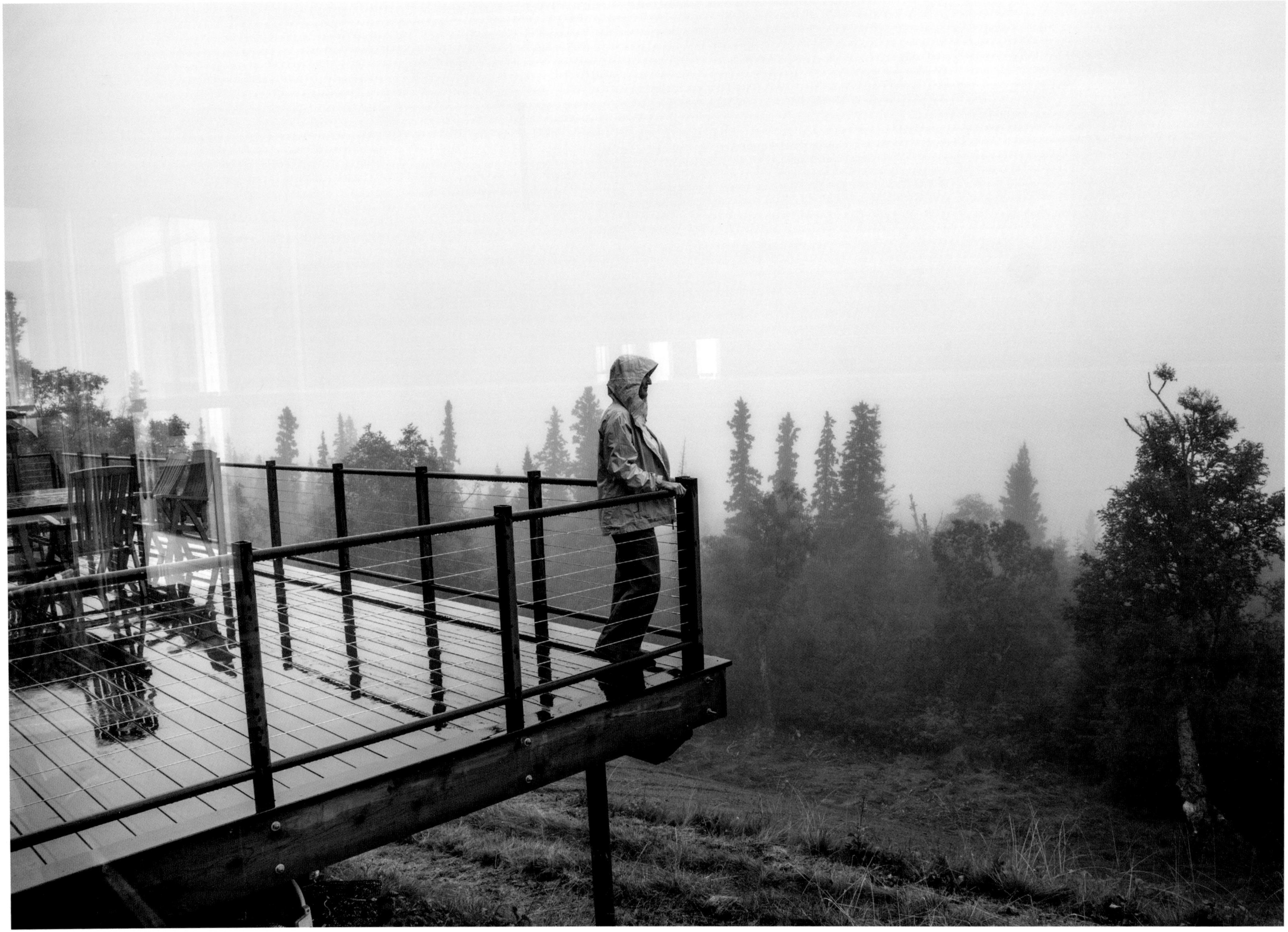

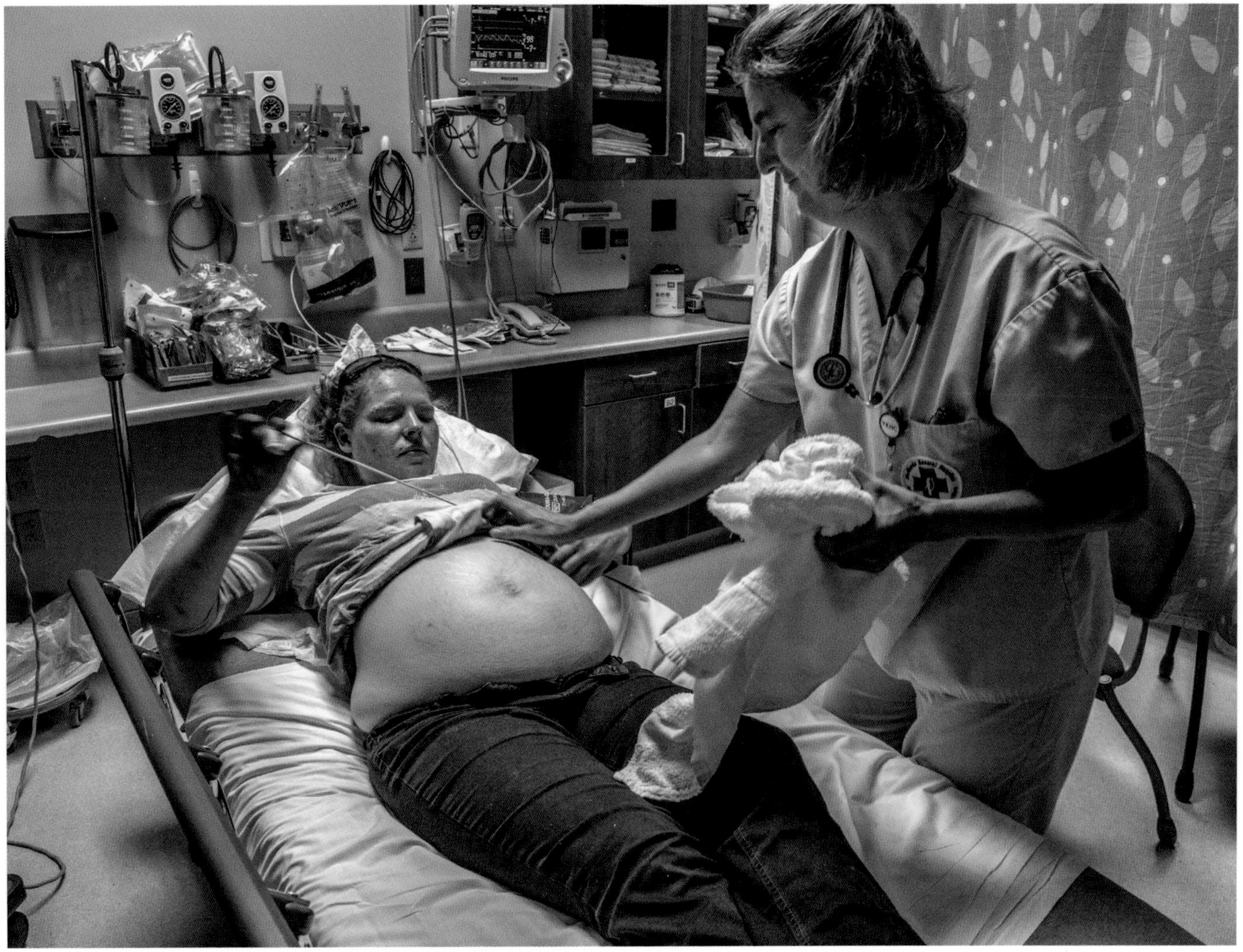

When you meet a patient, you get a window into their soul. I'm always surprised by how much people are willing to share with you, a total stranger. It's an honor to be in that position. I believe talking to patients is as therapeutic as medicine. *Where were you born? How did you end up in Anchorage? When did you get married?* I want to hear their stories. I know how to put in central lines . . . intubate patients . . . treat hypertension . . . but one of my most important procedures is *listening*.

When I was training on the OB service, a young woman came in with shortness of breath. She was only in her forties, but she was dying of gynecological cancer. My exam of her was cursory because I knew she needed to be admitted, and I just viewed her as additional work. I put in a bunch of orders and went back to what I was doing, but that night, she began to have trouble breathing. The third-year gynecological resident didn't know how to do a thoracentesis . . . it wasn't her specialty . . . so I stepped in and drained the fluid from the patient's lungs. It did seem to help. Then she died.

I think all physicians have a little graveyard in their hearts for the cases that didn't go as planned. We flagellate ourselves — wonder if we should have done something different, something better. I always knew part of the reason that patient died was because I was cavalier — I didn't take the time to investigate what was really going on.

When the gynecological surgeon would see me in the hallway, he'd point and say, "That's the girl who killed my patient." And I did. That's the story. But the lesson I learned from that early experience is every person you see deserves your full attention. ✚

Malinda Abbott, PA

Physician Assistant
Lexington, Kentucky

I was brought up on a twenty-acre farm in a little community outside of Lexington. We grew corn for our cattle and tobacco. We had an orchard and a big strawberry patch. We kept bees. My siblings and I would line up as soon as we got off the school bus, and Daddy would say, "You're on fence row. You're mowing." Or "You're going to weed the garden . . . and I'm gonna come check your work when you're done." Oh, man, the work ethic.

I just loved animals. I'd bring home every sick one I'd find . . . mostly cats and dogs, occasionally baby 'coons. My mama would help me tend to them. But every once in a while, she'd look at me and say, "We got to help this one go on," and Daddy would have to put it out of its misery. We lived down a little county road with a sinkhole in the way back . . . people would throw dogs and cats into it. As I walked toward the house, I'd hear the animals crying . . . and I'd sneak down and pull them out. I can't count the number of dogs we had. And there were so many cats. Cats *everywhere* — but never any mice left in the barn.

I really enjoyed taking care of animals, but that changed at some point . . . I wanted to take care of people, instead. My mama would tell me I was too kindhearted to go into nursing — thought I'd just get too attached. It made me sad, but I was afraid she might be right. After I left the farm, I kind of drifted for a couple of years — worked two jobs just to eat and pay rent.

My mama knew I was not happy doing the secretary thing, so she talked to her doctor. She told him, "Well, Melinda wants to be a nurse, but I'm worried that she's too kindhearted." Her doctor said, "You stop that right now! We have enough hateful, mean nurses — we need more kind ones." After that, she said I should do what I wanted to do.

I earned an associate's degree in nursing and gained a lot of experience, but I wanted to do more for my patients. The defining moment came when I was working in the ICU. A PA came in and asked me to share my notes about a particular patient. She then took my ideas to the surgeon and presented them as her own. I watched as he turned to her and said, "Oh, my. You really know this patient. You have really . . . I am impressed. This is. . . ." I pulled her aside later and said, "*What*?! Why would you do that? You stole from me. Those thoughts did not come from you. Why would you sell my ideas as your own?" She just said, "Because I can." At that moment, I thought, "Um, I don't think so. I can be a PA, too."

One of the best pieces of advice I've ever received came from an old nursing instructor. Every time we would go in for clinicals, she would stop us at the front door and say, "I don't care what's going on in your life right now; I don't care if you're fighting with your spouse; I don't care if you can't make rent. You set that down . . . you're not bringing it in here. These patients need *all* of you."

I was taught to never talk down to people. You always protect another person's dignity, no matter what. If they don't understand, *help* them understand . . . paint them a picture with your words. I probably aggravate doctors. Sometimes they'll say, "Hey, I just want the facts." I get that, but I'm trying to get them to see the patient as a whole person, not just a potassium level, or an x-ray, or a CT scan. If you've got someone from the hollers of eastern Kentucky, you can't just walk in, rattle off a bunch of numbers, and walk out. You have to sit down and say, "Hey, I'm very worried about your kidneys. Your creatinine level is high. Let me explain what 'creatinine' means."

I was raised in the church, and my parents always told me, "When you're at work, you're working for God. Give Him your best effort, make Him proud. Even if your boss doesn't like you . . . even if people are mean to you . . . none of that matters."

There's a verse in the Book of James that says, ". . . the wisdom that is from above is first pure, then peaceable, gentle, and easy to be entreated, full of mercy and good fruits, without partiality, and without hypocrisy." That's what I pray as I drive to work. Let me be fair in all my dealings. Let me be wise. Let me see past the façade. Let me treat my patients as myself. ✚

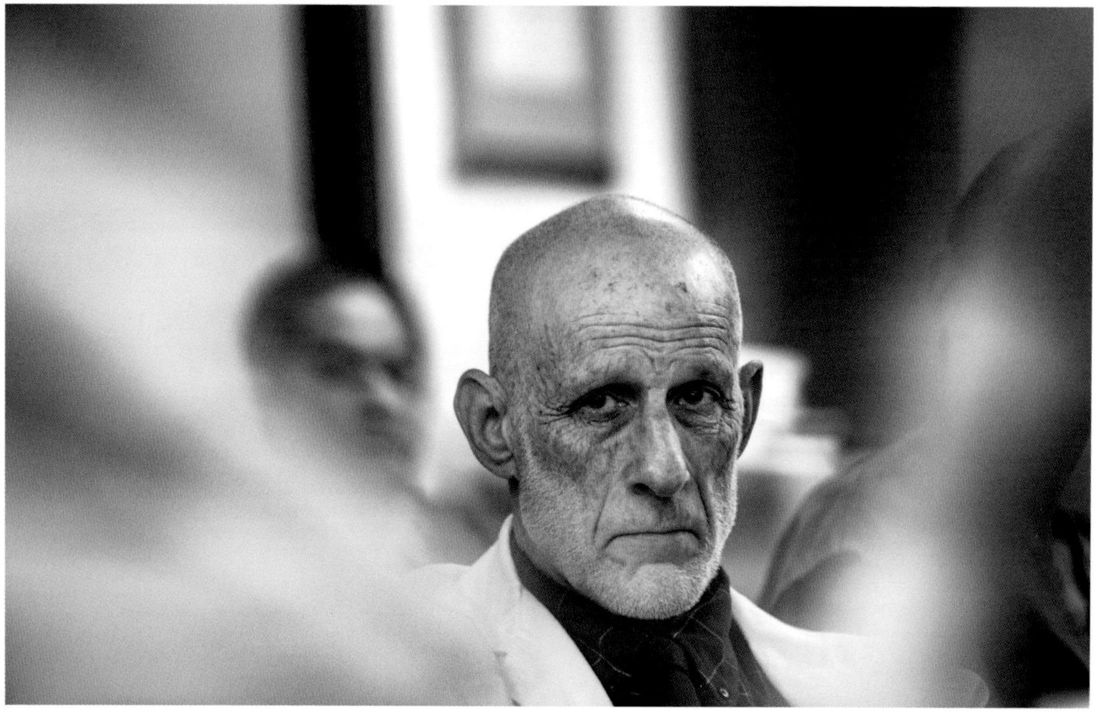

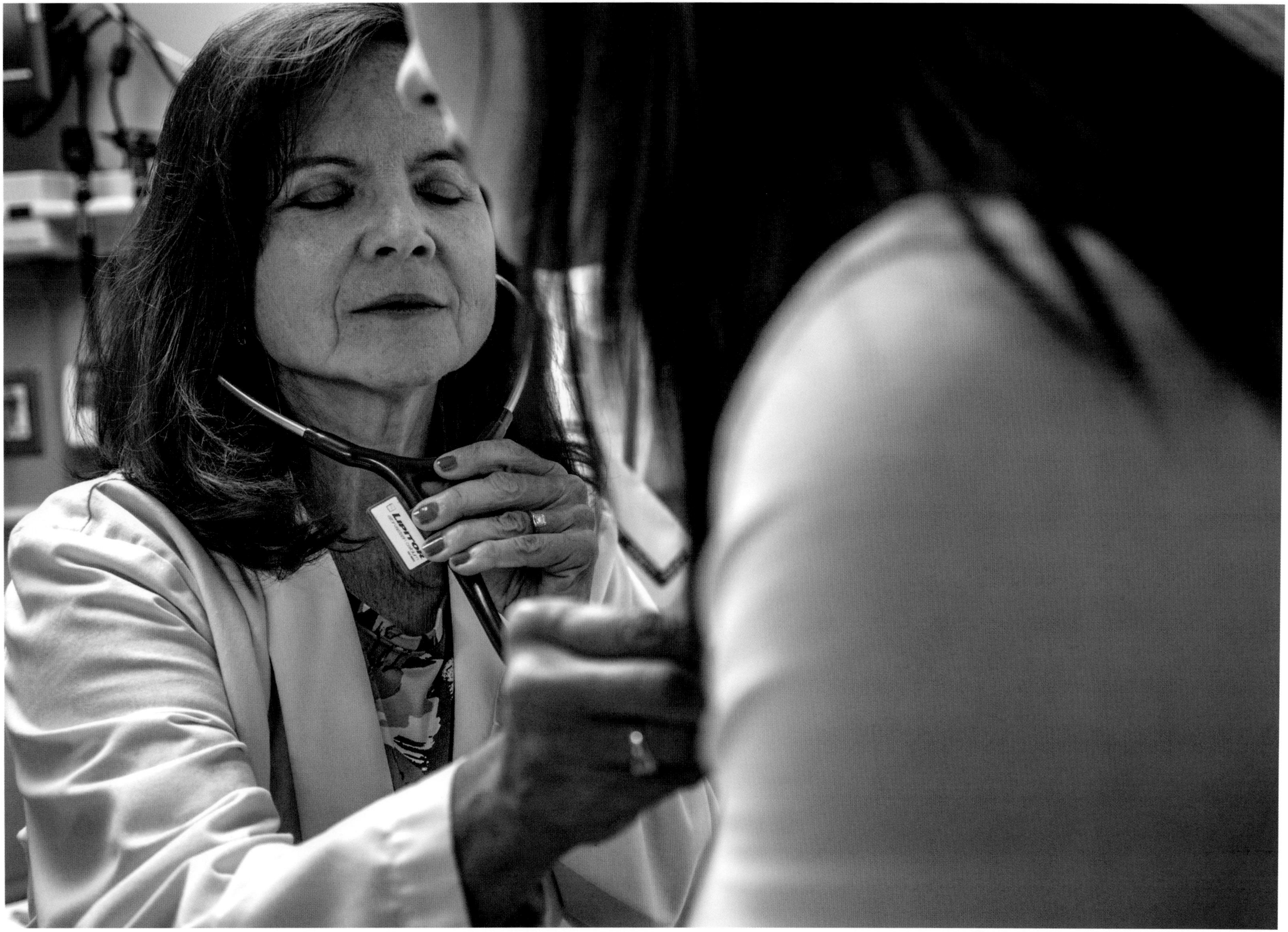

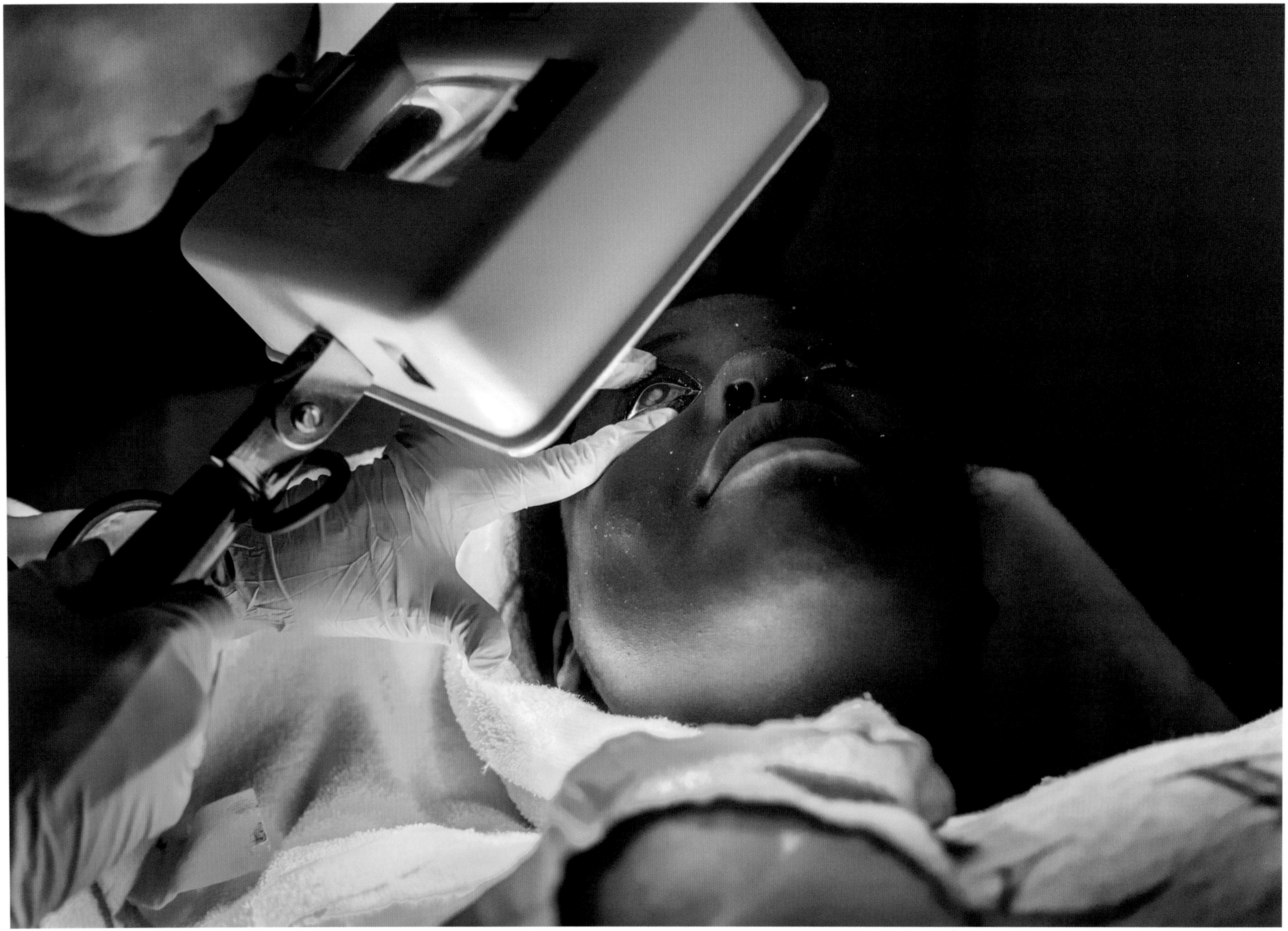

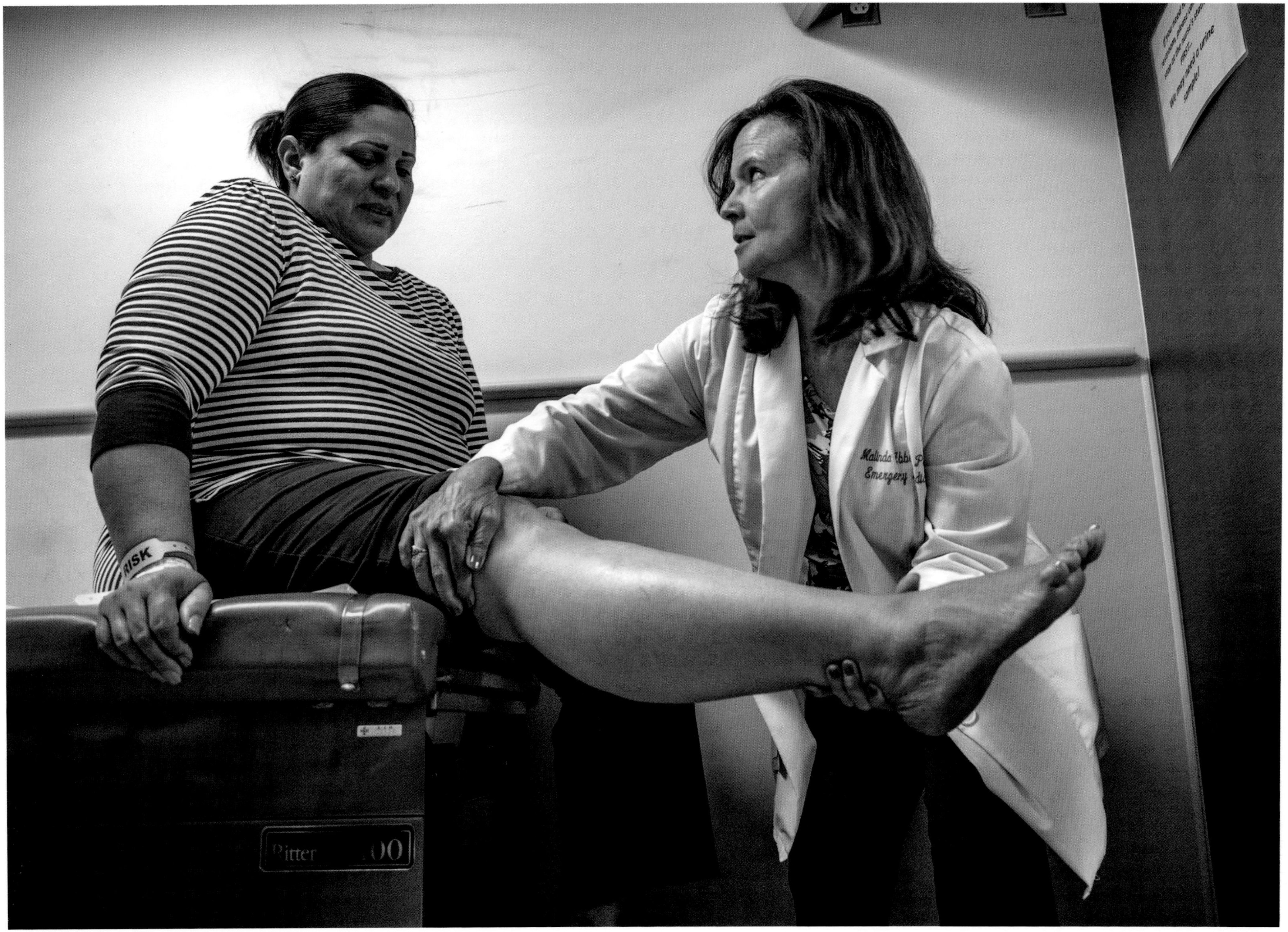
We may need a urine sample!
RISK
Emergency

Ralph Riviello, MD

Emergency Physician & Forensic Specialist
Philadelphia, Pennsylvania

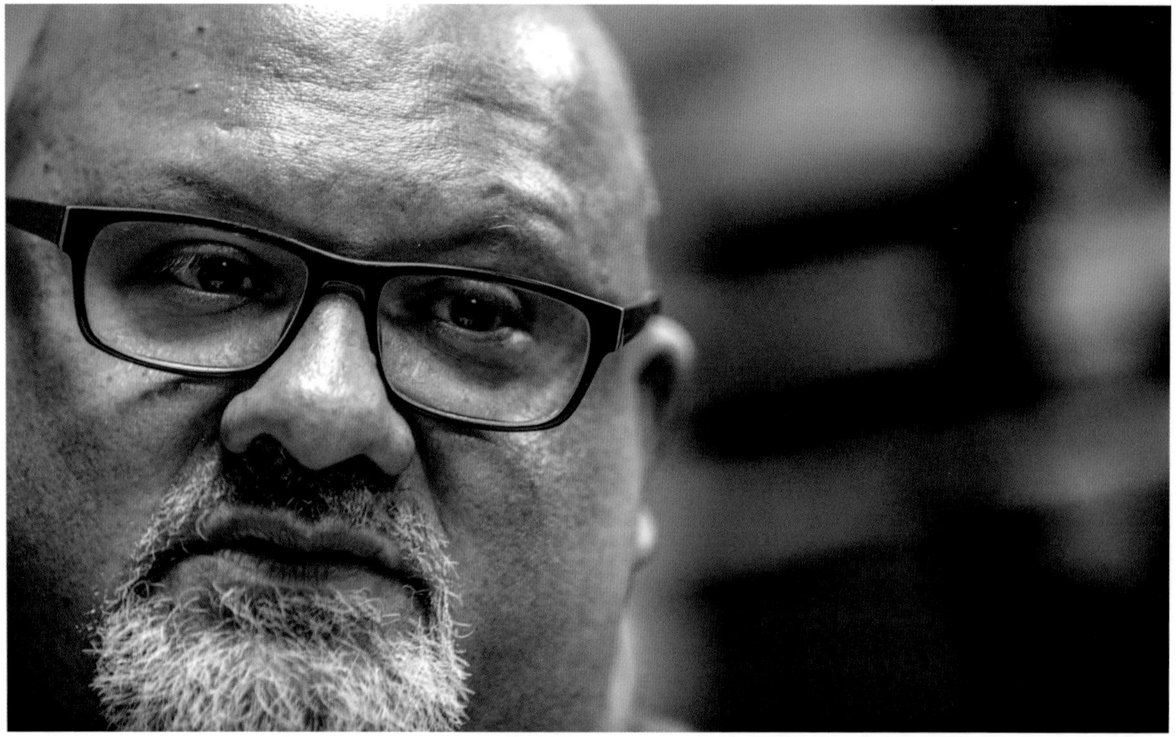

Sometimes it's detective work — piecing things together, catching a detail about an injury that doesn't make sense. This field is about knowing how to collect pieces of evidence, how to take a bullet out of somebody, and knowing what to do with that bullet so it can be introduced in court. A big part of the job is awareness, developing a sense of suspicion that enables you to interpret wounds differently. You have to ask yourself, "Does the story hold up?"

I'm always amazed how positively survivors react to their examiners. Most feel they're truly being helped; anything we can do for them is a great relief. I can tell when a victim is reassured by something I say or do, and I try to give them some peace in the aftermath of whatever horrific thing might have happened.

I remember a woman who came in after being physically and sexually assaulted by her ex-husband. It was during a hurricane. She had some pretty awful-looking injuries, things that were just beyond what you would normally expect in such a case. She looked a little grandmotherly, so I was struck by her history, which included drug abuse and that kind of stuff. When I looked at her chart, I realized she was only in her forties. Life had taken such a dramatic toll.

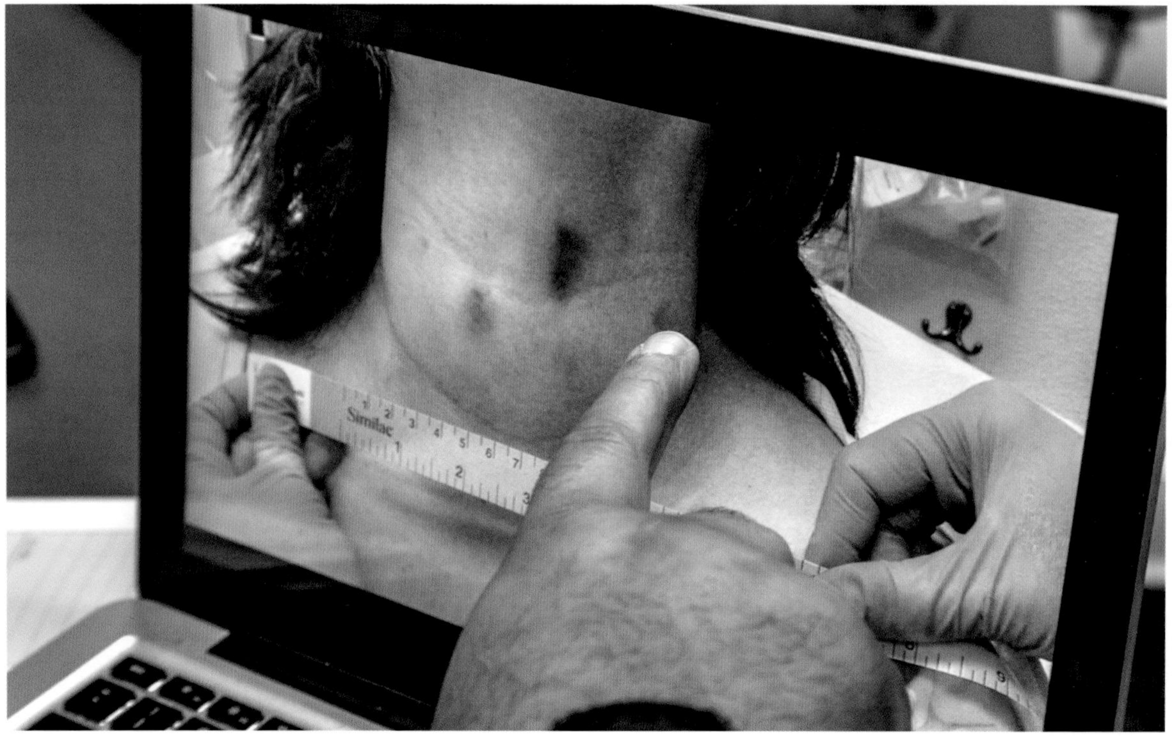

One of my most interesting cases involved a patient brought after a car accident. She was intoxicated. Somebody had died at the scene, so there were questions about whether she had been driving. She had an injury on her hand that looked like a bruise, but when I looked closer, I could see the letters "SRS" had been burned into the wound. I thought the mark might have been caused by the plate on the steering wheel, which popped off when the airbag deployed. I photographed her injuries for the police officers, described what I saw, and entered everything into the medical record. They eventually found the patient's DNA and blood on the steering wheel plate and concluded she had indeed been driving. She denied it, of course. In this environment, it helps to have a dark sense of humor.

Those of us in the field of clinical forensics try to teach our colleagues — physicians and nurses — how to work together so mistakes don't happen, so evidence doesn't get dropped, lost, thrown away, or mishandled. We teach them how to maintain a chain of custody, so everyone knows exactly where that evidence has been. It's very rewarding, especially when a success story comes along. Once in a while, someone will call to say, "Hey, thanks for your help. Because of what I learned from you, I was able to prosecute this case and I got a conviction."

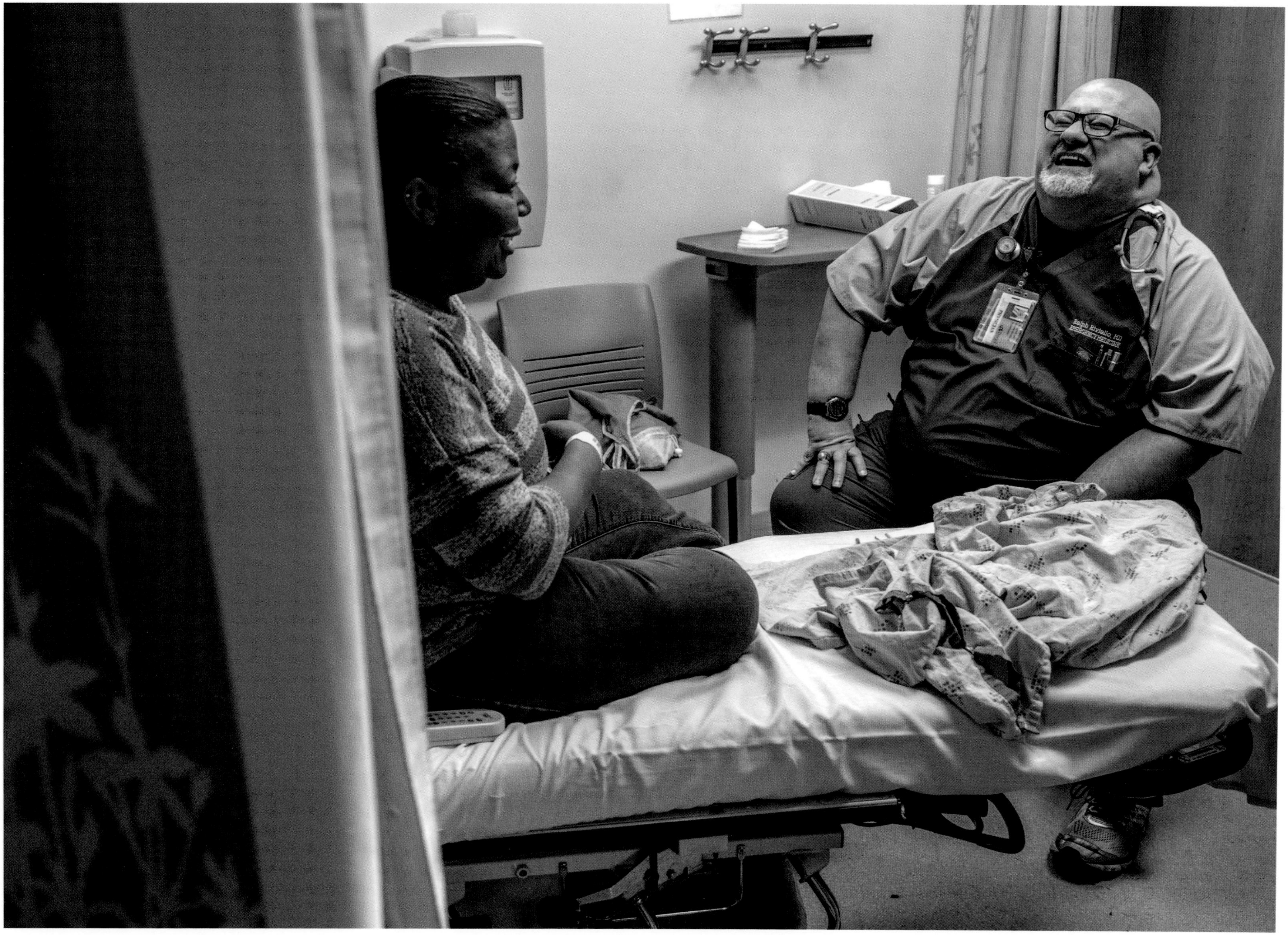

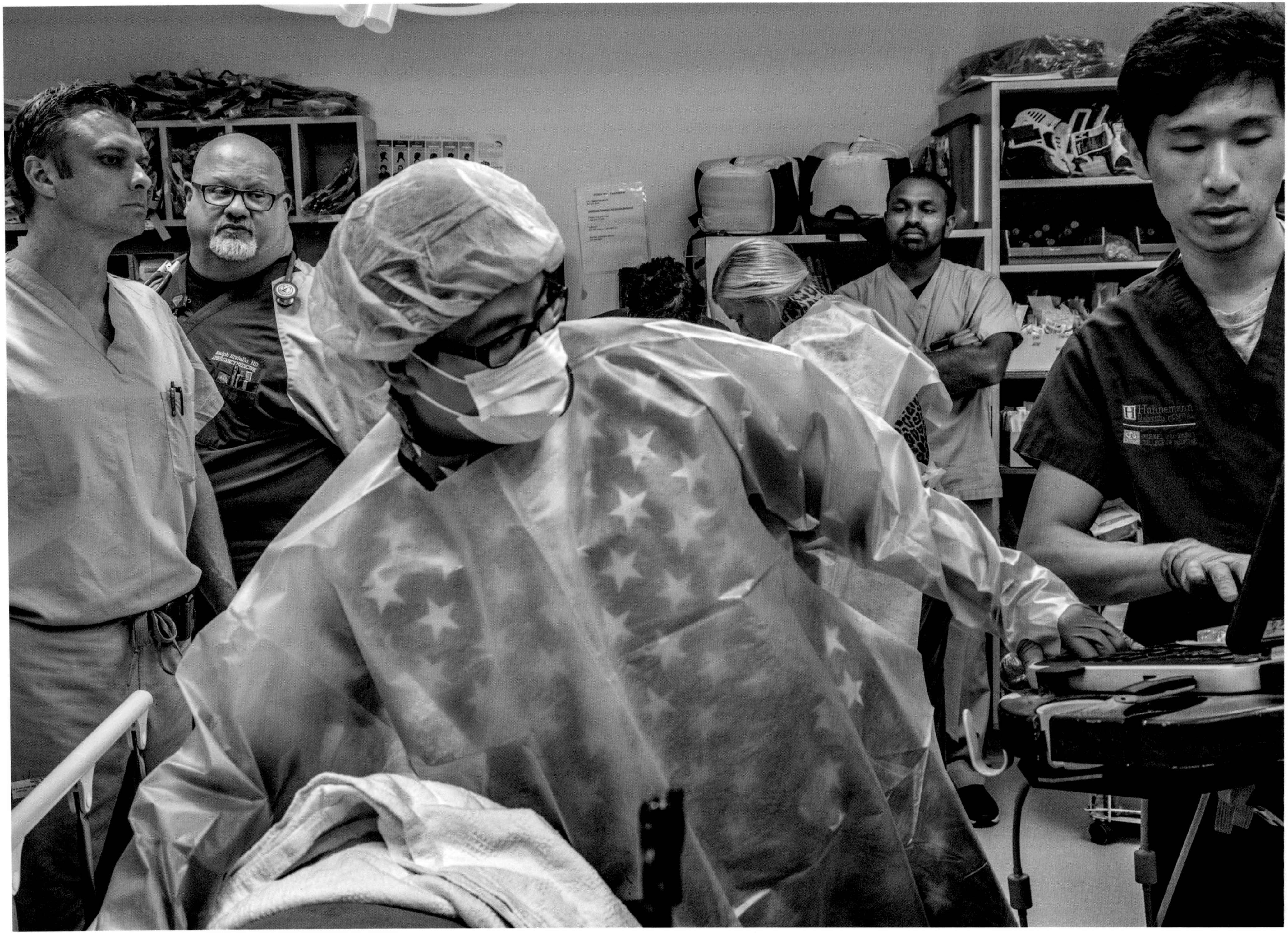
Hahnemann

I enjoy the work and, unfortunately, there will always be people who need to be served. The violence isn't going away, and I don't think our country's health-care situation is going to get better anytime soon. For now, I can provide a road to healing, and I can collect the evidence that allows the talented crime technicians, DNA analysts, and police officers to do their investigative work. Those of us in this line of work aim to create a bridge between the victim and the criminal justice system, but we are here for the victims, not for the police. If you're not doing this job for the patient, then you shouldn't be doing this job. ✚

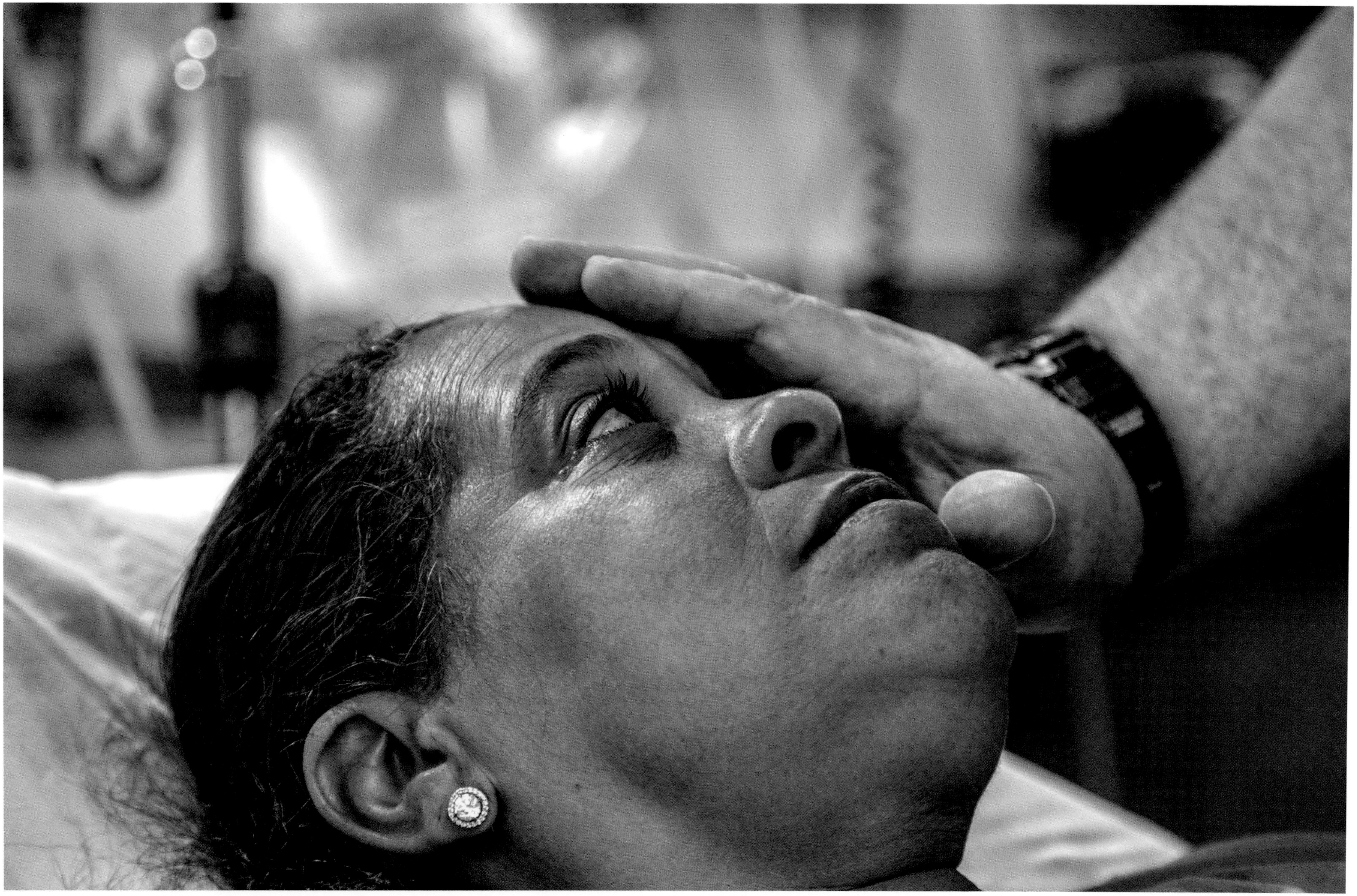

Jonny Kim, MD

Emergency Medicine Resident, NASA Astronaut Candidate & Former Navy SEAL
Boston, Massachusetts

I was always the last one picked for any sports team — the kid no one wanted. Growing up, I had a picture of the Apollo 11 crew on the wall above my bed. I always thought space was cool, but I never once thought about becoming an astronaut. I didn't think I'd ever really amount to anything, so I didn't entertain those kinds of dreams. The idea I could ever be an astronaut was laughable.

When I was sixteen, a friend of mine told me about the Navy SEALS. I was totally enamored with the way he spoke about it, and something just clicked inside my head. I didn't like the person I was becoming . . . meek and insecure . . . and I wanted a drastic change. So, I set my sights on joining the US Navy after high school. I knew it was something I was meant to do. I trained in the off-season . . . took long swims . . . ran on the beach . . . pushups . . . sit-ups. I began to reset my priorities . . . reset who I was.

I became a combat medic almost by accident, but it was enough to spark my interest in medicine. I dealt with injured civilians and, on at least one occasion, took care of a wounded enemy combatant. It's an intellectual exercise to imagine how you might feel or what you would do in a situation like that, and I often assumed it would be difficult. But when the time actually came, the medic's code of compassion took over. My job entailed treating patients with respect — *all* patients.

I served as a sniper during the Battle of Ramadi in 2006 and lost two friends . . . really good soldiers . . . in the Iraq War. I have their names tattooed on my arms — Marc Lee and Michael Monsoor. They both had a huge impact on my personal development and how I've come to view sacrifice. Those men would have continued to make great contributions, and their losses continue to fuel my desire to live life to the fullest. I owe it to them.

I left the SEALS in 2009 and matriculated to the University of San Diego. I earned a math degree and then started medical school at Harvard in 2012. During those years, I worked at a punishing pace, trying to be a good father and supportive husband and a rock-solid student. It wasn't easy. At some point, I finally realized I'm not a machine; there are only twenty-four hours in a day.

I think my studies were a good distraction from the culture shock, though. The transition from military life into civilian life was complex. It's a common story for a lot of veterans who return from war and struggle to adjust to the normal pace of things. But those experiences were essential . . . they helped me develop a more grounded view of the world.

I couldn't believe it when NASA called to tell me I'd been accepted into the space program. It was a surreal moment. I love being an emergency doctor. I was, and still am, passionate about it. But when I realized the impact my role as an astronaut could have on generations of kids, I thought, "Whoa, this is something I can picture myself doing." The opportunity to inspire others, lead my country, and be a force for good . . . a person who everyone can rally behind regardless of race or political affiliation . . . well, I'd never had anything else resonate with me quite like that.

My dream is to contribute as much as I can for as long as I can. I'm particularly excited about the medical research that comes from space. The human body goes through a lot of physiological changes in a microgravity environment, and we still have so much to learn.

I don't have to *be* the best, but I have to *give* my best. I also think it's very important to embrace your failures — as physicians, as friends, as parents. These experiences teach us how to be kind, loving, and confident human beings. Since childhood, I've been on a quest to figure out who I really am . . . what I'm capable of. It took the SEAL team, a war, and a whole lot of mistakes, but I think I finally found my identity — a version of myself who really wants to help the world. ✚

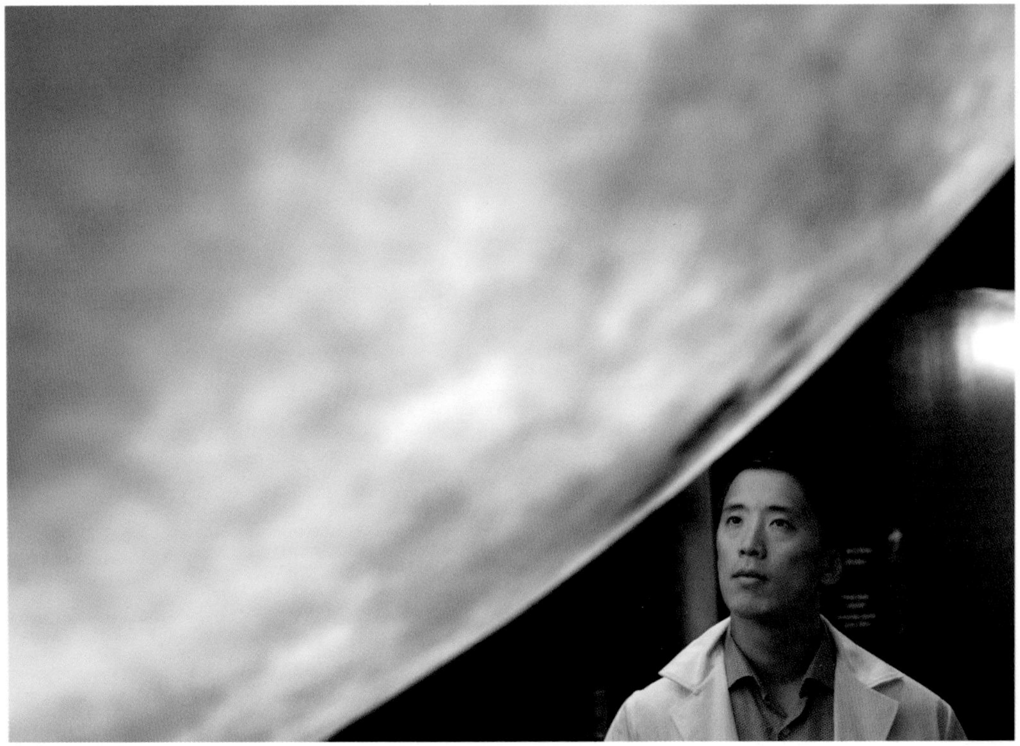

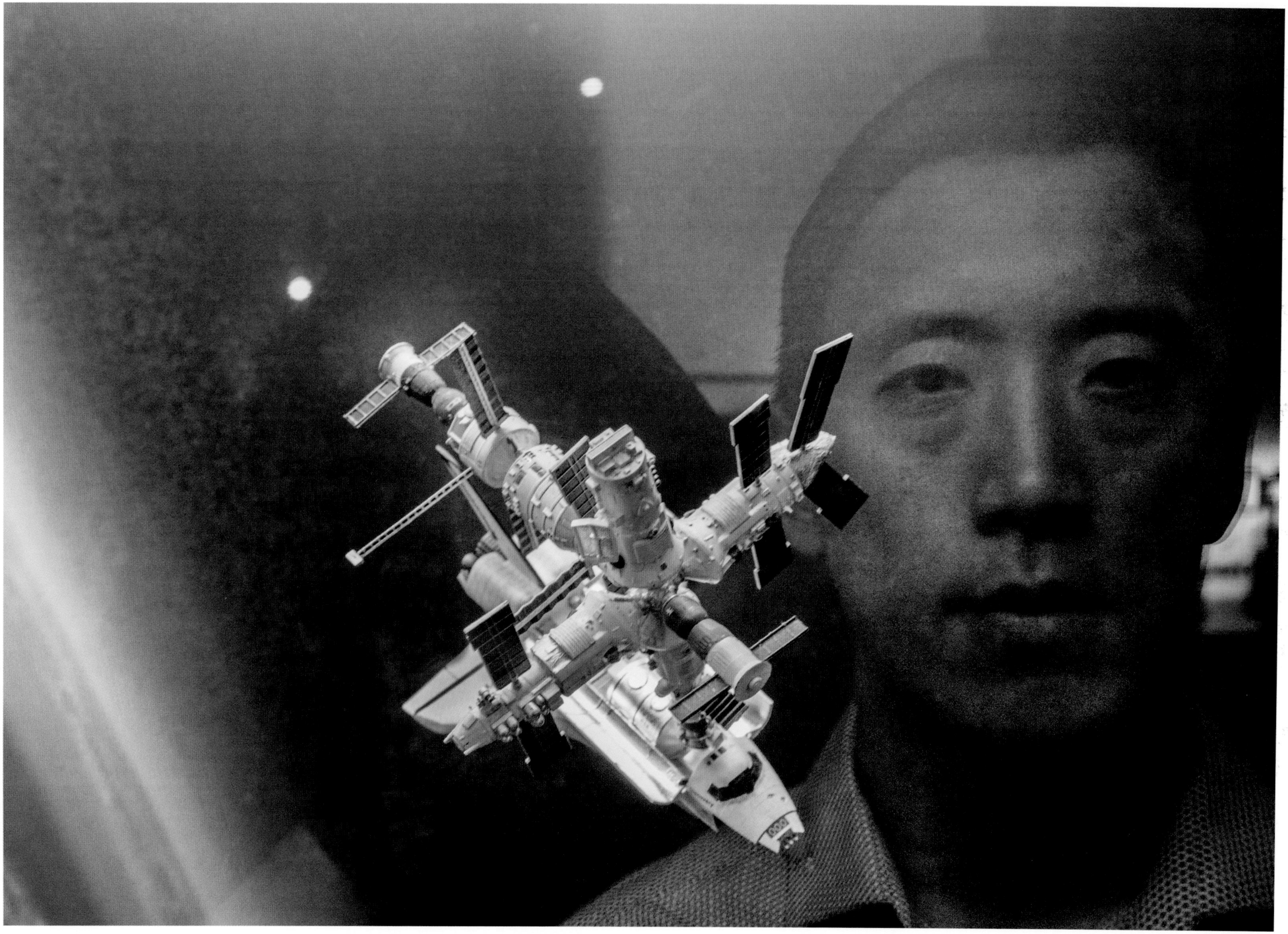

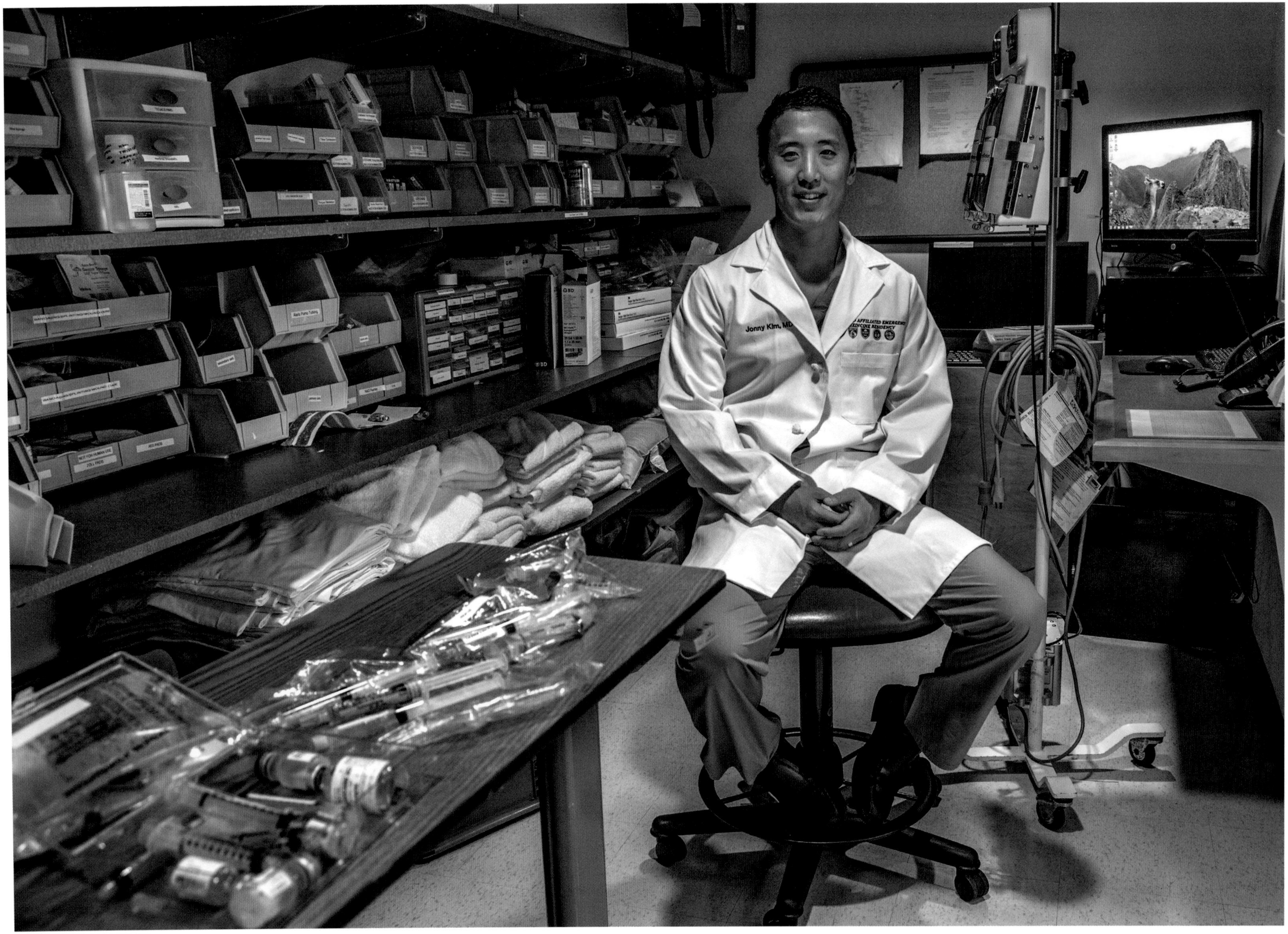
Jonny Kim, MD

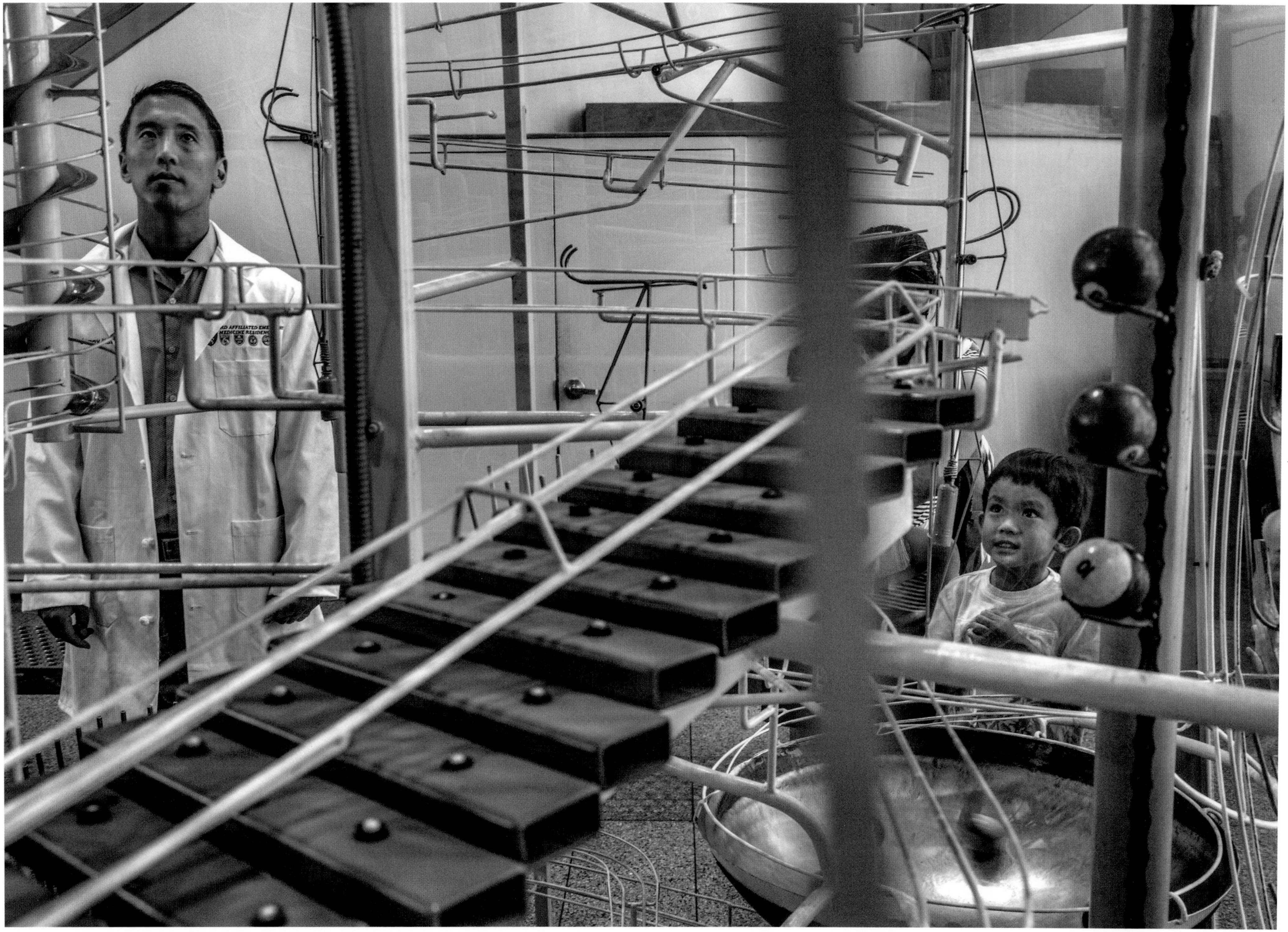

Judith Tintinalli, MD

Emergency Medicine Pioneer
Chapel Hill, North Carolina

I applied to medical school at the very last minute. It was a snowy day, and I remember wearing big boots and this drab, Polish-looking coat. I just walked down to the admissions office at Wayne State and said, "I want to go to medical school." I filled out some paperwork, and — as unbelievable as it sounds — the dean of admissions said, "You're in."

You couldn't even begin to do that today, but medicine wasn't as political back then. I was pregnant by the time classes started, which was very unusual for the times, but I was focused entirely on keeping my nose to the grindstone. Anyway, that's enough about the past. I have a lot to say about the future.

We must keep finding ways to treat patients faster and better without being limited by metrics. I was recently in Peru on a medical mission trip in the Amazon. We began receiving so many sick patients, but we had virtually no access to lab studies. I suddenly realized I didn't *need* to draw a blood test on everybody. I was skilled enough to make a presumptive diagnosis and treat the patient clinically.

In the United States, it's all about excluding pathologies . . . running test after test after test. This is the logic we've been taught. I suppose it's a by-product of our medical culture: *no mistakes, please*. But the quality of care should not be defined by how many CT scans you order for a headache. We can't forget the fact that every formula or algorithm comes with a disclaimer, ". . . not meant to substitute for the independent medical judgment of a physician." That really is the bottom line.

Everybody complains about the high costs of medical care . . . the growing number of people using the ED. But those things are never ever going to change until we have accepted the expectation that good health care is a right. We're a mobile society; when patients can't find primary care, they use the ED. The future is fragile, but if you want to work in emergency medicine, you will never be out of a job.

Most people associate emergency medicine with episodic care, but that isn't true. One of our jobs in the next ten years has got to be improving our message. You simply can't have an effective system of health care without emergency medicine at its core. We run the EMS system. We take care of an entire population. That's the information we need to get out to journalists, to legislators, to medical leaders. They need to understand the enormous value of what we do. The emergency department directly reflects the community itself — its illnesses, its citizens, its socioeconomic problems.

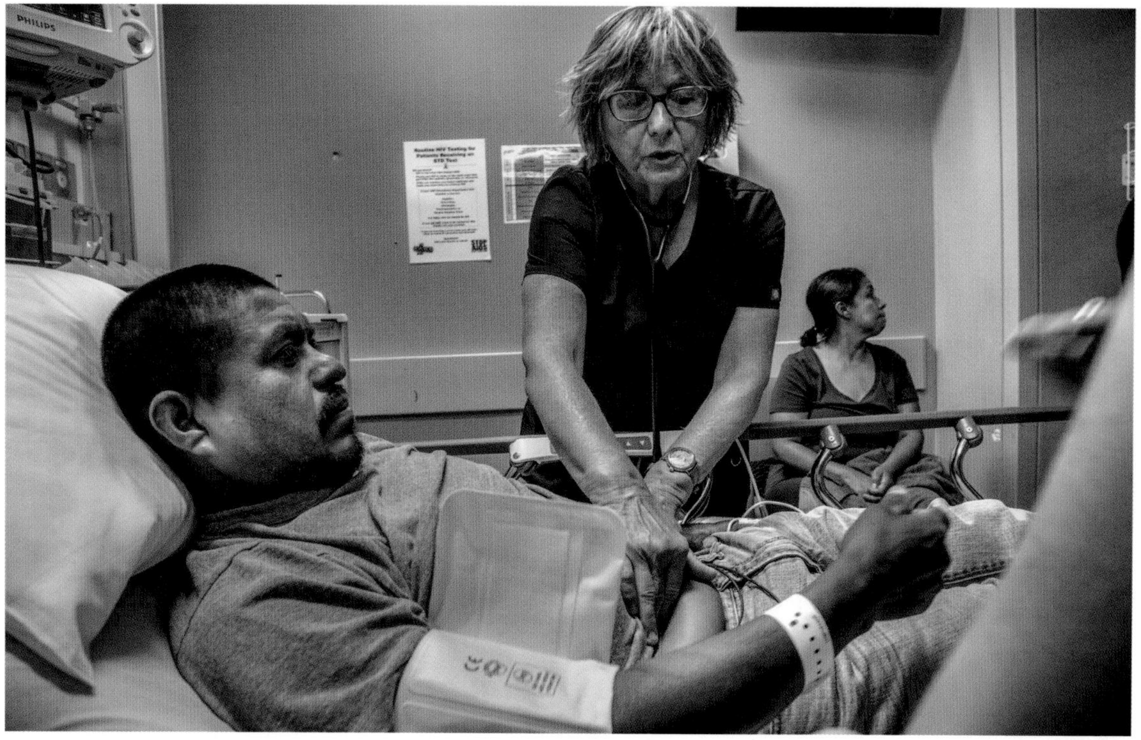

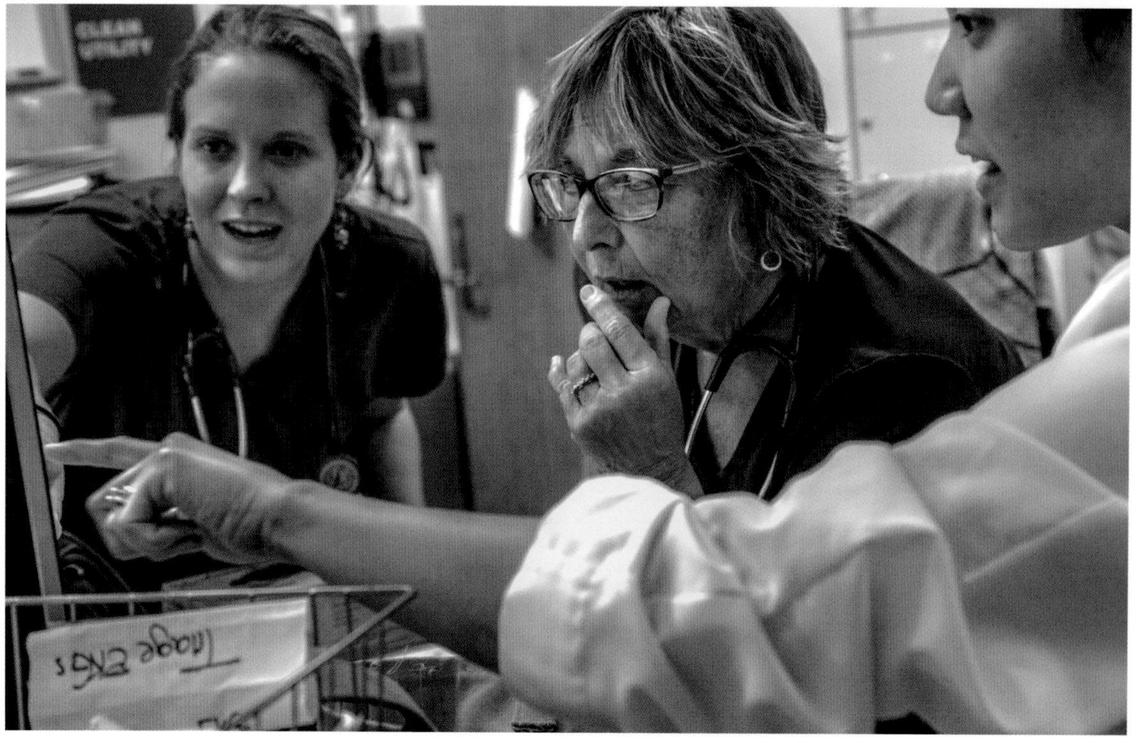

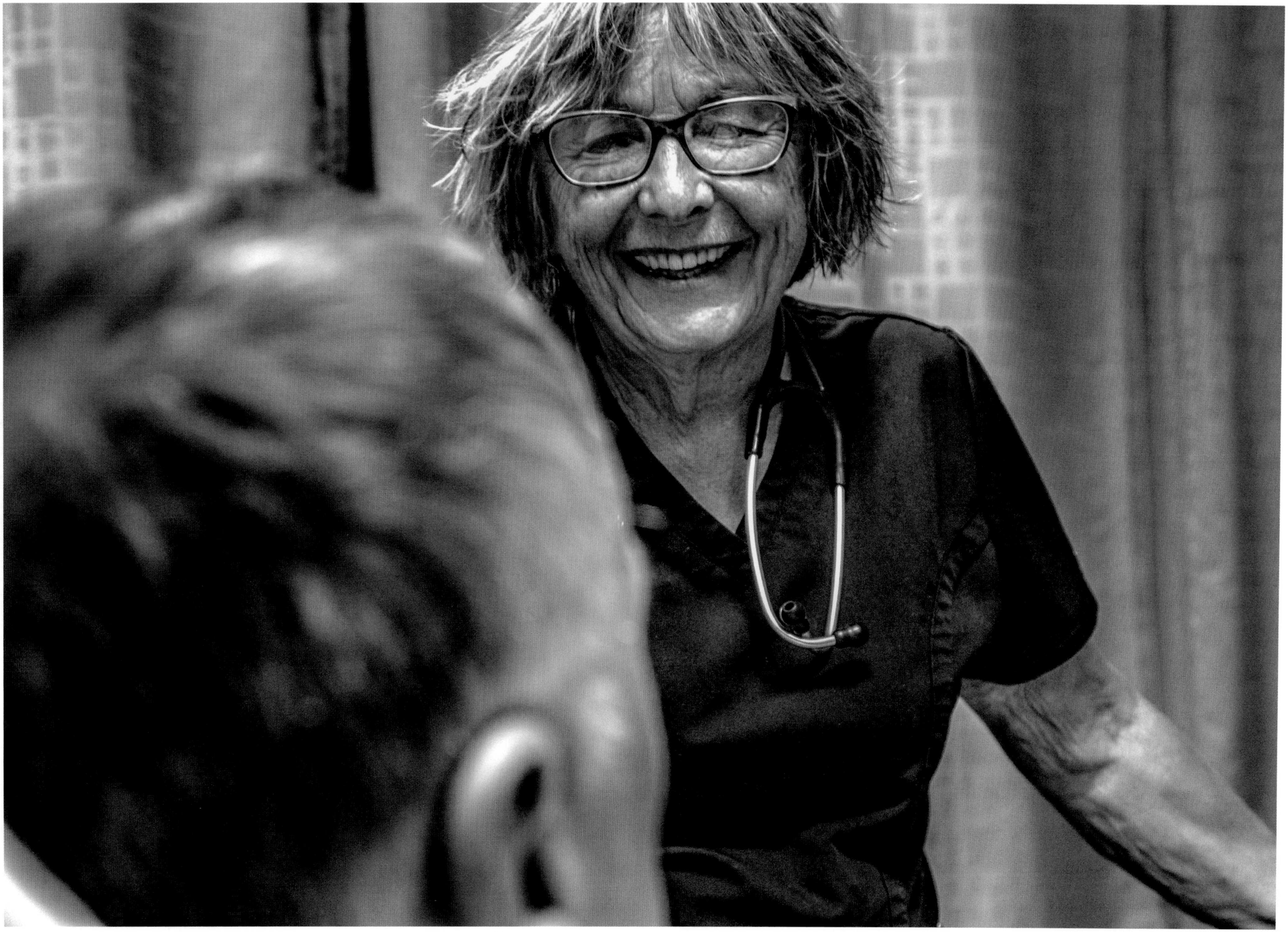

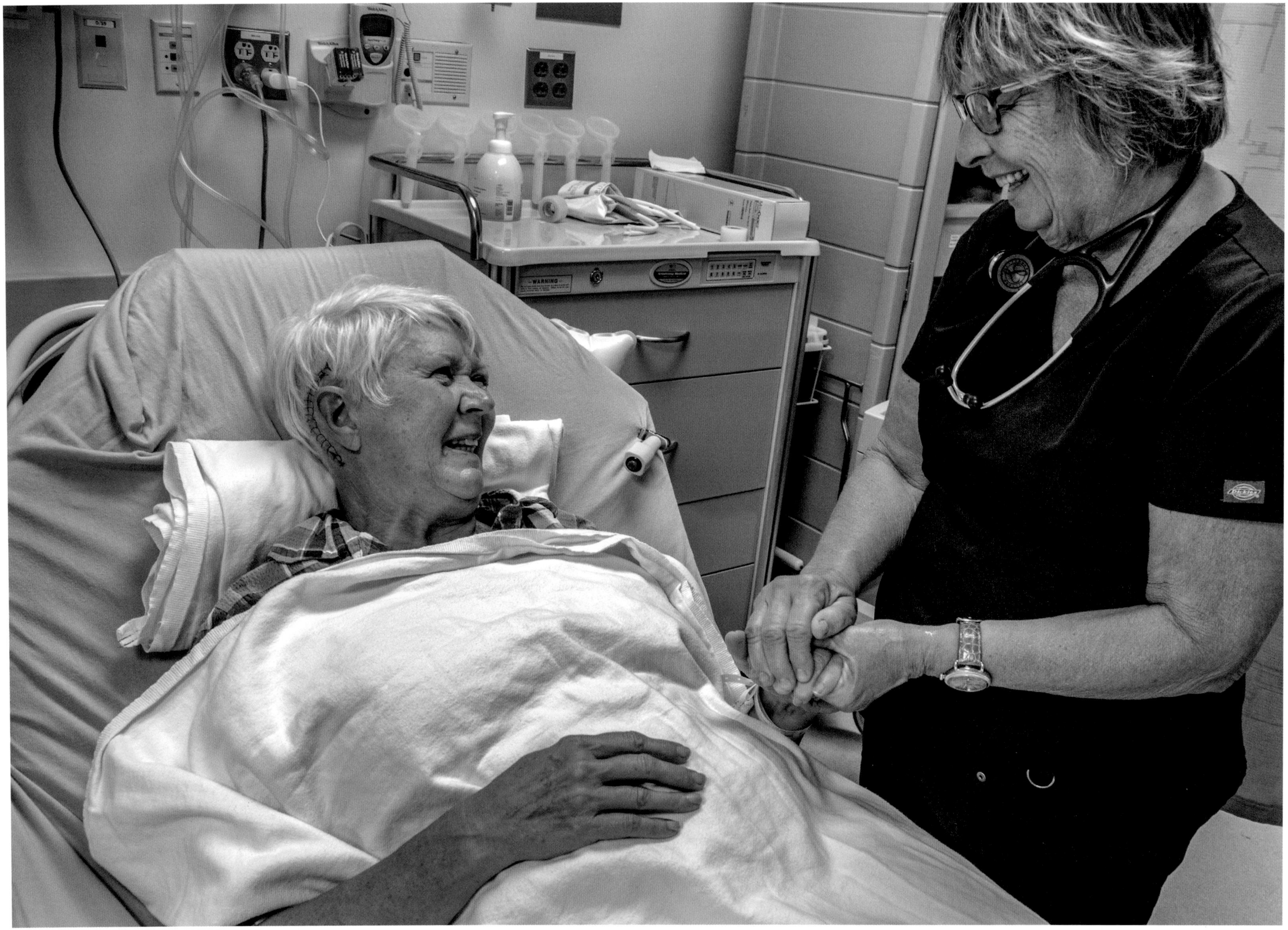
WARNING

You'll hear doctors using scientific terms with patients because they want to sound smart, or because that is the language of medicine. Let's just speak plain English. Physicians may think they need to establish a doctor–patient hierarchy . . . make it be known who's in charge. If anyone mistakes me for a nurse, I say, so what? It just doesn't matter. We should be connecting to patients as ordinary people.

Do I have a life outside of medicine? It's a question every physician needs to answer and work out for themselves. I love being a physician . . . it's an honor. I've studied all my life . . . I devote a lot of time to reading, editing, trying to communicate the newest information to the practitioners of our specialty. But you have to have some time apart for yourself, time apart for your family. I play the piano, I exercise, I bike. I have ten chickens. If you want to be happy in your specialty, you've got to find a way to free your mind. ✚

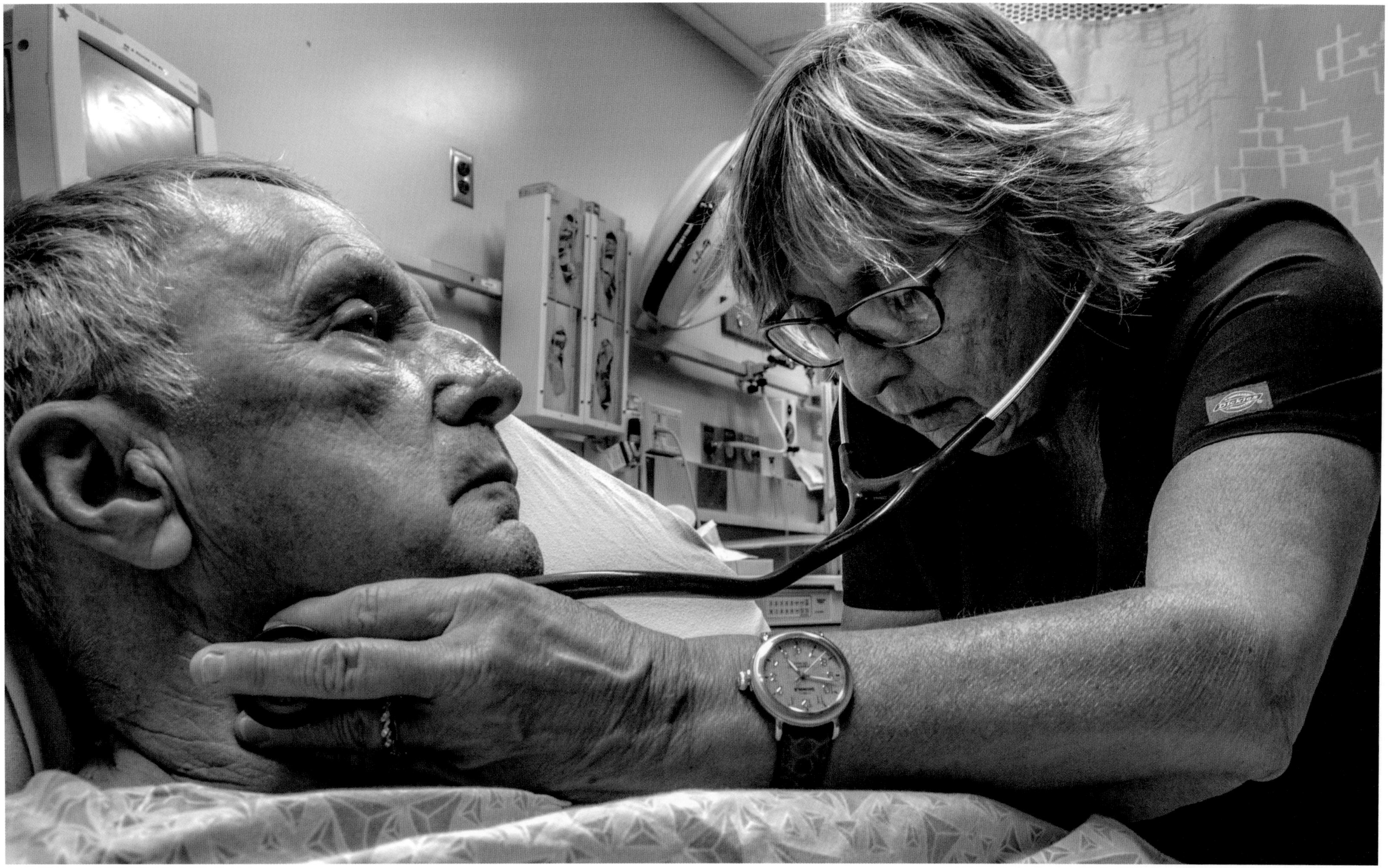

Adam Levine, MD

Emergency Physician & Global Medicine Specialist
Providence, Rhode Island

When I came back from Liberia, I was half hero, half pariah. I was interviewed by CNN and MSNBC and even met the president of the United States, but my friends didn't want anything to do with me. It was very isolating. And I was scared . . . every time I felt a tickle in my throat, I'd wonder, "Is this the beginning — am I getting Ebola?" I was required by law to check my temperature twice a day and report it to the Department of Health, but there were days I checked it twenty times. The fear followed me everywhere.

I'd been traveling back and forth between Liberia and Sierra Leone for more than a year, running the Ebola research team for the International Medical Corps. It was hard — fifteen-hour workdays with very few resources, no hot water, not enough food to go around, primitive working conditions, horrible sleep. Constant fear.

I've done earthquake relief in Haiti, I ran a clinic and a refugee camp in South Sudan, and I managed a trauma field hospital in Libya. In all those settings, the primary goal was caring for patients. Those situations were so dire . . . anything you could provide was better than nothing. We would pitch a tent and start seeing patients even before we had the right medicines or supplies.

But Liberia was completely different. When you're in the middle of an Ebola crisis, the primary goal isn't patient care — it's protecting your staff from the disease. To do that, everything must be in perfect order. You don't know if that patient who just came in has Ebola or not, so you've got to keep a meter's distance. We had to create a no-touch triage system — the doctor and nurse on one side of the fence and the patient on the other. It could get up to 130 degrees inside the protective "spacesuits" you had to wear, so you could only work for about forty-five minutes at a time before passing out. Rough.

The world seems like a pretty horrible place to a lot of people. They watch the news and feel overwhelmed by what they see — epidemics, pandemics, war, refugees all over the place. But the truth is, the last fifty years have been marked by constant improvements. Thanks to the effects of globalization, a huge proportion of the world's population has been lifted out of poverty. I've seen these things firsthand, so the current wave of US nationalism saddens me. I hate to see our country turning inward, cutting funding for humanitarian aid and abandoning the rest of the world.

I often think about the local staff I worked with on the front lines of the Ebola crisis. They saw what the virus was doing to their neighbors and loved ones and yet they still agreed to do the job. Over and over again they would say, "We are doing this to save our country." It was truly amazing. *They* are the true heroes of the epidemic, but that isn't to say they weren't afraid.

Courage is not the absence of fear. It's doing what's right, even though you're terrified. ✚

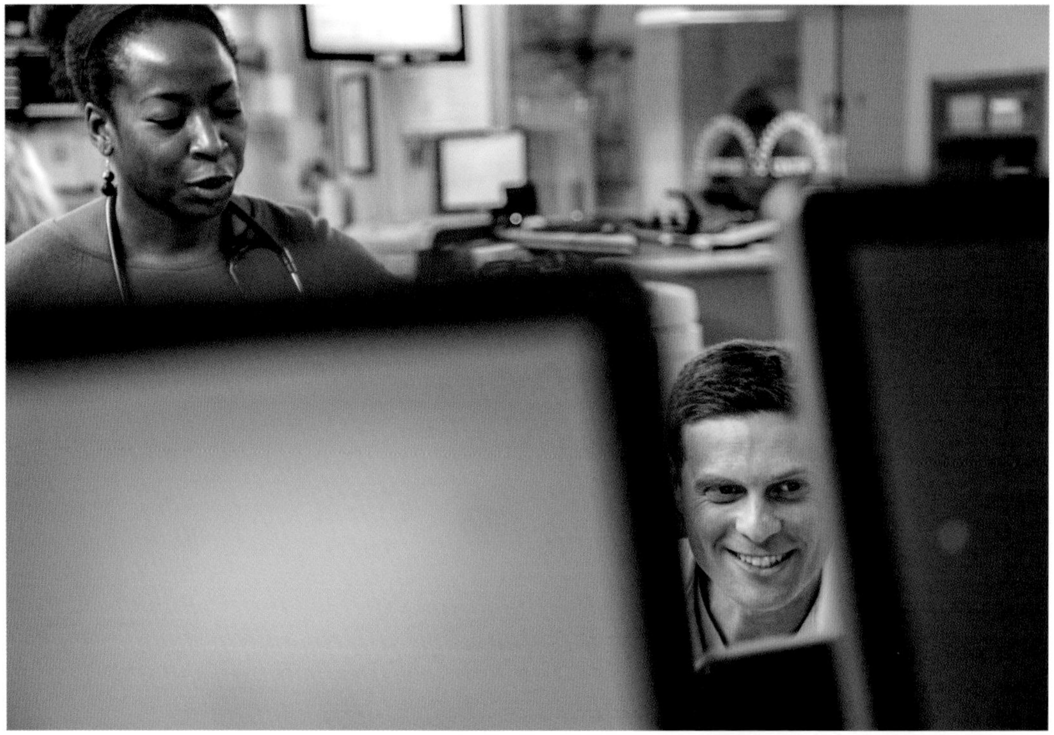

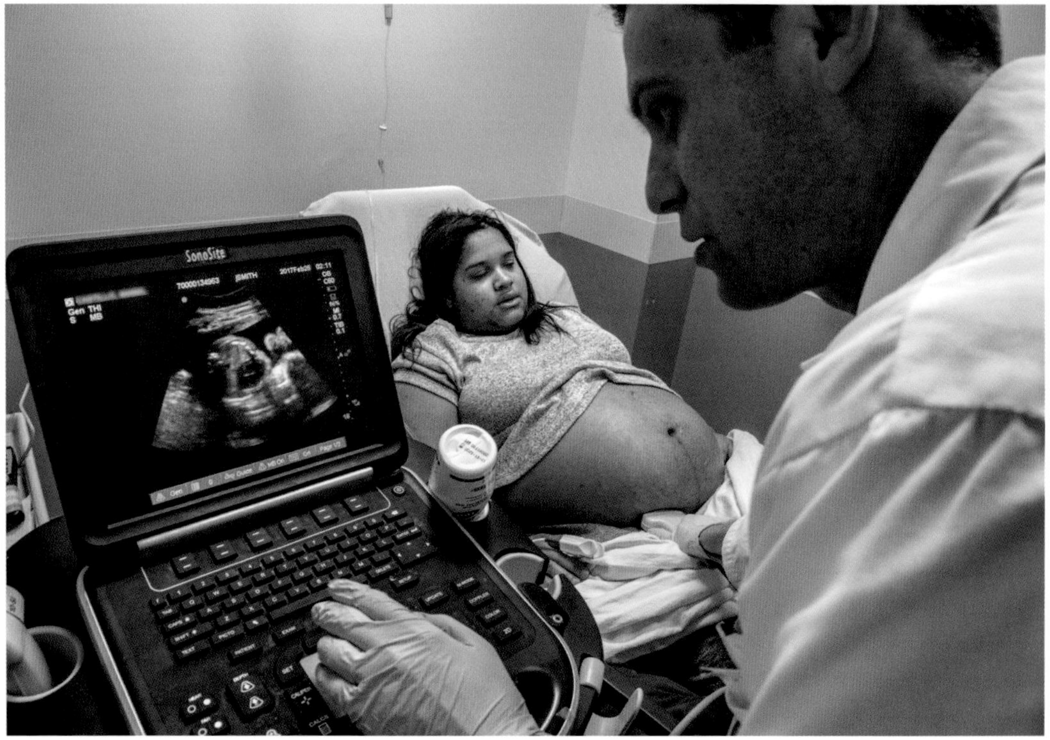

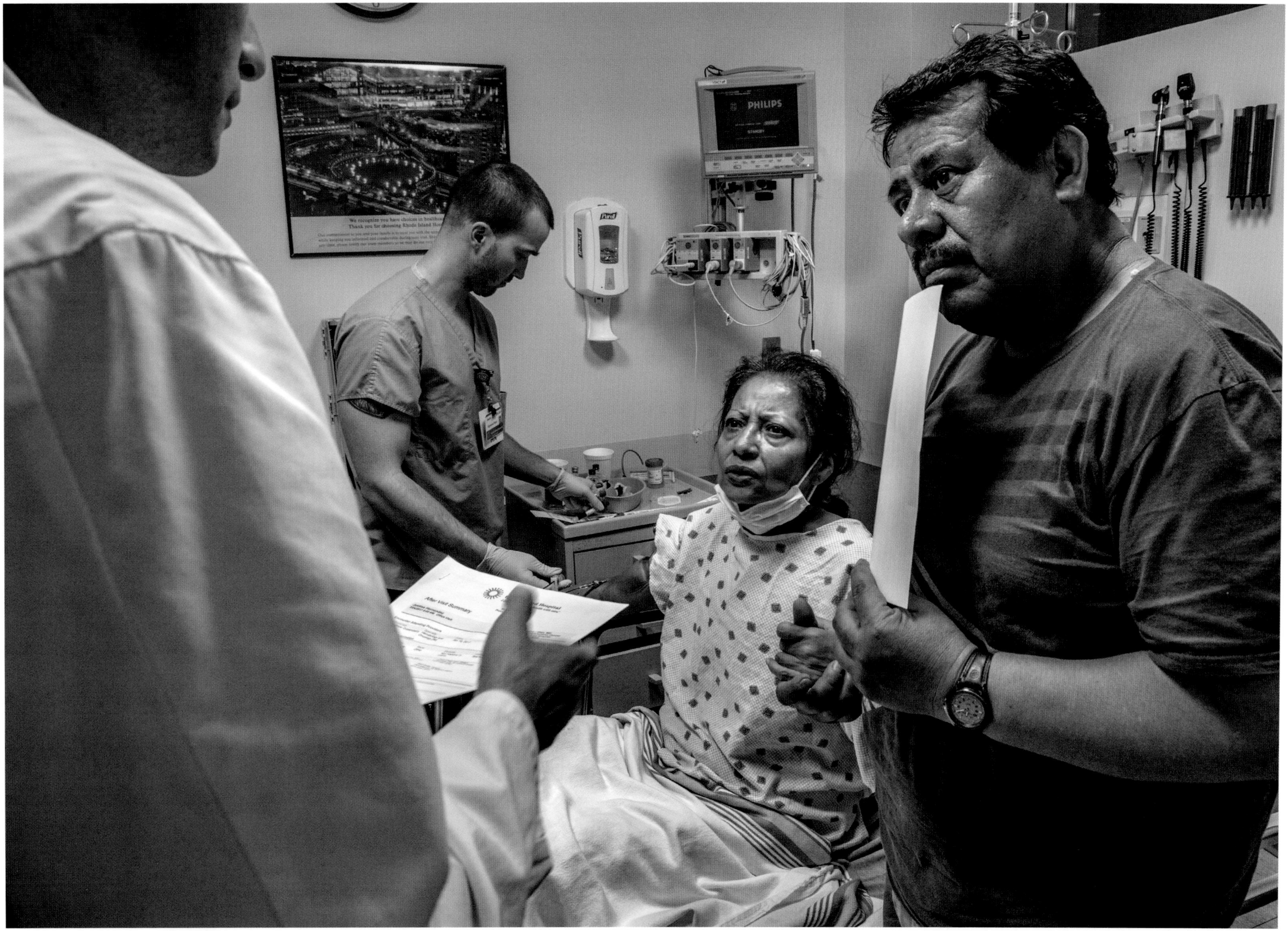
PHILIPS
After Visit Summary

John Ma, MD

Emergency Physician, Emergency Department Chair & Ultrasound Specialist
Portland, Oregon

Our patients are strangers. We have no relationship with them. They're vulnerable; they're naked. I don't know if you've ever worn a hospital gown, but it's pretty degrading — there's not a whole lot there. They're being asked very intimate questions about their lives and whatever condition has brought them to the ED. It's important to connect with them and gain their trust right away, yet you're under pressure to get to the point very, very quickly. You have to pretend you've got all the time in the world, even though you don't.

I worked as a sportswriter for a while, and I can think of no better training for emergency medicine than that. The initial meeting with a patient is a lot like a locker room interview after a game. The athletes are standing there with towels around their waists . . . or less. They may be on a high because they've won. Or they may be down, depressed because they've lost. I remember interviewing a University of Colorado kicker; he'd missed four field goals that game and his team had lost by three points. He was just devastated, but *he* was the story — no way to skirt that. I had to find a way to basically say, "Hey, why did you blow it? What happened today?"

I'll tell you the other thing that helped prepare me for this job . . . waiting tables. I worked at a restaurant called Bananas — everything was banana themed, everything. The concept didn't really take off, but I learned a lot of skills that apply in the ED. Now I always end every visit by asking my patients, "What can I do to make you more comfortable?" Sometimes they're cold — they could use a blanket. Great, I can do that. Just like in the restaurant business, if they want ketchup, bring them ketchup.

I trained back in the days when it was acceptable for instructors to berate their medical students. Surgeons would throw instruments in the operating room, and people would just duck. I mean, you'd be making rounds in the hallway, and some guy would get up in your face. You could feel the spit against your cheek; his finger would be jabbing you in the chest. That's just how it was. After a while, I realized they were trying to impart knowledge between the screams.

I trained under an amazing general surgeon; we called him "Stanley the Steamer" because he was always blowing up. I would start telling him about a case, and he'd say, "John, John, John, I don't want to hear that! Tell me what I really want to hear." So, I would start again, and he'd yell, "Nope, tell me what I *really* want to hear!" After about ten days of this abuse, he started to treat me like a normal person. He was like, "This guy gets it."

I actually flourished in that environment, probably because I grew up playing sports. I was used to coaches telling me I sucked. The experience really gave me a lot of confidence. I thought, "If I can survive *this*, I can make it in this field. I can overcome almost anything."

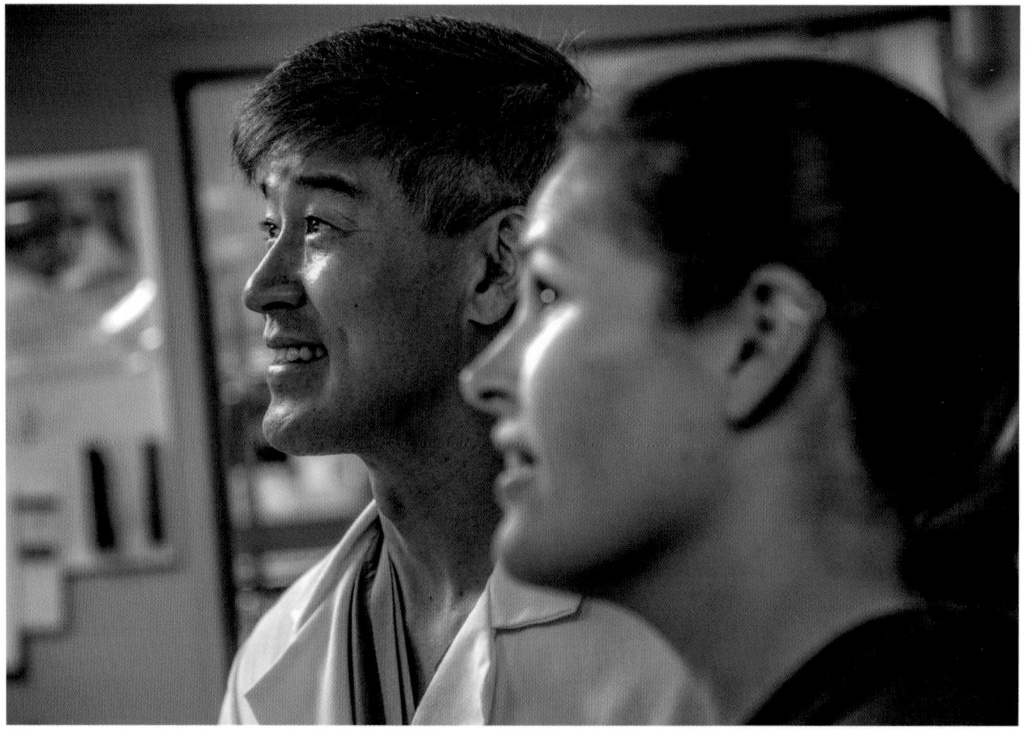

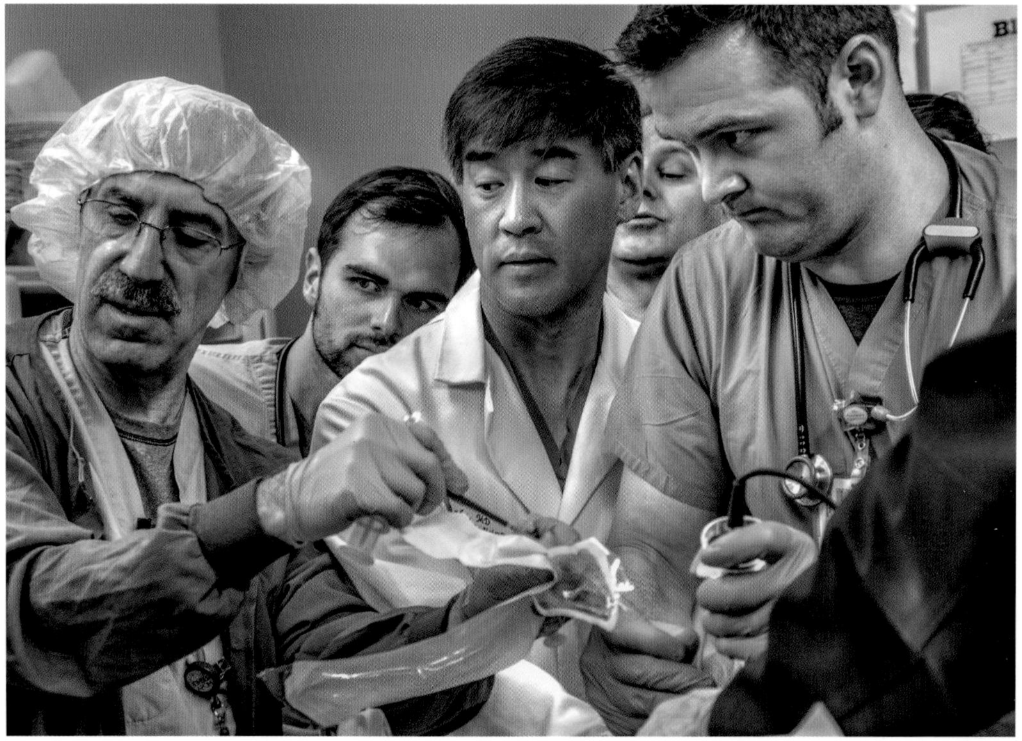

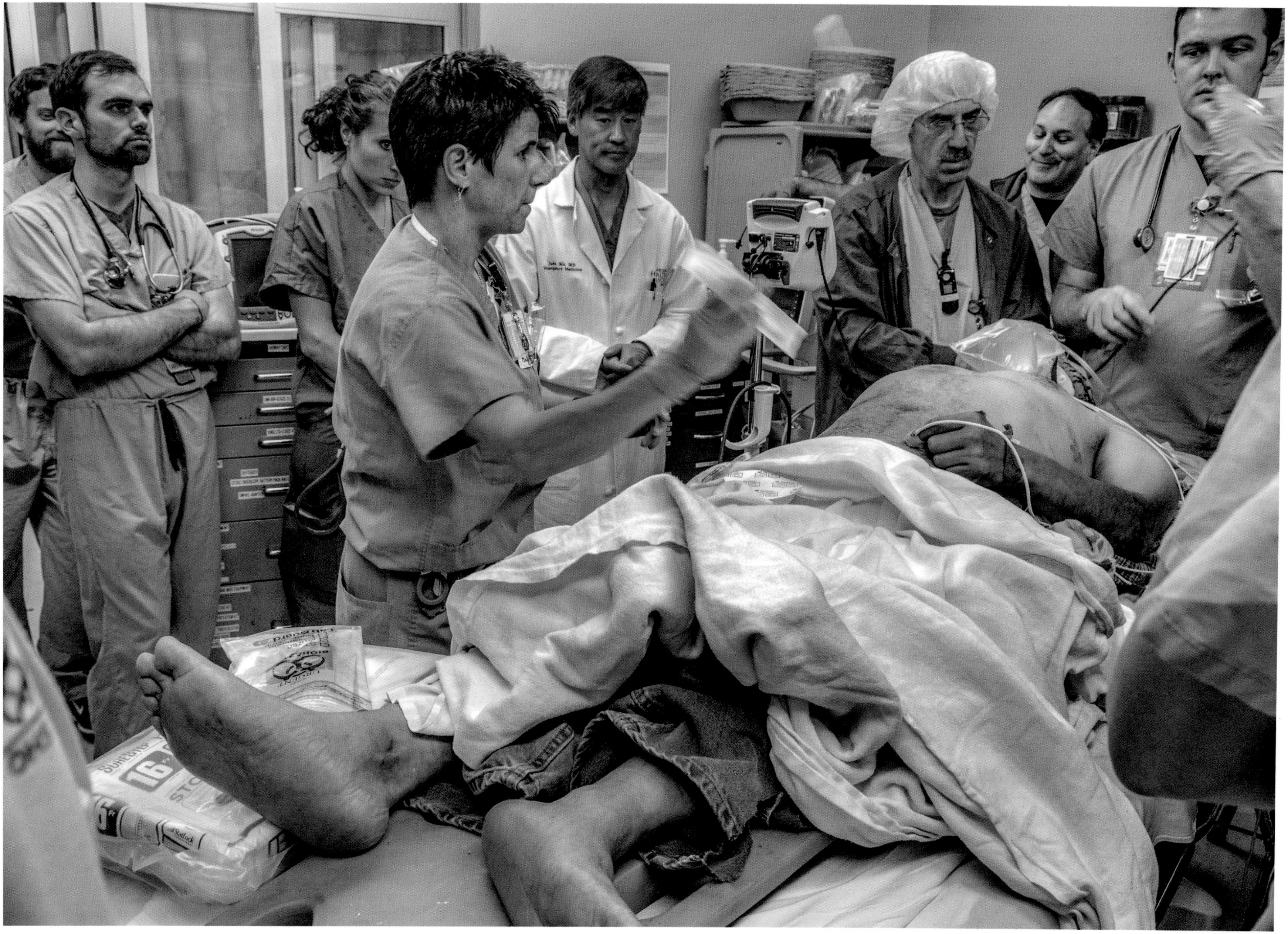

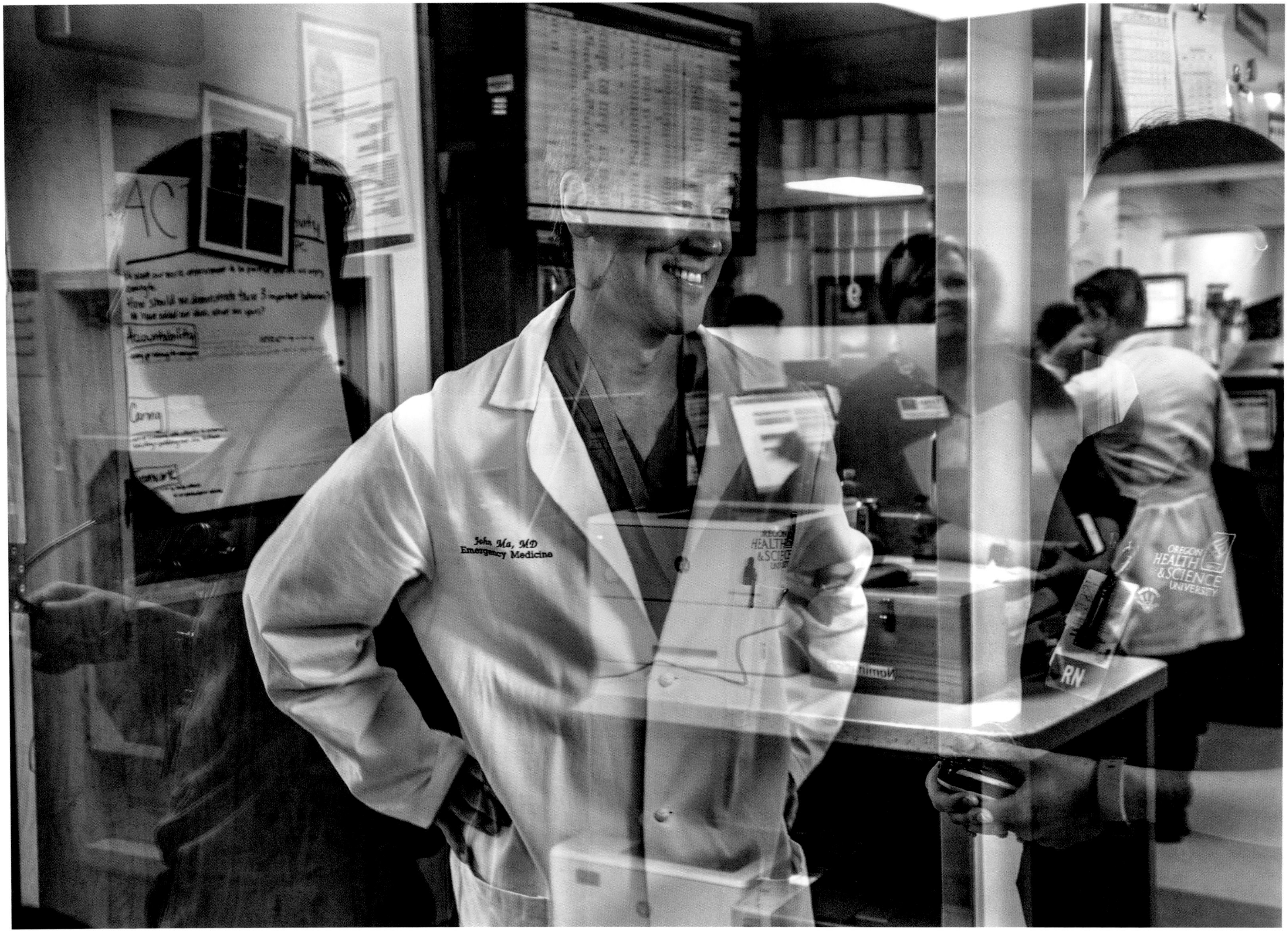
John Ma, MD
Emergency Medicine
OREGON
HEALTH
& SCIENCE
UNIVERSITY
RN

The things that intrigued me about emergency medicine got me interested in ultrasound, too — the detective work, the variety, the need for speed. And I love the procedures — getting my hands dirty. You've got blood, you've got guts . . . you get to dive into all kinds of stuff.

I had a job in Milwaukee in the '90s when the drug trade was in full force. I'd work a twelve-hour shift and get home in time for the eight o'clock news. They'd always start off with a string of shootings . . . this person got shot last night on 39th Street . . . this guy got killed on Broadway . . . I knew every single one of them. I'd think, "Hey, I put a chest tube in that patient . . . I intubated that guy . . . that one got a central line." It was bizarre.

There have only been a handful of times I've cried on the job. One time, we got a twelve-year-old boy who had been hit by a car. He had a serious head injury, and we were not able to resuscitate him. I notified the mother and walked her back to the trauma room. I stayed with her . . . looking at this woman with her dead son. It was overwhelming. But what still haunts me is watching her walk out of the room. She was just wobbling . . . like a drunk person. That's when I lost it. Still to this day, it's one of the most powerful things I've ever seen.

Does it ever get easier? I'm not sure. Last summer, we lost a young girl who'd fallen asleep behind the wheel. We pronounced her dead, and the trauma surgeon had to notify her parents. This surgeon had already seen everything — I mean, he's a Vietnam vet, gray hair, tough guy. But when we start to talk, he chokes up and says, "I'm just so fucking tired of having to tell families that their loved one has been killed." So, there we are, two seasoned clinicians just standing together, tears rolling down our faces. ✚

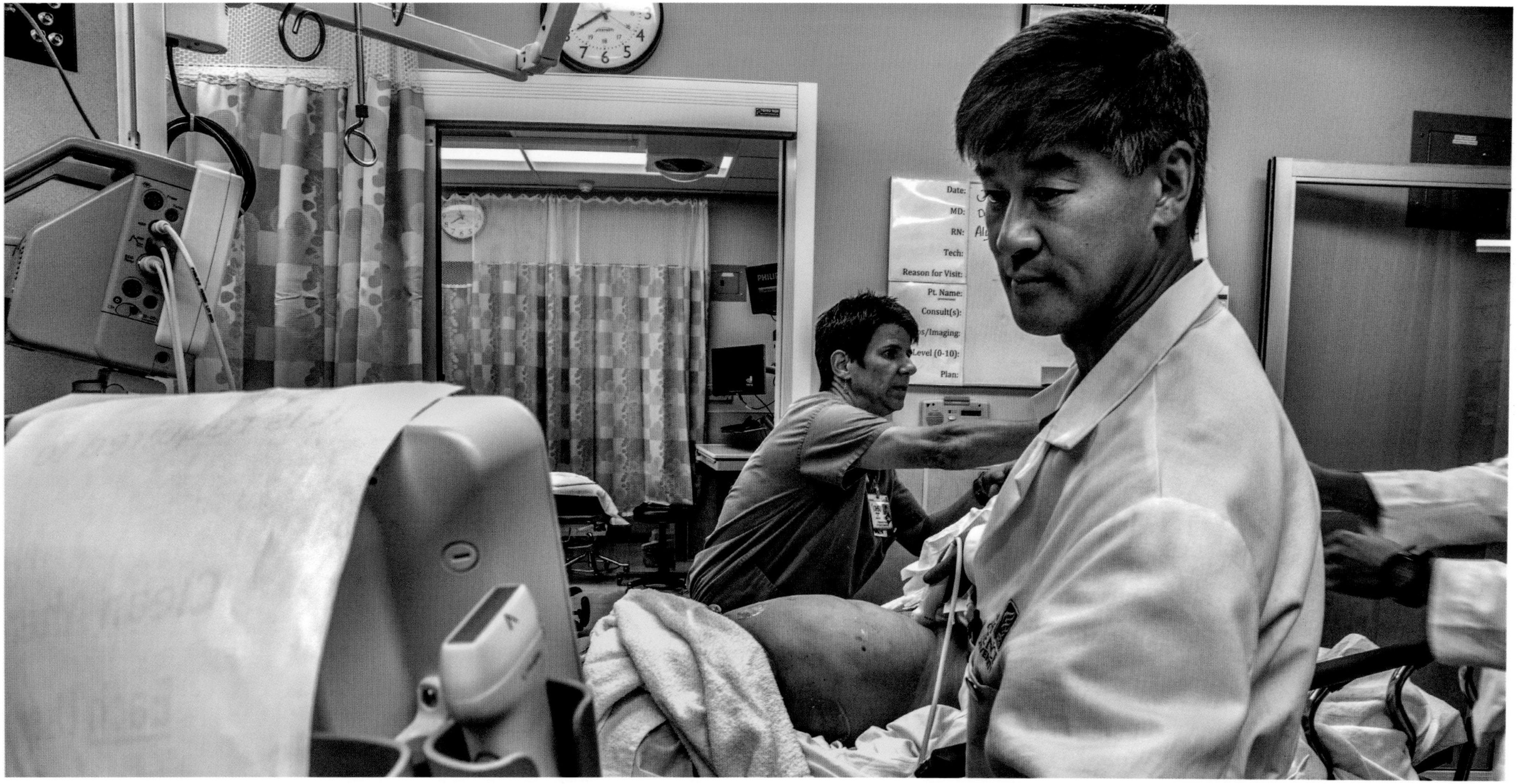

Elizabeth Nestor, MD

Emergency Physician
Providence, Rhode Island

Out of the 180 students in my medical school class, only three chose emergency medicine. One was a former craps dealer, one was a random guy who made a late choice, and then there was me. I remember an internal medicine doc who told me, "You people represent everything that is wrong with medicine today." They just couldn't understand what we were doing at all — couldn't get behind it.

In those days, most emergency departments were staffed by doctors who had bombed out of other specialties, and many thought of the ED as nothing more than a last resort for poor patients. We've developed our own body of knowledge in the years since, and the field has become quite competitive, but it hasn't always been that way.

After college, I worked as a church secretary for an Episcopal parish. I admired the priest and thought he had a fabulous job, so I decided to go to the seminary. I became a deacon in '79; the following year, I was ordained as a priest. It was a great experience, but it wasn't exactly what I was looking for. I learned I'm not someone who does well with open endings. I like to start something, finish it, and move on, so my favorite parts of the job were the weddings and funerals. The long, ongoing relationship doesn't appeal to me that much, which is one reason I was drawn to emergency medicine. At the end of every intense little shift, a new doctor comes in to take over your chair . . . and it's time for you to go.

The language people use — the speech of everyday life — is very different from the language of medicine. The conversations we have with patients often require translation. *Where do you hurt? Can you describe the pain? What are you experiencing?* I want to understand what they need, and I want them to know I'm listening . . . I'm paying attention . . . I have a reasonable plan for dealing with their conundrum. I don't want to challenge anybody. I don't want to condemn what they're doing. I don't want to enter a negotiation. Really, I just want to hear their point of view . . . and then I want them to hear mine.

A lot of emergency docs really like the blood and guts . . . the screaming and cursing. There's something about that atmosphere that's really stimulating to some people. Personally, I like to keep a quieter department, but you never know what you're going to get around here. Things will be going along just fine and then — *splash* — an intoxicated patient hurls a full urinal at your head. Yeah, the urinal bomb . . . definitely my least favorite weapon.

There are many, many patients I'll never forget — cases that have changed my practice. But I think longevity in this field partly depends upon your ability to pull back on your emotions. You can't allow yourself to brood continually, but that can be difficult when a case has gone very badly. I've had patients wreck my sleep.

If you have a case — especially one in which a patient has died — the lawyers tell you to keep your mouth shut. Don't talk to anyone about what happened. But how can you really get things right in your head if you don't get the story off your chest? When you get right down to it, though, who can you *really* talk to anyhow? When I'm walking with friends on the bike path, do I say, "Hey, let me tell you about this terrible case. . ."? No, they're not prepared to hear it.

My commute is thirty minutes from the hospital. If a case is still alive in my head when I get home, sometimes I'll go out to the back yard. It's a very quiet place . . . where I can look up at the stars. ✚

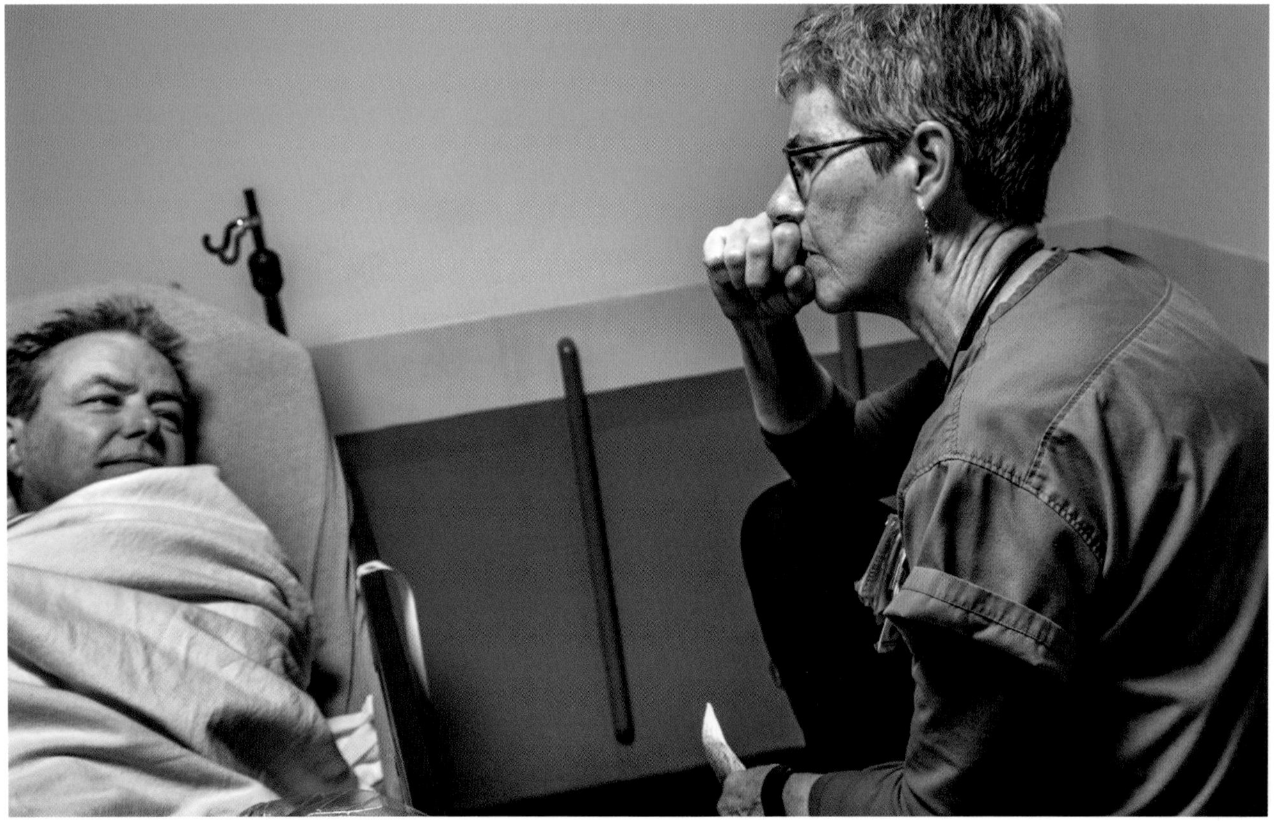

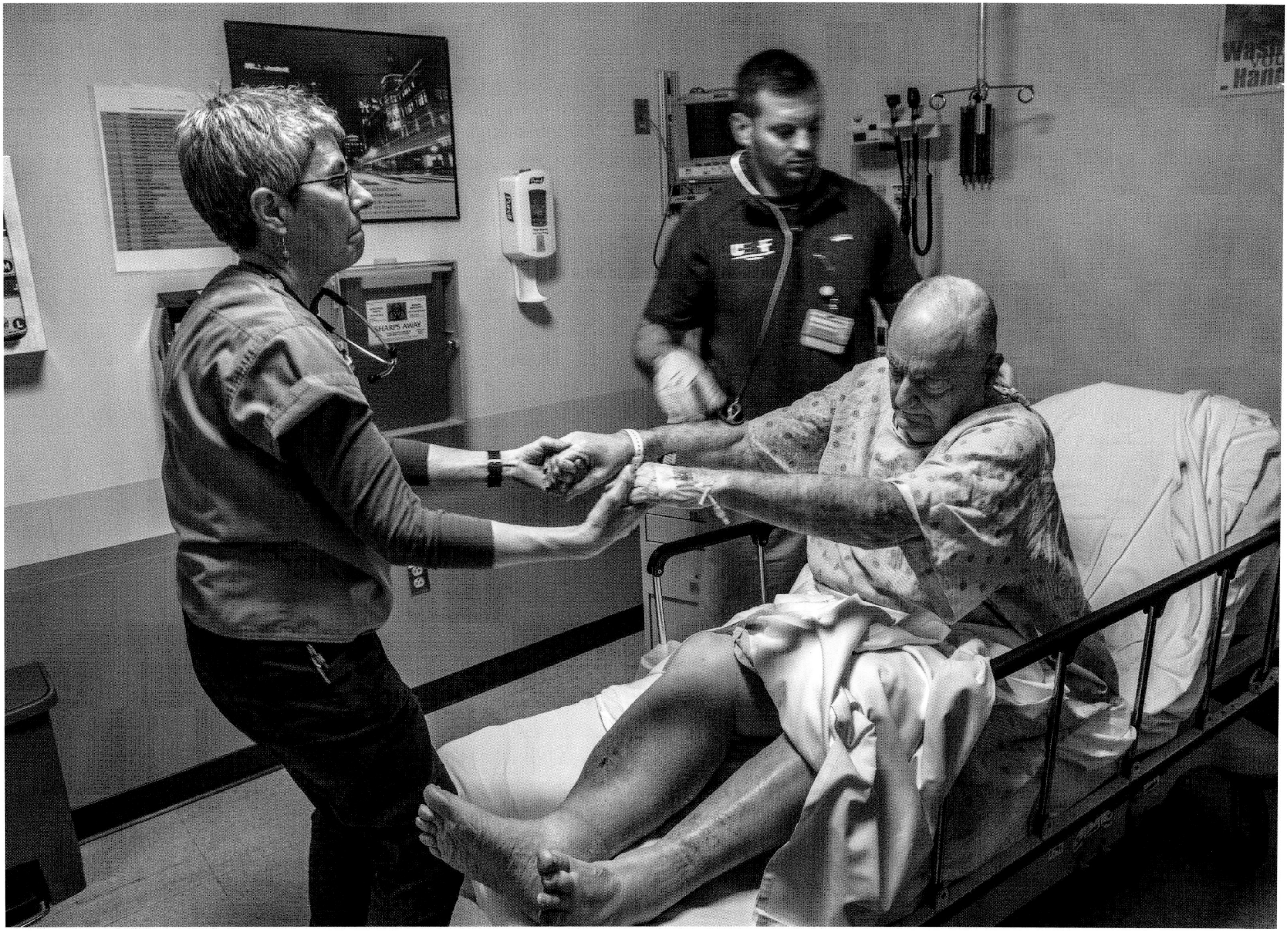
SHARPS AWAY

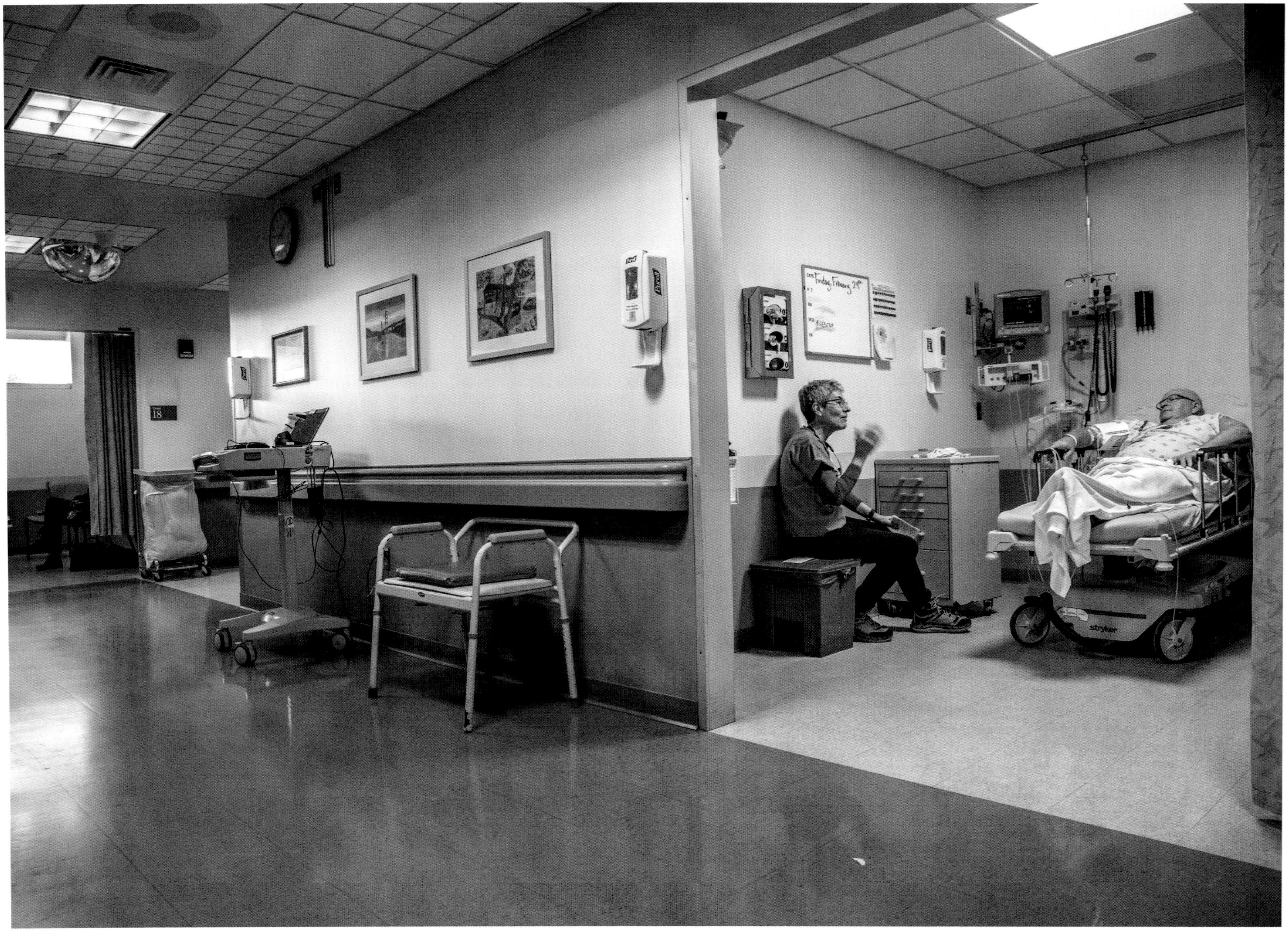
Purell
stryker

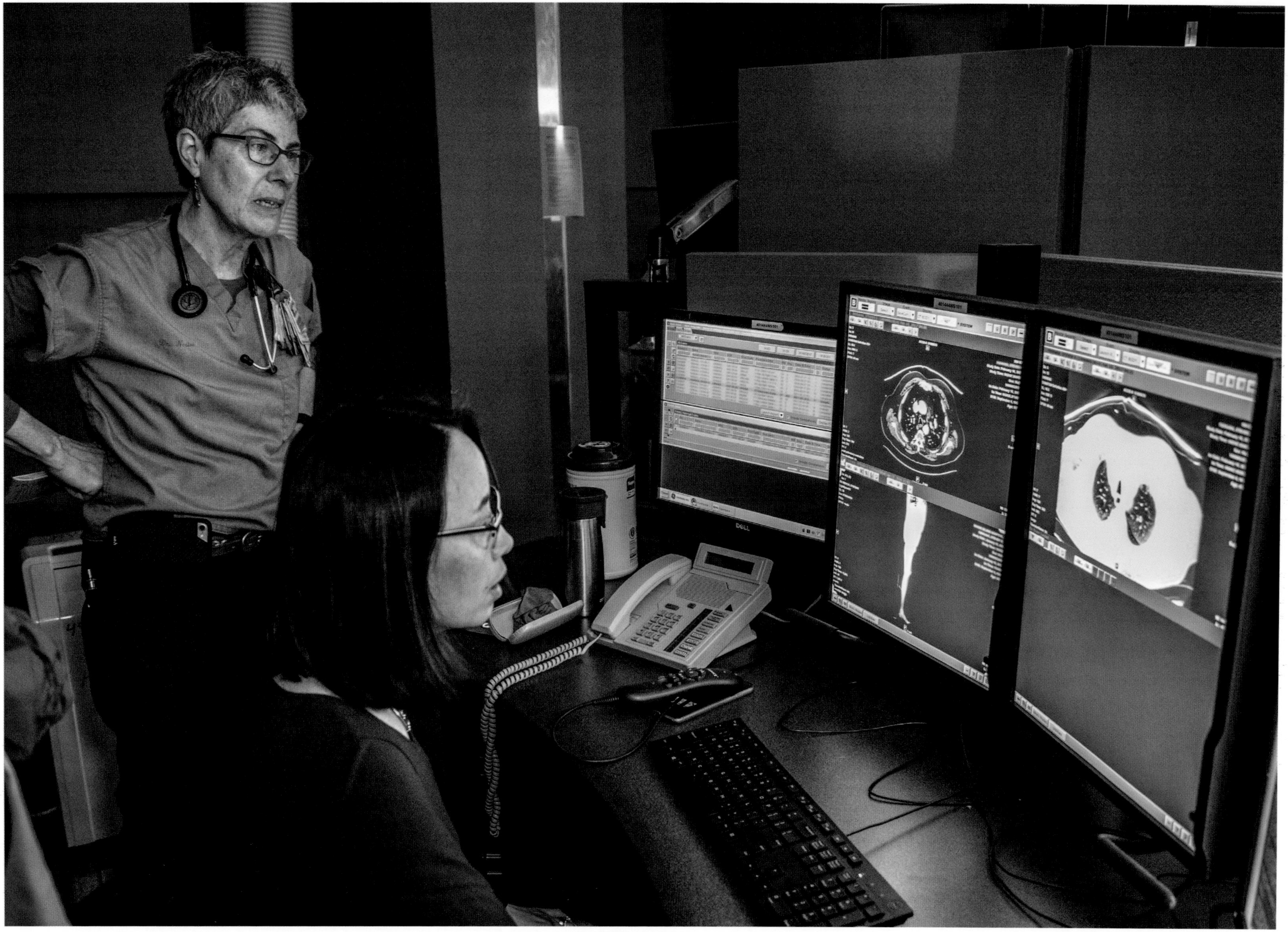

Bruce Janiak, MD

Emergency Medicine Pioneer & First Emergency Medicine Resident
Akron, Ohio

I have a passion for civil disobedience. I get joy from arguing my position. I'm somebody who likes to question everything . . . and gets frustrated when there is no answer. I like to go back to the microcosm, the minor parts, but I'm also interested in the bigger issues — like why did we used to paint every emergency department ceiling black? The answer usually is that somebody over here heard somebody over there, and somebody over there heard a rumor. . . . I don't want to comply for the sake of compliance.

In my third year of medical school, I started seeking out people who would tell me about emergency medicine. I loved the ER — loved that I could experience something different every five minutes. I could see and react to stuff I'd never even heard about. It was the most action-packed place . . . there was so much to learn.

I was offered an orthopedic residency, but I turned it down. I said, "Hey, I want to do emergency medicine. What do you think?" Cincinnati General Hospital eventually said if I agreed to stay there as an intern, they would work with me to create a curriculum. I set up my twenty-four-month program and became the first emergency medicine resident in the country. I didn't ask about my future or what kind of certificate I would get. I just wanted to do the training. Of course, people would ask, "Why would you waste your life doing that?" But my answer was always, "Look, if I were a stock, I'd buy me." I never doubted.

In 1974, I was hired to manage an emergency department in Toledo. Back then, there were no emergency specialists. You could find doctors who had done a little work in the ER, but their skills were variable — extremely variable. Some were horrendous. I had one physician who was treating ear infections with the highest-powered antibiotics available. I called him in and said, "I've been reviewing your charts, and you've been using an inappropriate medication. It's too expensive — and it's just *wrong*." He walked out, and I never saw him again. It took long hours and many shifts over several years until I found enough good doctors to staff the place.

My wife and I were making decent money and had three children of our own, but we thought it might be nice to share the wealth. Over several years, we became the foster parents to a lot of kids — I say sixty, my wife says over one hundred. We used two triplet strollers and three buses that looked like airport shuttles. I had to get a commercial driver's license to be able to take the kids to lunch. Eventually, we decided to adopt. Catholic Social Services initially turned us down because there was a waiting list and we already had kids of our own. But when I asked about children with special needs, their answer was, "Can you come in tomorrow?" We had three new kids within six months! We started with a few from Ohio, then added two from Paraguay, and two more from Chile.

Our last child came from Brazil. We took a taxi ride out to a small town where people were dipping water out of a dirty artesian well and were led to a tiny cinder-block building. Three hundred roaches scattered in every

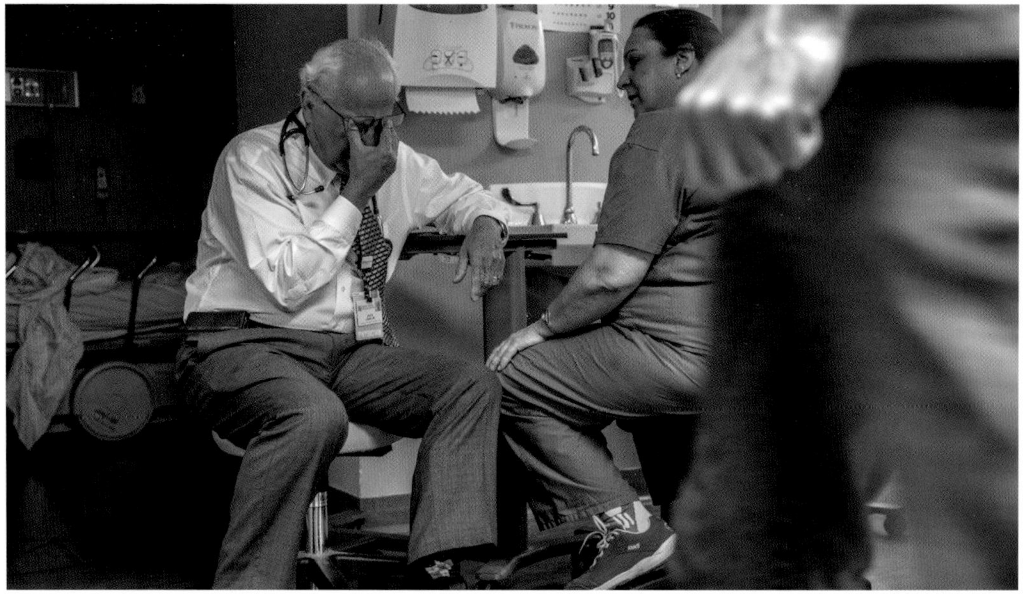

direction when the curtain was pulled aside, but there sat six or seven women holding babies. We were told, "Pick one." That was it. I think it took half a dozen trips between Toledo and Recife before the adoption was complete. It was a brutal process.

We had black kids, South American kids, even a Guarani Indian. It was like the United Nations. Now, I laugh at these college diversity programs — they don't have any idea what diversity really is. We had bumps — kids with severe medical problems, kids who got into trouble, girls who got pregnant — but they've all grown up. They go to work, pay their taxes, and raise their kids the best way they can. Our house is empty.

I enormously enjoy the work I do now, teaching residents, but I'm not happy with medical education in this country. It's got its head on backwards. I see residents from other services just checking boxes and blindly ordering tests. When you question their reasoning, they'll say, "My attending wants me to do that, and I'll get in trouble if I don't." Here we have a system that wastes billions and billions of dollars on unnecessary procedures, yet young physicians are punished if they don't comply with that approach. That should stop.

Unfortunately, we live in a zero-error society. The only acceptable outcome is to never make a mistake, but that way of thinking is a luxury we can't afford. Medical professionals should be empowered to take personal responsibility for doing what they think is best for the patient — and society as a whole. These decisions shouldn't be based on fear. No one should undergo a test just because you're trying to protect your own butt from a lawsuit.

I guess you have to have a fair amount of self-confidence to push back, but the older I get, the easier it becomes. I've had pretty good luck with personal resistance. I've seen change . . . I know it can happen. ✚

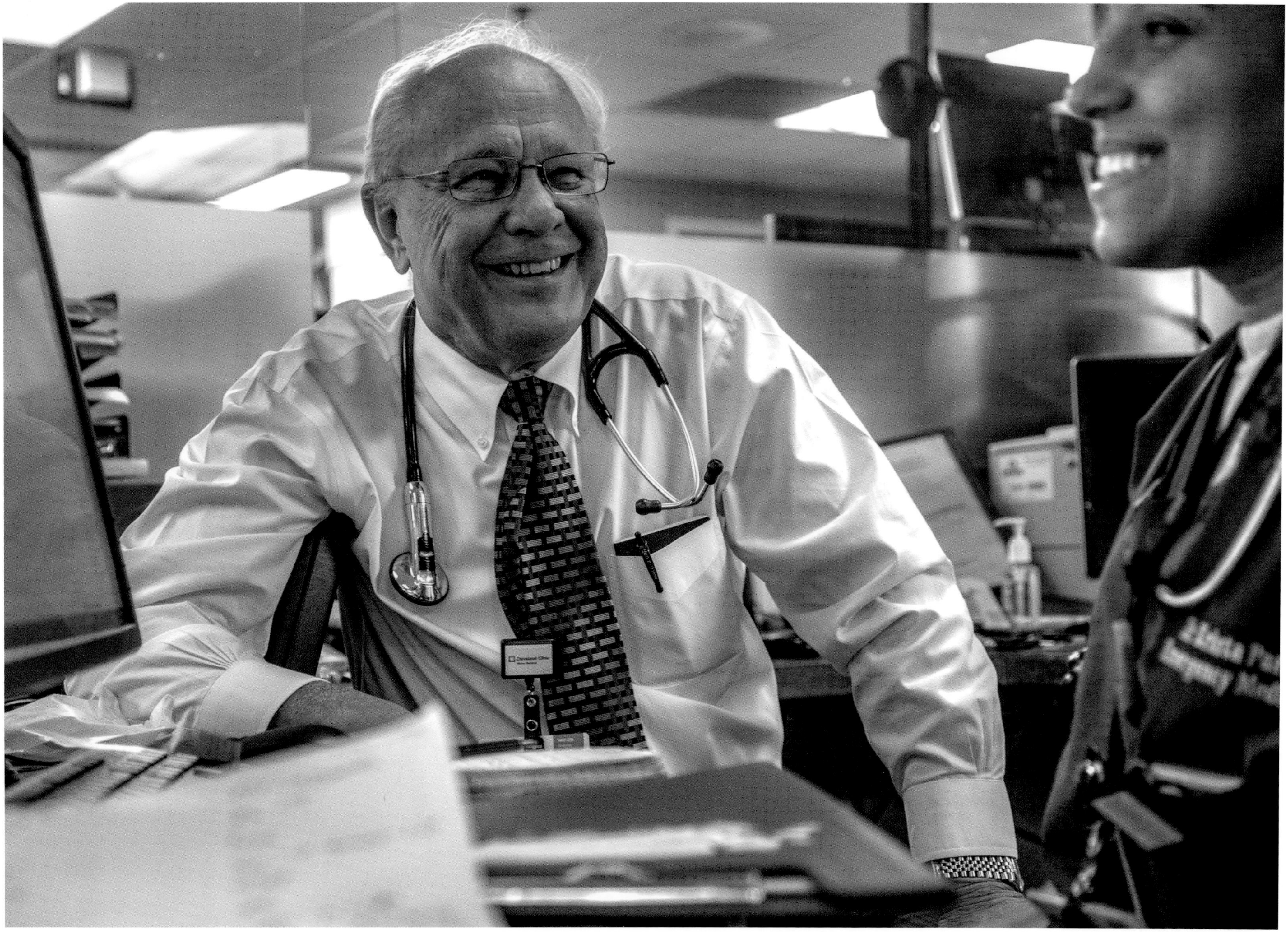

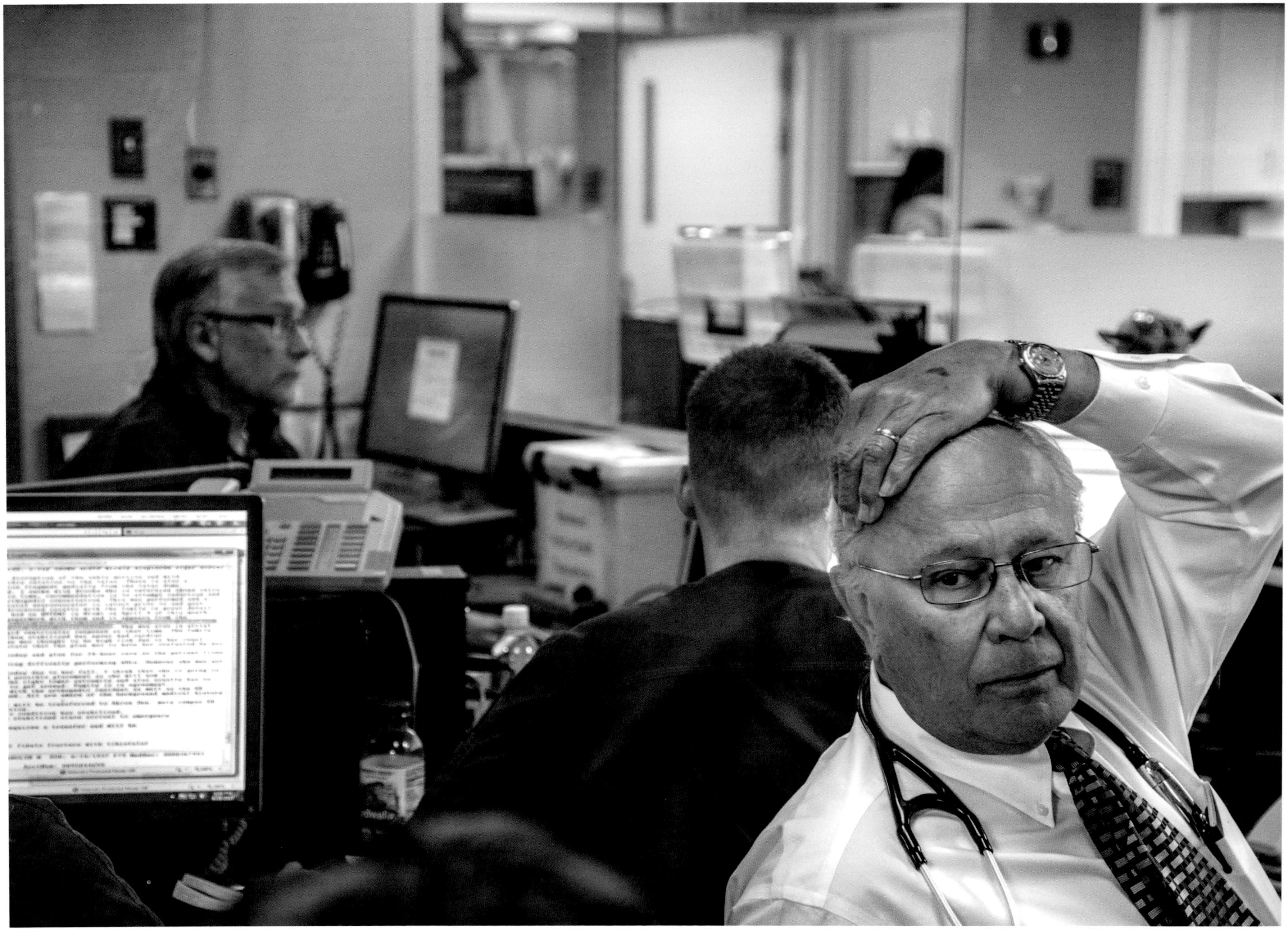

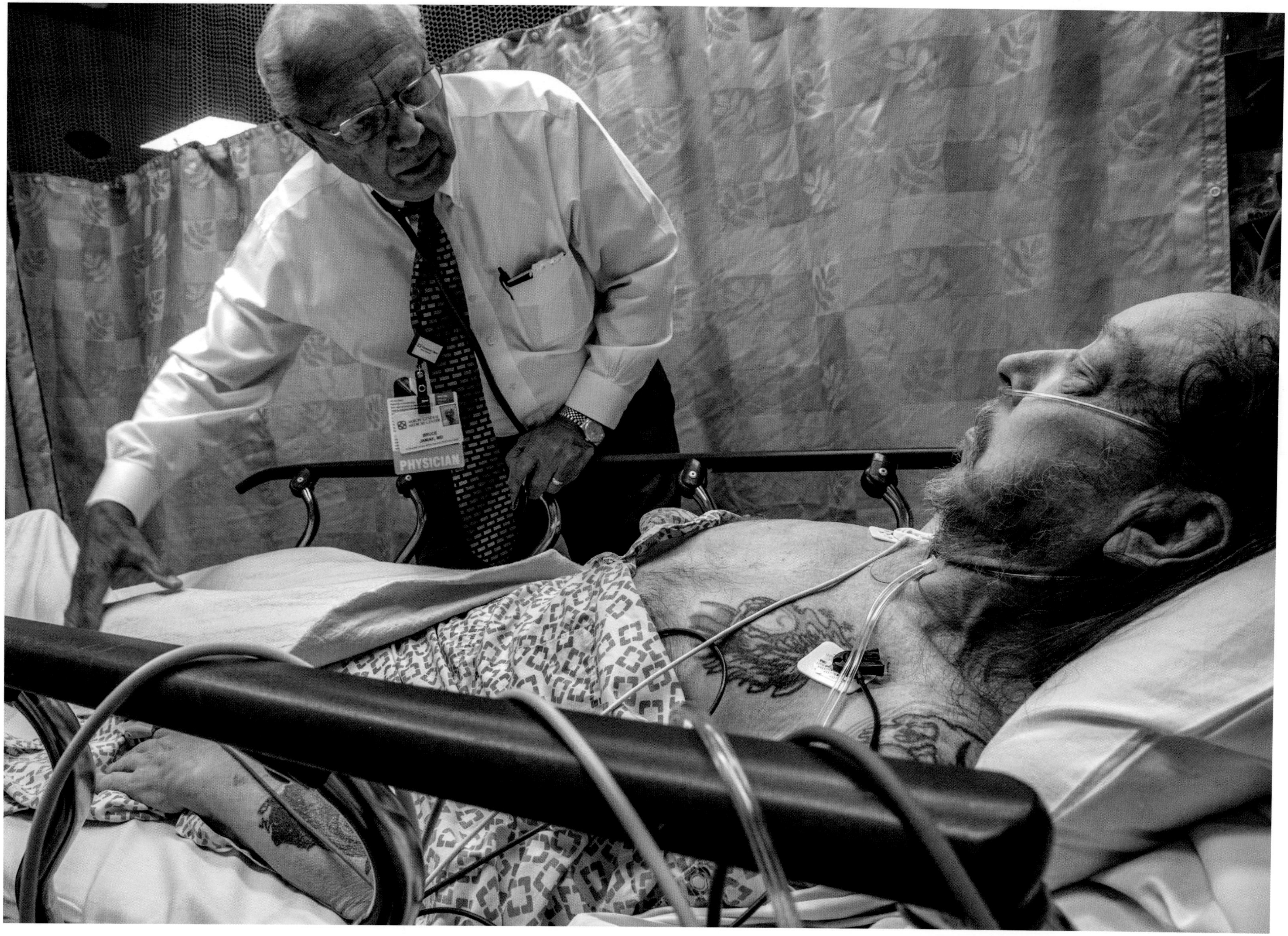
PHYSICIAN

Tom Stoffer

Paramedic
Denver, Colorado

I've got all kinds of stories — patients who have swung and spit and shoved. When you've been doing this job as long as I have, the list of things you *haven't* seen keeps getting shorter and shorter. When cell phones first came out, people would report every little thing they saw. Some poor guy from the suburbs would come into the city and dial 911 because he saw someone passed out on the sidewalk. We'd be like, "Welcome to Denver."

But we've seen serious violence, too. In the early '90s, northeast Denver was hot — bullets were flying. We had a lot of gangbangers — Crips and Bloods. I was sitting in City Park one night. It was slow, and I nodded off in the front seat of the ambulance. All of a sudden, I heard "bam, bam, bam" on my window and a guy tells me his buddy has been hit in a drive-by shooting. I called dispatch to request cover, and my partner and I ran over to take care of the patient, who — sure enough — had been shot in the head. We loaded him up in the ambulance, but the patient's friends followed us in their car . . . that's never a good thing. We alerted the cops, and they stopped the car a few blocks down.

After we'd dropped the guy off at the hospital, we got called back to the spot where his friends had been pulled over. The cops peeled back the carpet in the rear deck of this Cadillac. . . . it was stacked with custom-built boxes full of submachine guns. Turns out, *they* were the ones doing the drive-by. One of their guys had pulled out a gun, pulled the trigger — pop, pop, splat — and hit his own driver. Had tensions gotten high, they could have turned on us, too. You just never know.

Whether you're wearing the uniform or not, you remain very aware of perceived threats. When our family took a trip last summer I felt like a guard dog. I'm looking through doorways . . . I'm looking down sidewalks . . . I'm looking at people approaching . . . I'm checking around every corner. Is there anybody coming up behind us?

I've had some dark days — times when I was burned out, times when I tried to be a cowboy. But I've always found a way to embrace what I'm doing and the people doing it with me. I take a lot of pride in this job and feel a responsibility to maintain the standard set by the guys who came before me.

When I get crusty, I check my own attitude first. I've learned there's not a lot I can control, but I can change my approach . . . look for ways to move the needle. If I become bored, I'll dive into medical books, retrain myself, and get psyched up again about the clinical aspects of what we do. I'll have conversations with doctors and read about new things to look for or apply. Learning gets me back in that groove.

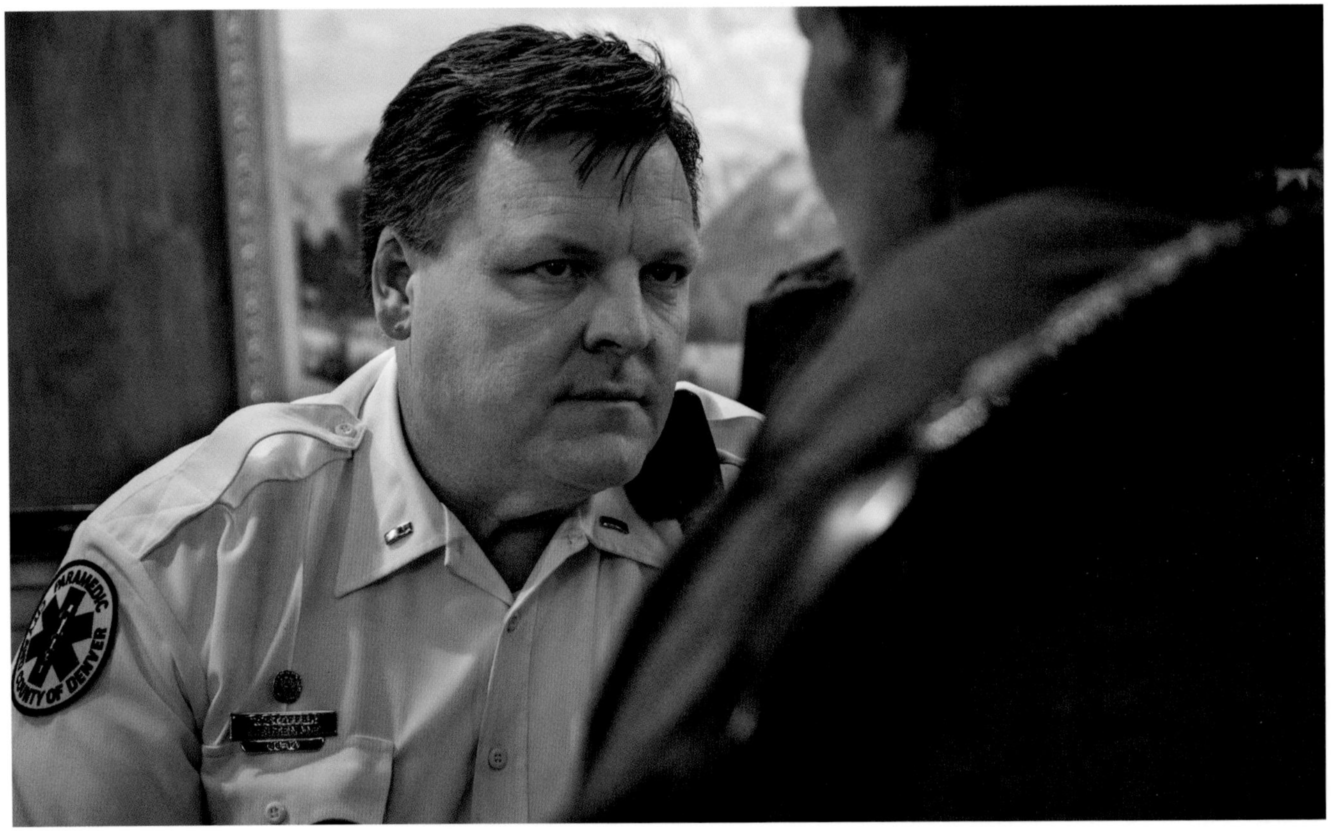

My job is easier when the patient is on my side . . . it's important to find that commonality. If you're always standing there acting official and using medical terminology instead of plain speak, it's very hard to gain their trust. We're caring for patients who may be irrational, who may not even want treatment. You're constantly making these little concessions. "Ok, I won't start an IV . . . as long as you'll let me take you to the hospital." It's like negotiating a deal with North Korea.

We're practicing street medicine. I remember getting called to a rough industrial area one day. As we were slowly pulling up to the scene, we saw a small group of guys. They looked like they might be homeless . . . they'd definitely seen better days. As we passed them, my partner said, "Ahh, these are my people." And I just thought, "Yeah, they really are." ✚

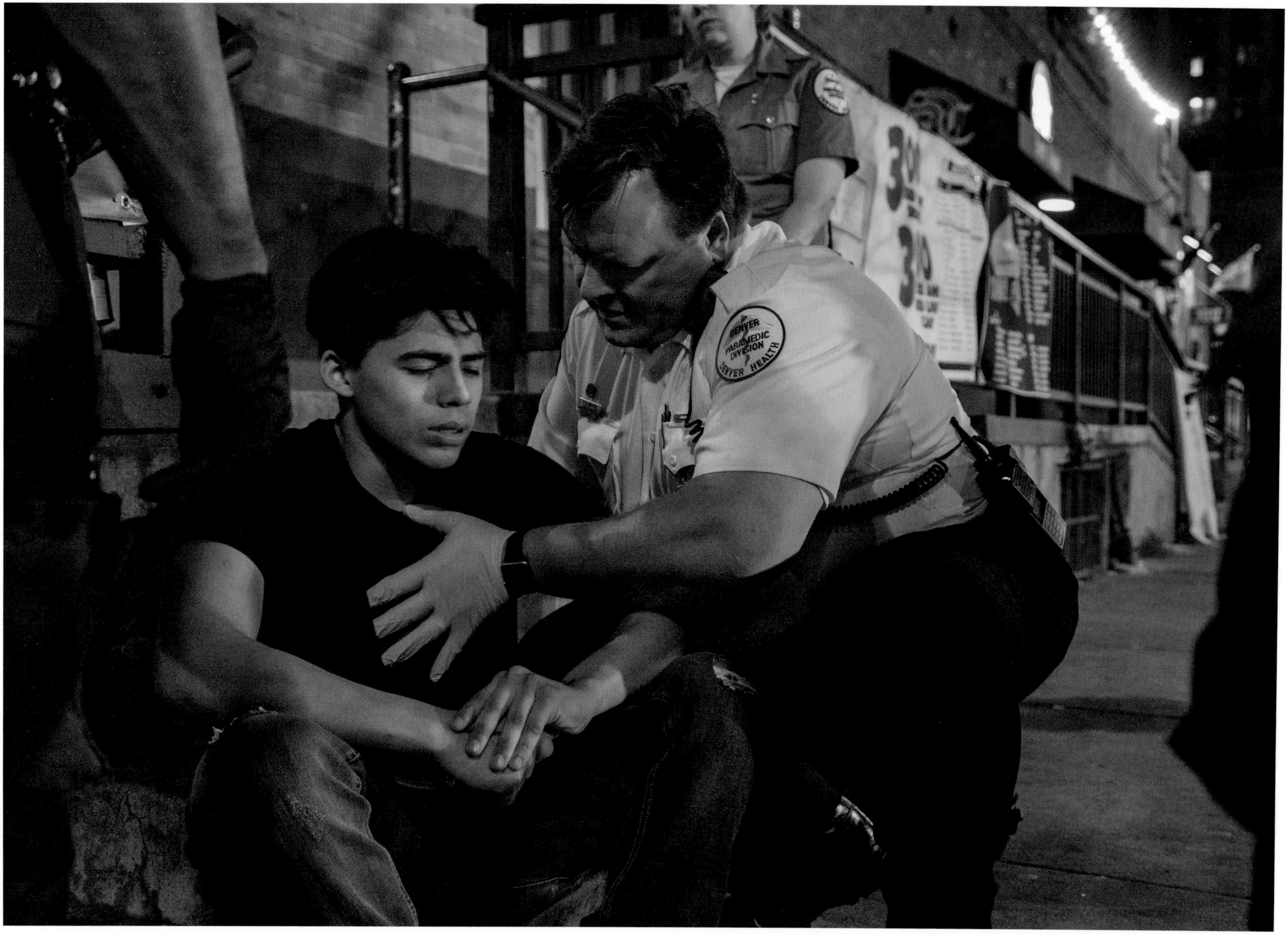
DENVER
PARAMEDIC DIVISION
DENVER HEALTH

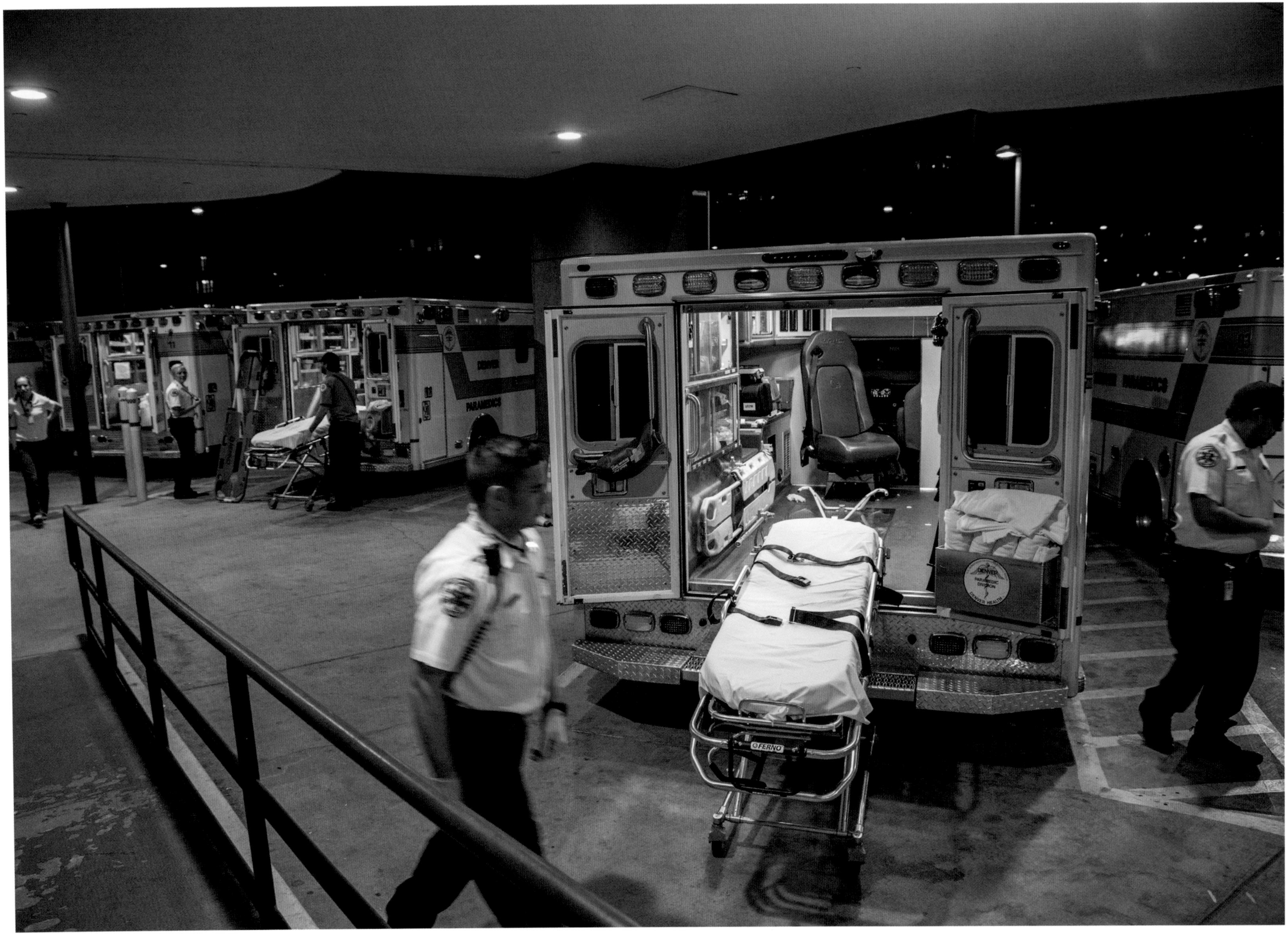
DENVER
PARAMEDICS
FERNO

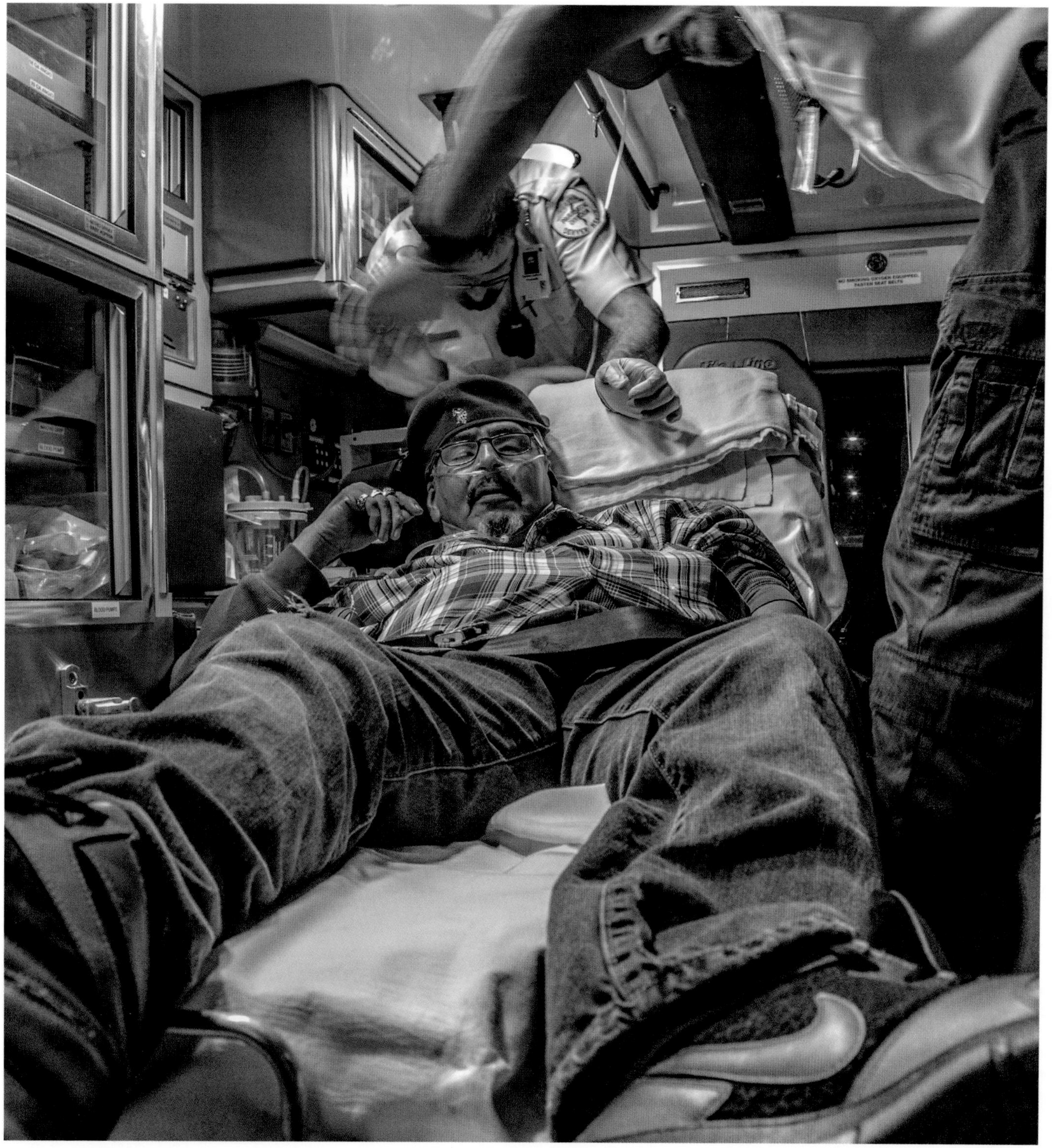

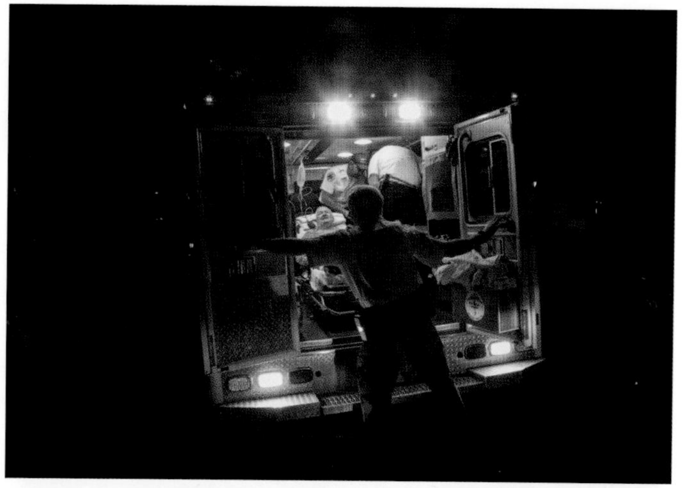

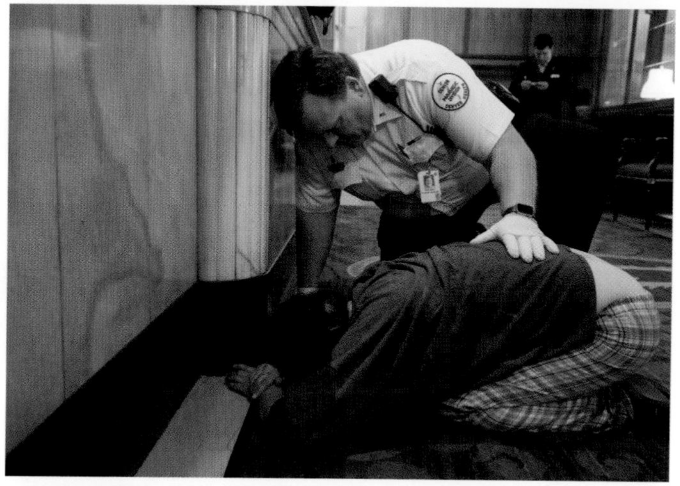

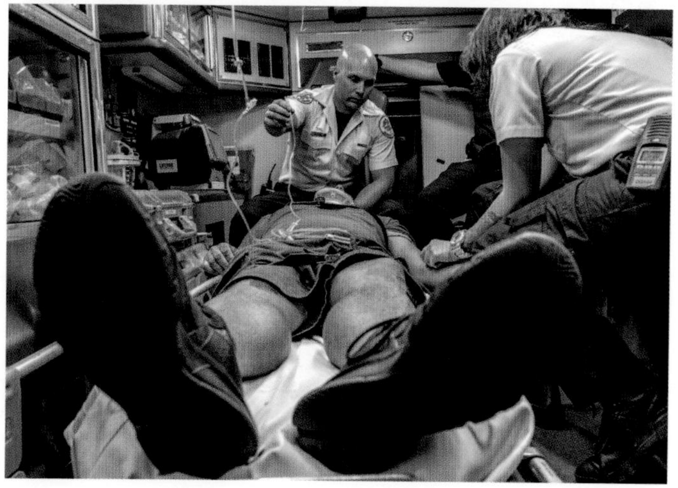

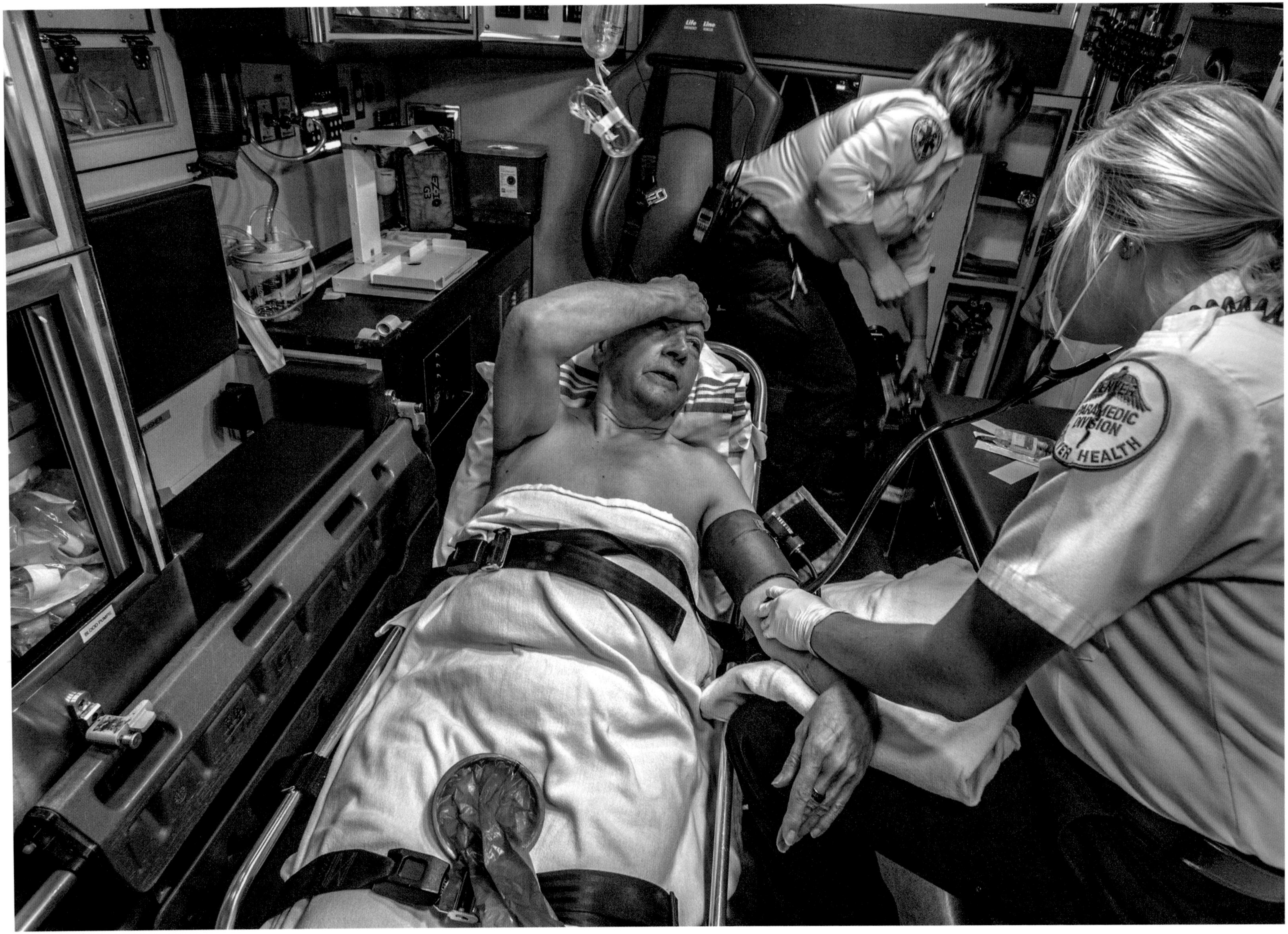
PARAMEDIC
DIVISION

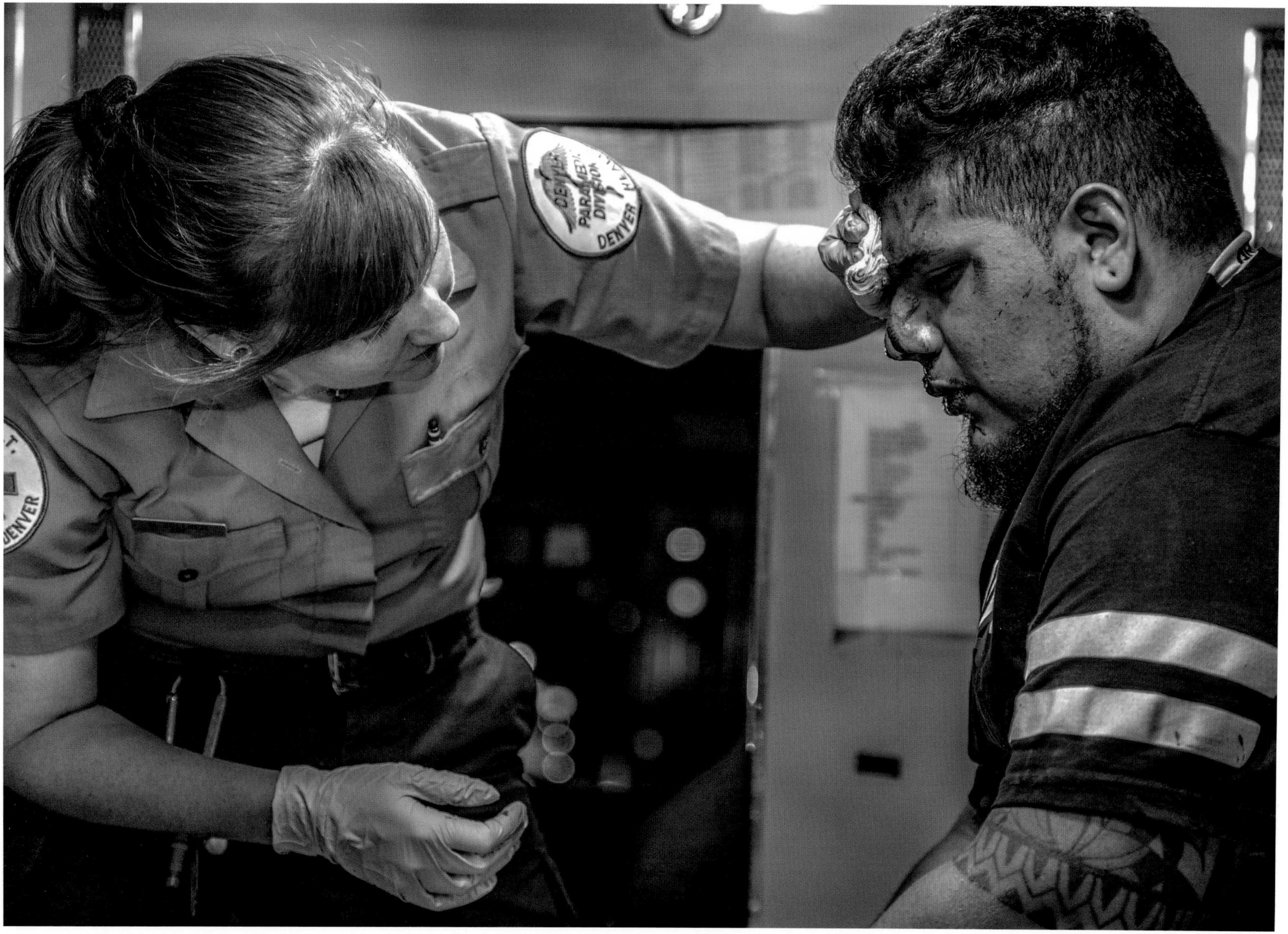
DENVER
DENVER

Peter Rosen, MD

Emergency Medicine Pioneer
Tucson, Arizona

I had a rather stormy relationship with my father, which is the kindest way of describing it. He didn't like losing to anybody, especially to me. I think I was the wrong son for him. He was a general surgeon, but he tried to convince me not to go into medicine. That's probably one of the things that pushed me into it.

My mother died of breast cancer when I was twelve. She came down to dinner for the first time in months — I was sure she was getting better — and died that night. My father sent me to school the next day and told me not to tell anybody. But when another kid asked how she was doing, I let it out that she had died. When I got home, my father punched me in the face. That's how things went.

I didn't get into medical school the first year I applied, so I felt lucky to be there when I finally did get accepted. I eventually ran out of money and planned to drop out for a year. But the dean offered me a big scholarship to stay and said, "By the way, your insane father called and told me to throw you out of medical school, so I hung up on him." I told him, "Right, he doesn't think I should be a doctor." But the dean said, "I do." That piece of encouragement made an important difference in my life.

I fell in love with surgery, but some of the surgeons I trained under were consummate instrument-throwing, verbally obnoxious bastards. They used to hit residents . . . smash you over the hand with bone spreader and scream, "Pull harder! More traction!" I eventually moved to Wyoming where I was the only surgeon within eighty miles . . . I drove about two hundred miles a day. It was terrifically exciting . . . until I had a heart attack on Christmas Day and became a patient in my own critical care unit. I was only thirty-five. Six weeks later, I had a second one, which ended my career in surgery. I decided maybe I should try a different specialty.

In hindsight, I think my dad's aggressiveness helped prepare me for the future. I ended up in emergency medicine — a field that wasn't very highly respected by other physicians — but I was used to older people not having much faith in me or my accomplishments. I knew how to figure things out for myself.

In those early years, emergency care was abysmal but not because those guys weren't trying. They were well intentioned but often terribly sleep deprived . . . and faced with an unbearable workload. There was no backup . . . no teaching . . . and some of the sickest patients anywhere on the planet.

I've enjoyed teaching because it has enabled me to transfer the knowledge I've acquired to others with the hope they won't have to put up with some of the things we did. I'd like to think I've been a father to a lot of residents and students . . . maybe the father they never had . . . that *I* never had.

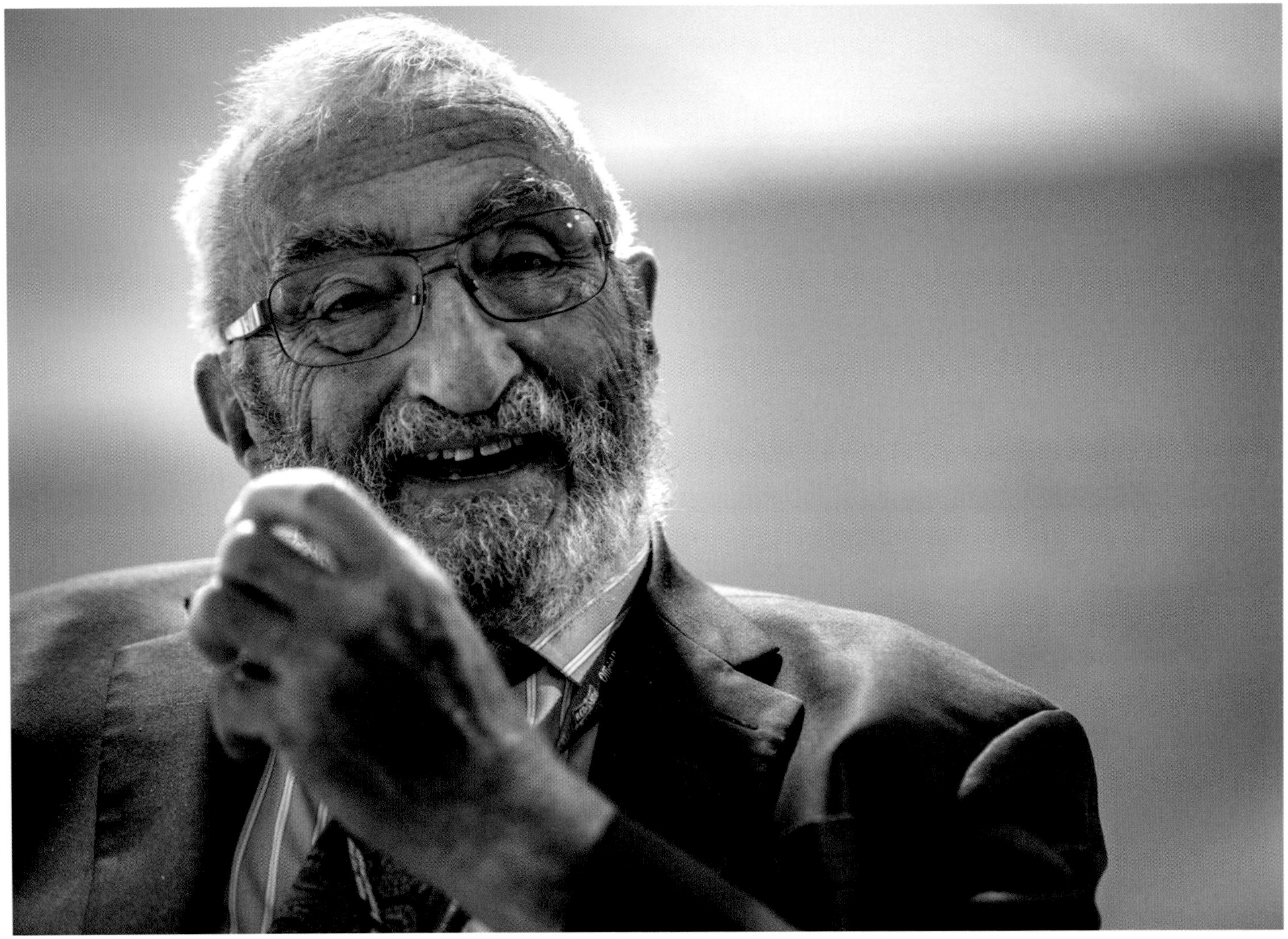

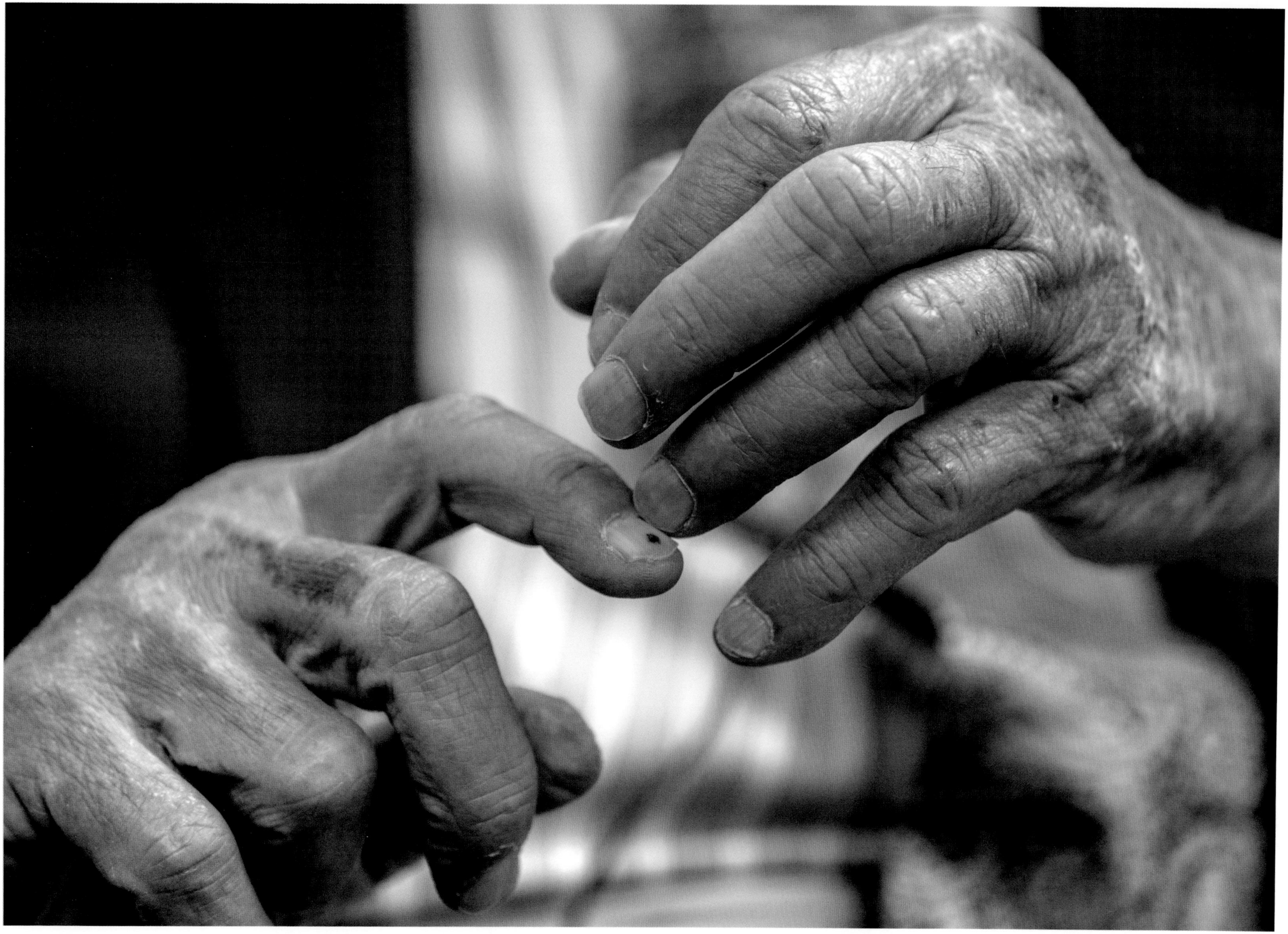

I inherited a very short fuse from my old man, but you don't accomplish anything when you really lose control of yourself — other than making a lifelong enemy. Over time, I've learned it's all right for a doctor to have emotions, but there are times when you have to control them. One of the things that has saved me throughout my career is I really like people. They amuse me. They satisfy my curiosity. They amaze me. They're just fun to get to know and to take care of . . . even the ones I don't initially like.

I took care of a guy one night who had a gunshot wound to his belly . . . and a swastika tattooed on his forehead. He took one look at me and said, "Get outta here! No fuckin' Jew is gonna take care of me." I told him, "Your choice. Death — or the fuckin' Jew." His choice? The fuckin' Jew.

After I met my wife, my father threw me out of the house for dating a shiksa. But she and I have been through a stunning number of years together, and she has been unfailingly generous with her emotional gifts. I've spent my life trying to make her laugh . . . I love the sound of her laughter. I got very depressed after a recent back surgery because — overnight — I lost the ability to take care of myself. My quality of life was just gone. But my wife stepped in . . . she took me to the park and patiently walked laps with me until I could do it on my own. She got me out of the darkness. She told me she knew I was depressed and hoped it would go away soon. And there was something so wonderful in the tone of her voice . . . she wasn't just sick to death of hearing me whine . . . she had a genuine wish for me to be better. She's a lovely lady.

The second law of thermodynamics says without an ever-increasing infusion of energy any closed system will assume maximum disorder. This applies to both atomic particles *and* life. You have to fight . . . you have to struggle . . . but it begins to take more and more energy to do the same thing, year in and year out. Eventually, you reach a point at which you can't create enough energy to salvage the system, and then it fails.

One of the truisms of life is there's an end to it — and it's called death. So, we shouldn't spend a lot of time on things that don't matter. What happens after death is unknowable. You may conjure up your own imagery or, if it helps, you can accept another person's version of the hereafter. But the reality is we just don't know. So, why worry about it? I consider myself an atheist, but I have a friend whose rabbi says, "It's all right to be an atheist as long as the God you don't believe in is Jewish." I can live with that.

I like to think I'm a pretty good doctor. I did respect my father as a clinician, and I guess I always subconsciously hoped I'd finally win his approval. But I have a bad heart now, and nobody wants a doctor who's having an anginal attack. It has been very hard for me to give up clinical work. I just didn't want to quit, but I eventually realized it was the intellectually honest thing to do. I can't physically get through a shift anymore . . . I can't stand up that long . . . I can't walk that far . . . and when I get tired and weak, I can't think about anything other than how my body is feeling. That's not fair to the patient.

But I dream about the emergency room. In my dreams, I'm still there. I'll always be there. ✚

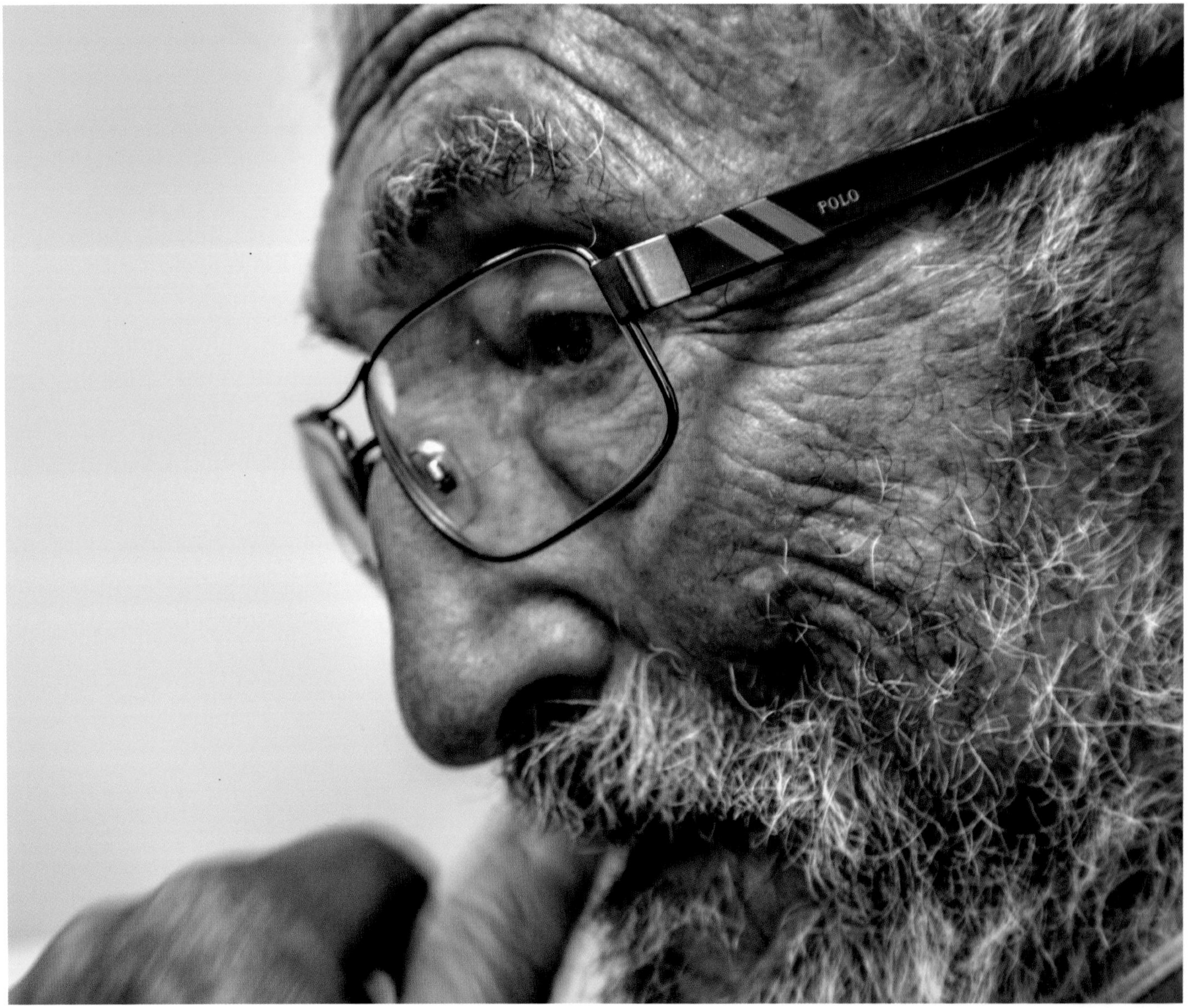

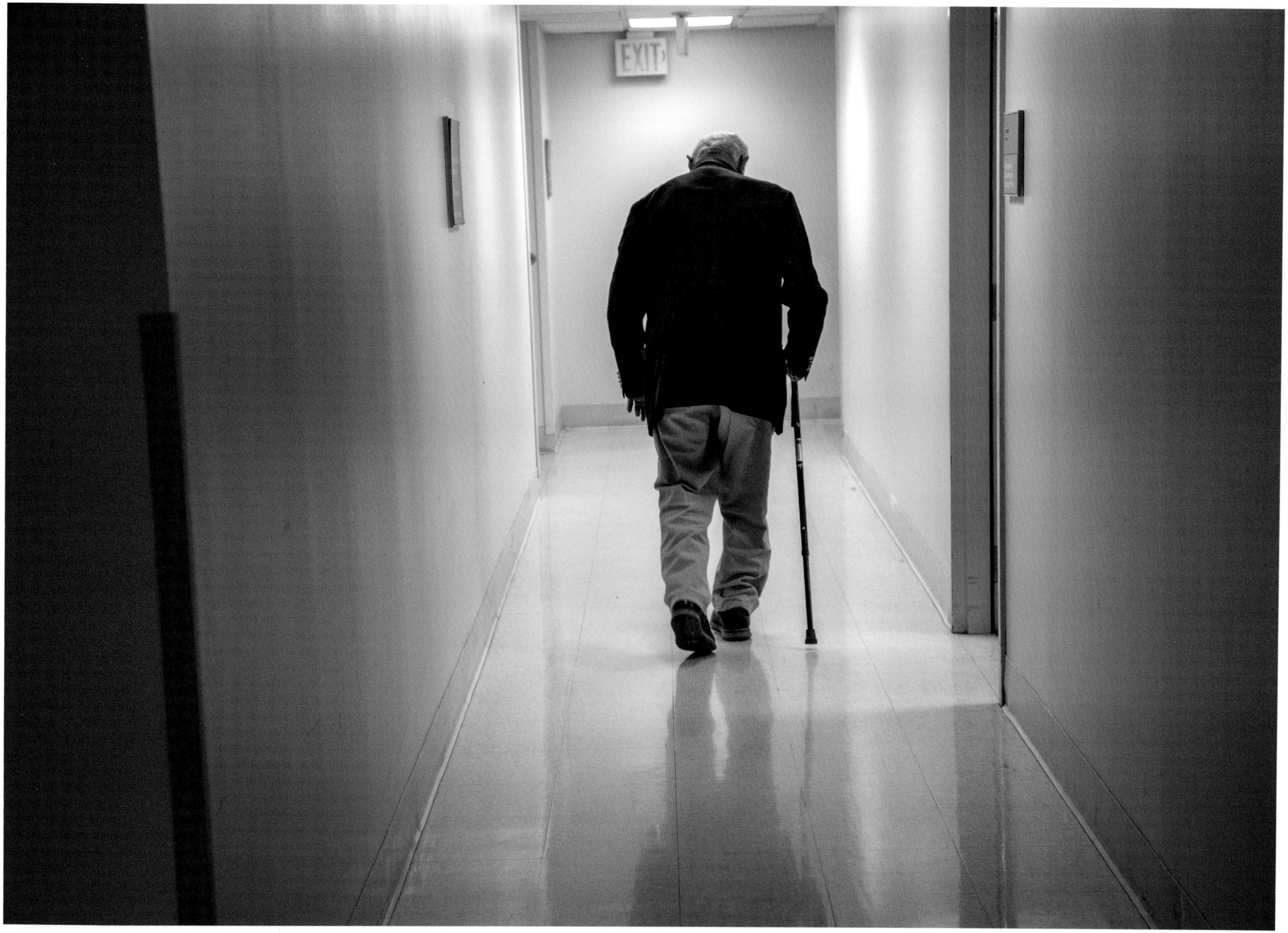
EXIT

Afterword

Emergency medicine was absent in organized health care when John Wiegenstein, MD, and a small group of colleagues formed the American College of Emergency Physicians in 1968. The fledgling organization's logo — a checkerboard of squares with one missing piece — expressed this critical dearth, as well as ACEP's ambition to fill it.

Now, five decades later, the specialty once maligned as "the weakest link in the chain of hospital care" serves as the front door to the American house of medicine. The stories within this book illustrate just how far we have come. While diverse, the fifty clinicians featured on these pages are unified by a common passion: they embody the heart and soul of emergency medicine. We hope they inspire the next generation of caregivers drawn toward the chaos, fires, and flashing lights.

As ACEP celebrates its golden anniversary, we can take pride in the progress we have made, but we cannot rest. We are compelled to look outward to address the other missing pieces in our fractured medical system and apply our talents to shape and improve care for a new generation of patients.

America is changing. The "silver tsunami" has brought an older and more medically complex patient population to our doorsteps. Our society has been ravaged by the opioid epidemic that continues to claim the lives of a staggering number of young people. EMS organizations and emergency departments face regular funding challenges and must fight constantly to maintain the viability of our "safety net" systems. State support for mental health resources are inadequate, a shortfall that puts both communities and patients at risk. And while new technologies constantly dazzle with the promise of breakthrough treatments, the driving technological imperative threatens to weaken the doctor–patient relationship.

By providing an important bridge between the community and the hospital, emergency clinicians are well positioned to address some of medicine's most pressing problems. Emergency medicine research is growing at an unprecedented pace, fostered by innovative alliances with subspecialties and resulting in ever-better treatments for conditions such as stroke, substance abuse, and sepsis. The number of emergency physicians engaged in federal advocacy efforts continues to grow, bolstered by a commitment to ensuring the nationwide availability of lifesaving care.

John Wiegenstein was tragically killed in a car accident in 2004, but he lived long enough to witness the specialty he championed come nearly full circle. He was there to help the "emergency room" transform into a robust system of care.

While the future is certain to present obstacles that rival the ones we have already faced, those of us on medicine's front line are ready for the challenge. Bring 'em all. We can't wait to see what comes next.

Mark F. Brady, MD, MPH, FACEP

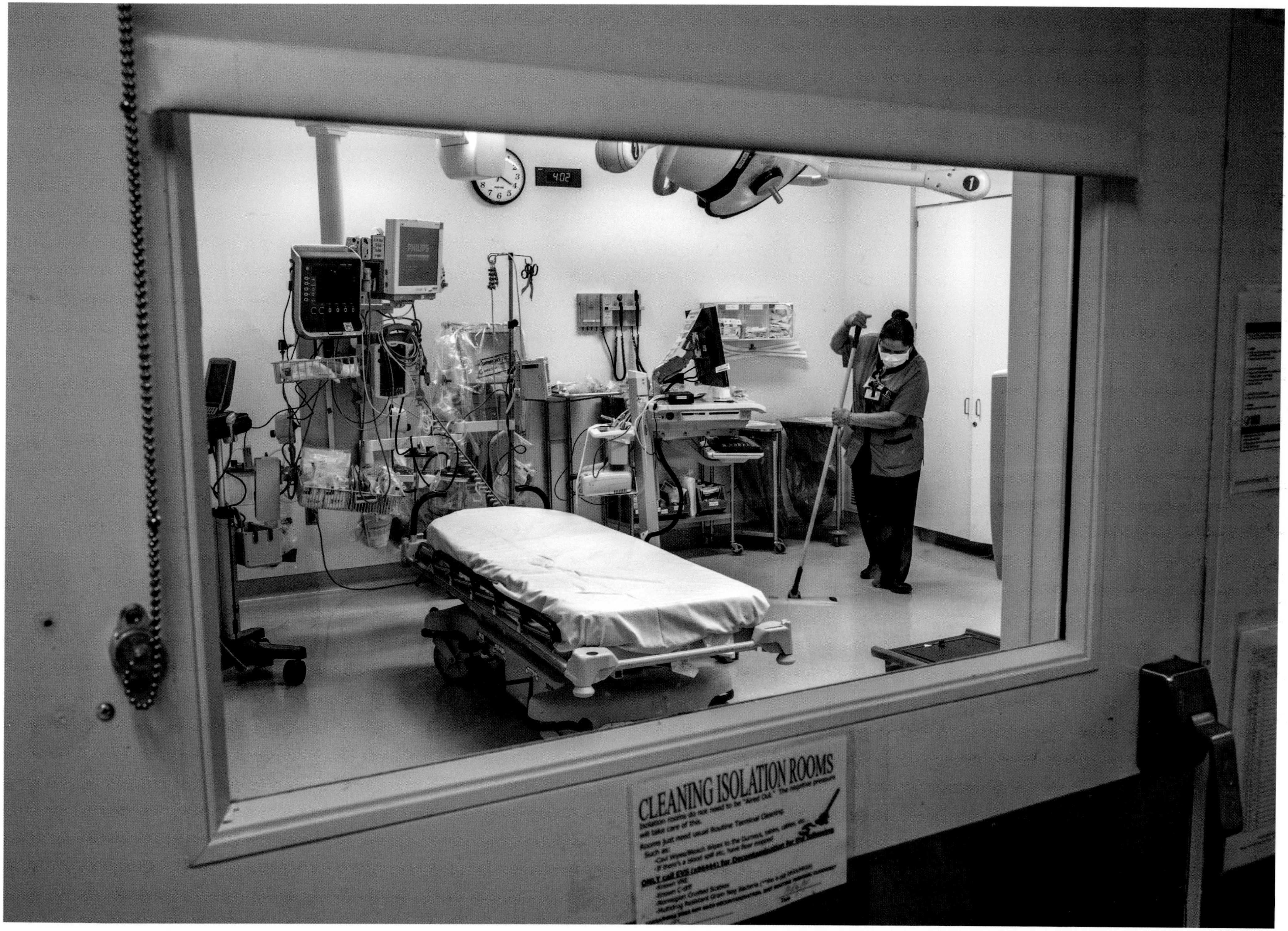
PHILIPS
CLEANING ISOLATION ROOMS

ACEP extends its deepest gratitude to the following supporters, who so generously helped underwrite this project.

Wiegenstein Presenting Sponsors

Schumacher Clinical Partners
TeamHealth
Vituity

Pontiac Plan Sponsors

Brault
Emergency Medicine Residents' Association (EMRA)
Envision Physician Services
FUJIFILM SonoSite
Hagan Barron Intermediaries
Janssen Pharmaceutical Companies of Johnson and Johnson
MultiView, Inc.
Teleflex®
United States Army Medicine

About the Artist

Eugene Richards

Born in Dorchester, Massachusetts, Eugene Richards earned a bachelor of arts degree in journalism and English from Northeastern University. After a year of studying photography, he joined VISTA — Volunteers in Service to America — and was assigned to eastern Arkansas, where he later helped found a social service organization and a community newspaper that reported on black political action and the Ku Klux Klan. His first publication was *Few Comforts or Surprises: The Arkansas Delta* (1973) followed by *Dorchester Days* (1978), a portrait of the inner-city neighborhood where he was raised.

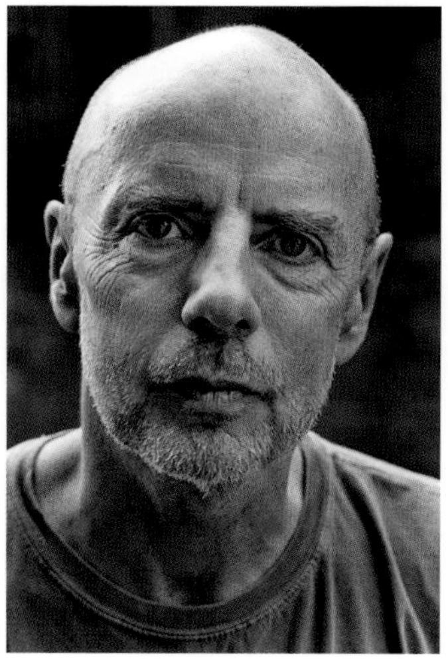

Photo by Jocelyn Bain Hogg.

Richards's subsequent books include *Exploding Into Life* (1986), which chronicles his first wife's struggle with breast cancer; *The Knife & Gun Club: Scenes from an Emergency Room* (1989), which explores issues of life and death in an acclaimed, inner-city health-care facility; *Cocaine True, Cocaine Blue* (1994), a study of the impact of hardcore drugs on American cities; and *War Is Personal* (2010), a chronicle of the consequences of the Iraq War. His most recent book is *The Run-On of Time* (2017), a comprehensive retrospective of his photographic work to date. His feature-length film, *Thy Kingdom Come*, premiered at the 2018 South by Southwest Film Festival.

Richards has earned numerous honors, including a Guggenheim Fellowship, the W. Eugene Smith Memorial Award, and the Robert F. Kennedy Lifetime Achievement Journalism Award. A retrospective of his photographs, "The Run-On of Time," opened at the International Center of Photography in New York City in September 2018.

About the Editors

Don Stader, MD, FACEP

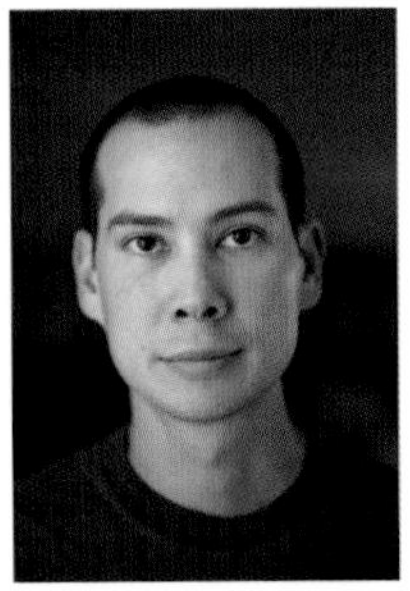

Don is an emergency physician with CarePoint Health and practices at Swedish Medical Center in Englewood, Colorado. He earned a medical degree with honors from Baylor College of Medicine in Houston, Texas, where he was an Albert Schweitzer Fellow and completed a residency in emergency medicine at Carolinas Medical Center in Charlotte, North Carolina. Don is the co-executive producer of the Emmy and Telly Award-winning documentary *24|7|365 - The Evolution of Emergency Medicine*. He serves as the president of Colorado ACEP and is the former president of the Emergency Medicine Residents' Association (EMRA).

An expert on the opioid crisis and opioid addiction, he is the editor-in-chief of Colorado ACEP's *2017 Opioid Prescribing & Treatment Guidelines* and the senior pain management and opioid policy physician advisor for the Colorado Hospital Association. Don is also the founder of two nonprofit organizations, the Emergency Medical Minute and the Last Words Project.

Mark Brady, MD, MPH, FACEP

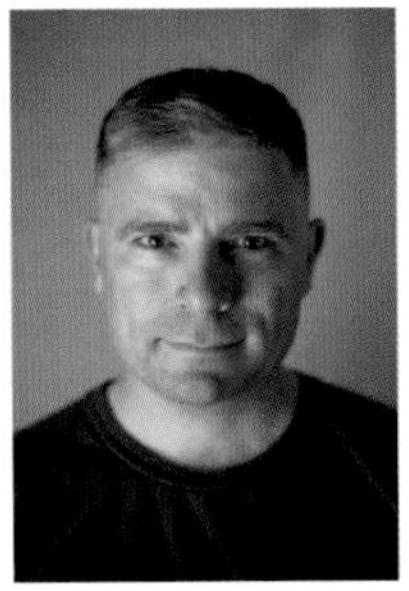

Mark is a faculty physician in the Department of Emergency Medicine at the University of Tennessee Health Science Center in Memphis. He earned his medical degree from Brown University and completed a residency in emergency medicine at Yale New Haven Hospital. He also completed a National Institutes of Health-Fogarty Clinical Research Fellowship in Lima, Peru. Mark holds a master's degree in public health from Harvard University and a tropical medicine diploma from the London School of Hygiene and Tropical Medicine. He has taught and done research in Africa, Asia, and South America.

Mark has served in Europe and Asia as an officer in the United States Navy and has deployed with the United States Marines in the Middle East. He has written for the Discovery Health Channel, an experience that fueled his interest in telling stories about medicine. He also was the co-executive producer of *24|7|365 - The Evolution of Emergency Medicine*.

Rachel Donihoo

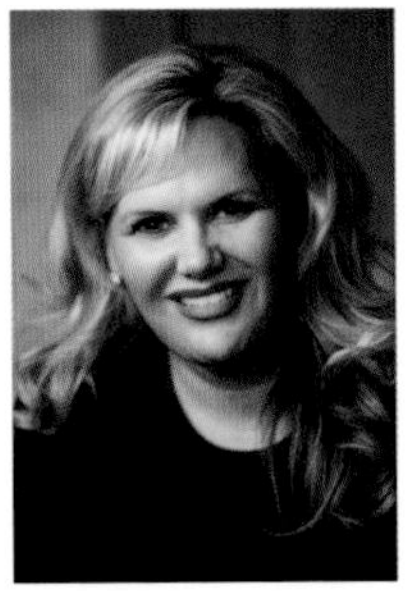

Rachel is the manager of educational publishing at the American College of Emergency Medicine (ACEP) and the managing editor of *Critical Decisions in Emergency Medicine.* Over the course of her twenty-five-year editorial career, she has earned numerous journalism awards from the Council for the Advancement and Support of Education, the International Association of Business Communicators, and the Press Club of Dallas. Prior to joining ACEP, she managed publications for the University of Texas Southwestern Medical Center and the Emergency Medicine Residents' Association.

A seasoned writer and medical editor, Rachel's editorial credits include a number of distinguished books, including the second editions of *Anything, Anyone, Anytime – The History of Emergency Medicine* and the *Emergency Department Resuscitation of the Critically Ill*. In addition, she was an associate producer of *24|7|365 - The Evolution of Emergency Medicine.*

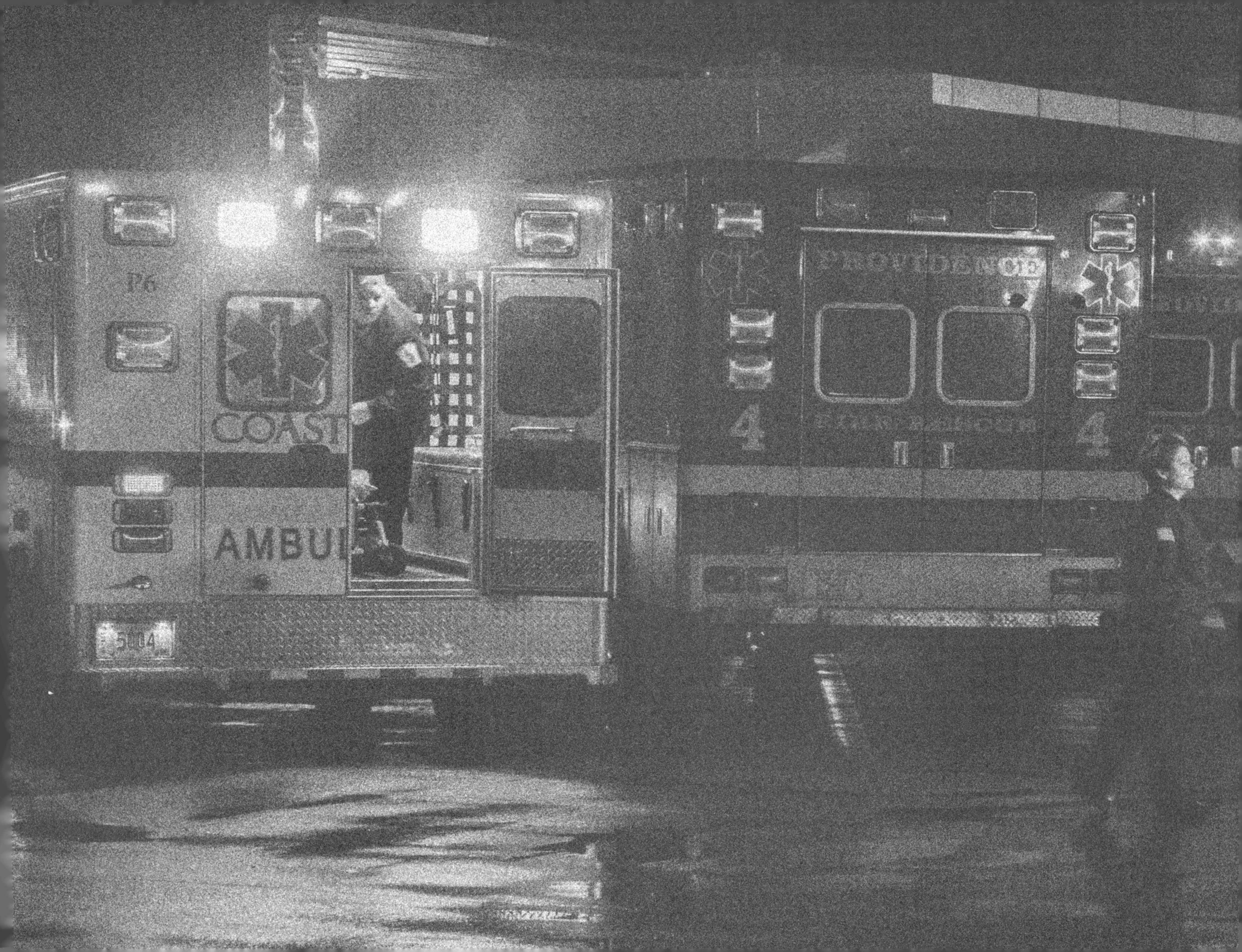
P6
COAST
AMBUL
5004
PROVIDENCE
4
4